MODELS OF COLLABORATION

MODELS OF COLLABORATION

A Guide for Mental Health Professionals Working with Health Care Practitioners

DAVID B. SEABURN,
ALAN D. LORENZ,
WILLIAM B. GUNN, JR.,
BARBARA A. GAWINSKI, AND
LARRY B. MAUKSCH

BASIC
BOOKS

A Member of the Perseus Books Group

New York

The Library of Congress has cataloged the hardcover edition as follows:

Models of collaboration : a guide for mental health professionals working with health care practitioners / David B. Seaburn . . . [et al.]. — 1st ed.
    p.   cm.
   Includes bibliographical references and index.
   ISBN 0-465-09580-1
   Consultation-liaison psychiatry—United States. 2. Managed mental health care—United States. 3. Psychotherapy—Practice—United States. 4. Psychiatric referral—United States. 5. Medical referral—United States. 6. Holistic medicine. I. Seaburn, David B.
RC455.2.C65M63   1996
616.89'023—dc20   96-15804
                                                CIP

Paperback ISBN 0-465-07515-0

03 04 05 / 10 9 8 7 6 5 4 3 2 1

To our families, with love and affection
Bonnie, Rachel, and Emily Seaburn
Gaylinn Greenwood and August and Amylark Lorwood
Cynthia, Joshua, Sean, and Will Gunn
Phil Stern and Taylor and Dylan Gawinski Stern
Sally Kentch and Claire and Eli Mauksch

CONTENTS

ACKNOWLEDGMENTS

ANY BOOK IS a collaborative endeavor. But a book on collaboration may be even more so. We have been blessed with the wisdom and support of many colleagues, friends, and family who have shared their ideas and experiences generously and shaped our work significantly. Our interaction with them has added great richness to the adventure of writing this book. To them we express our deepest appreciation and admiration.

We would like to thank the departments, programs, and clinical settings in which we work for their support: University of Rochester, School of Medicine and Dentistry, Department of Family Medicine, and Highland Hospital, Family Medicine Residency Program; University of Rochester, School of Medicine and Dentistry, Department of Psychiatry, Division of Family Programs; University of Rochester, School of Nursing; Canal Park Family Medicine, Palmyra, New York, an affiliate of Clifton Springs Hospital and Clinic; Duke University Medical School, Department of Community and Family Medicine, and Department of Psychiatry, Family Studies Program, Duke University Medical Center; University of Washington, Department of Family Medicine, and the University of Washington Medical Center Family Medicine Residency.

We are deeply indebted to the following people who read portions of the manuscript or were interviewed about their experiences collaborating. Their openness and insight have been invaluable. In many ways the book is about them: Priscilla Adams, C.N.S., Bruce Amundson, M.D., Macaran Baird, M.D., M.S., Terrence Becker, M.D., Michael Bennett, M.D., Seth Bernstein, Ph.D., Gary Bischof, M.S., Donald Bloch, M.D., Buzz Bricca, M.D., Theodore Brown, Ph.D., Simon Budman, Ph.D., Judith Baggs, R.N.,

Ph.D., Thomas Campbell, M.D., Richard Chung, M.D., Kathy Cole-Kelly, M.S.S.W., Valeria Correa, M.A., Rick Cote, M.S.W., Kathryn Cruze, M.S., Deborah Davis, M.D., Robin Dea, M.D., William Doherty, Ph.D., Fred Donovan, Ph.D., Barry Dym, Ph.D., Michael Enright, Ph.D., Tillman Farley, M.D., Jerry Gale, Ph.D., Linda Garcia-Shelton, Ph.D., Michael Glenn, M.D., Gaylinn Greenwood, M.D., James Griffith, M.D., Richard Heinrich, M.D., Carrie Henderson, M.S.W., Jeri Hepworth, Ph.D., Jay Indik, M.S.W., Beverly Johnson, R.N., Wayne Katon, M.D., Charlie King, M.D., Jeremy Kisch, Ph.D., Reuben Lorenz, M.B.A., Jennie Lowery, M.S.W., Ross Mayberry, Ph.D., Susan McDaniel, Ph.D., Patricia Meadows, M.S.W., Louis Moffett, Ph.D., Susan Molumphy, Ph.D., Sherri Muchnick, Ph.D., Jo Ellen Patterson, Ph.D., C. J. Peek, Ph.D., Brad Pope, M.D., Douglas Rait, Ph.D., David Raney, M.D., Don Ransom, Ph.D., Mary Richards, M.S.W., John Rolland, M.D., Nancy Ruddy, Ph.D., Carolyn Schroder, Ph.D., Bill Schwab, M.D., John Sherman, Ph.D., Greg Simon, M.D., Jenny Speice, Ph.D., Stephen Tarnoff, M.D., Margaret Tichler, R.N., Jane Tuttle, R.N., Ph.D., Susan Walter, M.S.W., Marianne Wambolt, M.D., David Waters, Ph.D., Sanford Weimer, M.D., Margo Weiss, Ph.D., Peter West, M.D., Lorraine Wright, R.N., Ph.D., and MaryAnne Zabrycki, C.S.W.

Acknowledgment is made to the following for large doses of personal or professional support and assistance: Kathy Andolsek, M.D., John Dickinson, M.D., Al Ellsworth, D. Pharm., Jennifer Griffith, Jeanne Klee, Judith Landau-Stanton, M.B., Ch.B., D.P.M., David Losh, M.D., Ellen Rhinard, Roger Rosenblatt, M.D., Jean Sauvain, Ron Schneeweiss, M.D., Phil Stern, Karen Vane, and Pat Williams.

David Seaburn would like to express special thanks to Don Bloch, M.D., for planting the seed that became this project, and to Susan McDaniel, Ph.D., for her vision, encouragement, and wisdom; to Jo Ann Miller; and to Eric Wright of Basic Books for his editorial guidance.

Alan Lorenz would like to acknowledge his immediate family for their support and his "extended family" of obstetric patients whose slow labors provided an opportunity to write through the night.

William Gunn wishes to acknowledge his parents, William and Mary Hunter Gunn, who taught him a great deal about working collaboratively with others. He would also like to recognize his friend and colleague Dr. David Waters, who helped him adjust and thrive in family medicine.

Barbara Gawinski expresses her appreciation for her parents, Joseph T. Gawinski, Jr., and Florence F. Gawinski. Through witnessing their response to difficult times, she has gained the courage and strength to learn and offer new ways to work together with health care professionals.

Larry Mauksch would like to especially acknowledge six people: Richard Weinberg, his longtime friend who continues to teach him about writing, about people, and about himself; Scott Stevens, M.D., and William Phillips, M.D., who took him into their day-to-day life in primary care and taught him; lastly, and most importantly, his parents and sister, Ingeborg Grosser Mauksch, Hans Otto Mauksch, and Valerie Mauksch, who will forever influence him in their love, their personal and professional perspectives, and their desire to strive in life.

We want to express our gratitude to the family medicine residents, patients, and families we have worked with over the years, who have taught us more than they may realize.

MODELS OF COLLABORATION

PART I

Foundations of Collaboration

Learning how to work together for the benefit of patients and their families is one of the most important challenges facing mental health and health care professionals today. The traditional boundaries that have often separated these two areas are no longer adequate to meet the needs of patients and the requirements of an ever-evolving health care system. Change in how we work together is not just an opportunity, it is a necessity.

Our Western culture has been divided into two separate subcultures: one that cares for the mind and one that cares for the body. The first section of this book argues for integration. Our intent is to provide a framework for developing collaborative relationships that bridge the gulf that often exists between these two subcultures. To do so, we must reassess many of the basic premises upon which our current approaches to health and mental health care are based, especially those that unduly hamper efforts to collaborate for the welfare of patients and their families. This is both a challenging and exciting endeavor, one that will not only transform the way we think and practice but may also stimulate our own growth and development, professionally and personally.

To begin this process, part I of the book provides the most essential foundation for a collaborative approach to health and mental health care. Chapter 1 articulates a rationale for collaboration and defines critical terms. The "culture of collaboration" is described, and the basic tenets of collaboration are laid out. As is often done throughout the book, case material is used to illustrate critical concepts. Chapter 2 explores the most important historical trends and themes that have shaped how various professional disciplines deal with issues of mind, body, and collaboration. Chapter 3 outlines the key ingredients of collaboration and identifies six principles that apply to all forms of collaboration. A list of practical guidelines is provided for each area. Chapter 4 is both a comprehensive and succinct discussion of the current research on the efficacy of a collaborative approach. It provides the reader with important evidence to support the development of collaborative care designs.

The foundation for collaboration is established in part I. Here the collaborative venture begins. Each of the ensuing parts provides practical information and useful insights from health and mental health professionals who are currently engaged in collaborative approaches to care. We hope their experience will encourage the reader to create and implement his or her own model of collaboration.

CHAPTER 1

Foundations of Collaboration

THE COMPLEX NATURE of human suffering is the best argument for collaboration between health and mental health professionals. The human experience of illness, pain, or discord affects the body, mind, heart, soul, and relationships simultaneously. And just as the proverbial elephant cannot be understood by touching only its trunk or tail or ears or legs, the health and mental health problems of patients and families cannot be adequately understood or treated separately or in parts. Physical, emotional, mental, spiritual, and relational health are all parts of a whole.

No single view is broad enough to understand the intricate interaction of health and mental health difficulties. While each professional may be interested in the whole elephant, our professional training may prepare us to understand only tails or ears or trunks. To be effective, those who understand tails must talk to those who comprehend trunks, and those who comprehend trunks must converse with those who understand ears. Together we must look and listen and, in the process, see and grasp more. It is through collaborative dialogue among professionals, patients, and families that a picture of the whole evolves and directions for the most effective treatment are created.

This book focuses on what collaboration is and how it is being practiced by health and mental health professionals in a variety of contexts. We provide an overview of collaboration, its history,

3

nature, and forms. And we profile those on the front line of health and mental health collaboration and how they work.

In this chapter, we present the basic elements and ideas on which collaboration is based. We discuss the "culture of collaboration"—the broad factors that contribute to a collaborative milieu, including the patient in his or her family context, health and mental health care provider interaction, and the role that the larger health care delivery system plays in how professionals, patients, and families work together. We also present the basic tenets of collaboration. These include an integrative paradigm for thinking about health and mental health problems; an ecological perspective on how health and mental health professionals can work together; and a commitment to treating patients and families as full partners in health care and collaboration. In varying forms, these basic ideas are reflected in all the examples of collaboration in this book.

But before we discuss these concepts, we begin with a clinical case. We chose a case study as our starting point because at the heart of the need for collaborative approaches to health and mental health care are the dilemmas and difficulties faced by particular patients and families, day in and day out. It should be noted that all clinical material presented in this book has been disguised to protect the confidentiality of the patients and families who have been our teachers.

Linda is a 61-year-old woman. She lives alone in a low-rent apartment acquired for her by the department of social services. Linda was married but has been separated from her husband for 18 years. She reports that her husband abused her sexually and physically throughout their marriage. This is a very painful subject about which she is hesitant to talk. Her husband no longer lives in the same town, but Linda sees him from time to time at family gatherings. She continues to be fearful of him.

Linda has seven adult children, most of whom live in the area (see Figure 1.1). Her oldest daughter died of breast cancer over 10 years ago. Linda continues to grieve and experiences severe depression each year at the anniversary of her daughter's death. Several of her children are receiving public assistance. Two are employed, one of whom is in the military. Each of her sons has problems with substance abuse. Two of her daughters are currently in abusive relationships.

For many years Linda was employed in a local factory doing assembly work. She has been on disability for several years

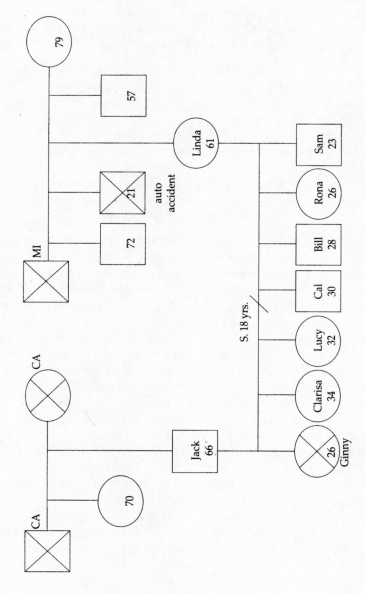

FIGURE 1.1

LINDA'S GENOGRAM

Note. ✕ indicates deceased.

owing to chronic back pain. She also reports a variety of other physical problems, including chronic nosebleeds, chest pain, persistent cough, vision problems, diabetes, and a history of depression, for which she has been hospitalized in the past. Linda currently is being treated in a medical clinic where she is followed by a primary care physician and a family therapist.

The importance of collaboration in such a complex situation may be obvious. The many different and challenging parts of the problem make it difficult to see the whole. Linda faces multiple medical problems; she has a painful family and psychosocial history; her two-inch-thick chart belies her frequent use of the outpatient health care system; she is somatically fixated, expressing many of her personal and interpersonal stresses through her physical symptoms; and persistent uncertainty surrounds most, if not all, of her problems. The importance of collaboration crystallized, though, when Linda's diabetes became uncontrollable.

Linda's diabetes had been managed for several years with oral hypoglycemics. Then Linda began to develop sores, and her blood sugar levels became greatly elevated. The treatment plan was no longer effective. Her children worried about their mother's health and wondered why nothing could be done. The recommendation was made for Linda to begin insulin treatment, which would mean giving herself daily injections. Linda was reluctant to take this step and continued to put it off. Her primary care physician was concerned that if she did not comply, Linda would need inpatient treatment to stabilize her diabetes.

Linda's physician learned about Linda's history of abuse during a routine pap smear and pelvic exam. That examination also led to an increased focus on Linda's abuse in psychotherapy, where it was discussed in greater detail. What Linda's physician did not know was that the abuse Linda experienced involved, among other things, being forced to sew into her own skin with needle and thread. The thought of insulin injections increased Linda's flashbacks and her anxiety. Once Linda revealed this detail of her abuse to her therapist, her therapist asked Linda for permission to discuss the matter with her physician. Linda gave permission because of the connection between her physical and emotional trauma and the treatment of her diabetes.

Linda's physician, a female, was very open to Linda's concerns. Together, Linda, her physician, and her therapist developed a treatment plan. Linda's children, who had been involved in her treatment before, were invited to meet about their mother's health, but they declined. Several were informed by phone of the plans for insulin treatment. They were glad that "finally something was being done."

The treatment planning process involved three or four hallway consultations between the therapist and the physician; they also held one conjoint medical visit in which the therapist met with Linda and her physician while Linda learned how to give herself injections; and they had one conjoint psychotherapy visit in which the physician met with Linda and the therapist to better understand how Linda's history of abuse affected her capacity to carry out the treatment plan. Linda was also referred to the diabetes education program at the hospital. The family was invited to attend these educational meetings but continued to decline. Their reluctance to get involved concerned the therapist and physician. They felt that without the family's understanding and approval of the plan, Linda might not follow through. It was decided that the therapist would make a concerted effort to contact Linda's children and explicitly ask for their help.

Linda succeeded in inviting one of her sons to a therapy appointment. At that visit, Linda tentatively talked about her diabetes and her abuse. To her surprise, her son was aware of what she had gone through and was supportive of her efforts at healing. In the meantime, plans moved forward for Linda to begin her injections. A date was set, and during the first week of the insulin treatment a nurse-practitioner was available each morning by phone to act as a coach.

In the next month, Linda's diabetes began to stabilize. During the same period, she heard from one of her daughters, who had learned from her brother about Linda's abuse. The daughter lived out of town but joined Linda by phone during a therapy visit. This daughter was very supportive of Linda and acknowledged that she had also recently entered therapy to deal with her own experience with abuse.

Linda continues to work on the terrible legacy of abuse. She also continues to give herself daily injections, although her diabetes has improved to the point that the injections may shortly be discontinued. Linda is gradually engaging her children more in the dark story that has cast a broad shadow across all of their lives.

This, case illustrates the rich blend of interactions common to effective collaboration among patients, families, health care providers, and mental health care providers. Collaboration is built on the quality of these relationships, the dynamics of which form what we call a "culture of collaboration" (Figure 1.2).

THE CULTURE OF COLLABORATION

Weber defined culture as a "web of significance spun" by humans themselves (Geertz, 1973). This "web of significance" includes the beliefs, values, attitudes, rituals, and behaviors of a people. By "culture of collaboration" we mean the web of significance, the sys-

FIGURE 1.2

THE CULTURE OF COLLABORATION

Health Care Delivery System

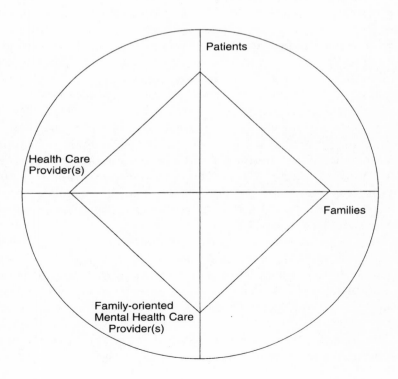

tem of interaction, that is created when health care providers, mental health care providers, patients, and families work together over time to treat illness and facilitate health. All of the participants play vital roles. Each brings experience, knowledge, skills, beliefs, and wisdom to bear on the task of resolving problems, stimulating change, and alleviating suffering. In the process, relationships are formed that affect each participant and through which the potential for healing is made manifest.

Dialogue provides the bridge between the relationships formed within the culture of collaboration. Through dialogue different strands of the "web" are connected and spun together. To collaborate is to create conversations in which people are joined together, meanings are fashioned, purposes are defined, roles are clarified, goals are established, and action is taken. Together the participants create a treatment culture in which the whole is greater than the sum of the parts.

In this section, we present the main components of the culture of collaboration, in particular, the patient in the context of the family, the health and mental health care provider interaction, and the larger health care system. We begin with some preliminary thoughts about the health care system. All collaboration occurs within this larger culture. The current health care system is in a dramatic state of flux at the federal, state, and local levels. Changes in the larger system will have a greater impact on collaborative family health care in the future than any other single factor.

The Health Care System

The health care system, like any other cultural system, is "anchored in particular arrangements of social institutions and patterns of interpersonal interactions" that are designed to integrate the components of health care (Kleinman, 1988, p. 24). These components include institutions (medical schools, hospitals, clinics), social roles (the sick, the healer), interpersonal relationships (patient-provider, nurse-physician), and beliefs about illness and health (the "will of God," the activity of "germs"), as well as economic, political, and social values and constraints (budgets, health care reform, pro life–pro choice positions on abortion). These larger systems factors influence how care is delivered at every level. When health and mental health care providers collaborate, they must be cognizant of the larger health care delivery system's expectations of how care is provided in even an individual situation.

In Linda's case, the physician and therapist are both aware of the larger health care expectations regarding cost. Linda matches the profile of the patient who utilizes the largest amounts of health care resources. She carries both a biomedical diagnosis and a psychiatric diagnosis. These problems are complicated by her somatic fixation, or tendency to focus on physical symptoms when dealing with emotional and interpersonal stress. Mauksch and Leahy (1993) note that high utilizers of health care tend to have both diagnoses. At Group Health Cooperative of Puget Sound, Wayne Katon and his colleagues found that the top 10% of medical utilizers accounted for one-third of outpatient resources and one-half of inpatient resources. Half of these high utilizers had mental health as well as physical health problems (Katon, Von Korff, Lin, Lipscomb, Wagner & Polik, 1990).

Linda had a prior psychiatric hospitalization owing to suicidality. Her therapist is concerned that the impact of her past sexual abuse might lead to another hospitalization. At the same time, Linda's physician is concerned that Linda might need to be hospitalized owing to her wildly fluctuating sugar levels. A collaborative approach not only provides the best method of care for Linda's complicated problem but in all likelihood will save money and resources that might otherwise be spent on inpatient treatment.

Like Linda, the majority of patients and their families turn to primary care physicians, nurses, nurse-practitioners, and physician's assistants for not only their health care but their mental health care as well. Eighty percent of all psychiatric diagnoses are made by primary care health providers, who also treat 50% of all patients with mental illness (Schurman, Kramer, & Mitchell, 1985). As reform efforts expand the number of citizens receiving health care, an ever-increasing number of patients and families will be turning to primary care providers to meet their complex needs. Even with an influx of new primary care providers, it is unreasonable to expect them to treat all the health and mental health problems of a majority of their patients and families. New methods of providing care and paying for it are needed.

What is called for are health care delivery systems that encourage a collaborative approach based on a partnership between health and mental health professionals and patients and families (see chapter 13). For example, in fully capitated health care delivery systems, a specified amount of money is provided for the health and mental health care of each patient in the system. Providers must decide how to organize and utilize the resources available to meet the needs of patients and families. Such a model discourages expensive treatment in hospital settings. It encourages preventive care and treatment that can be provided less expensively on an outpatient basis. This revolution in how health care is delivered has created anxiety among all health and mental health care providers, especially specialists and subspecialists who are not delivering services at the primary care level. For many mental health professionals, this change has been conceptualized as one more attempt of the larger system to control what they do.

Any revolutionary change breeds anxiety. Old ways of operating are suddenly called into question, and new ways seem foreign at best. What is called for in such situations is vision. The health care revolution is focusing on the macro level of how to arrange systems and utilize money and other resources. It is not providing a vision for delivering clinical care. Herein lies the most important opportunity for health and mental health professionals. Managed, capitated health care must not be viewed as "doing the same with less"; it must be viewed as "doing the best with the resources we have." From that perspective, it is incumbent upon health and mental health care providers to come together, creating collaborative partnerships that are both care-effective and cost-effective.

The Patient in the Context of the Family

At the heart of such a health care partnership are patients and families, who will bear increasing responsibility for the health of all family members in the future. Their needs will only expand in the coming decades. The population as a whole is aging. With age comes an increase in health problems. Half of all people over the age of 65 and one-quarter of those between the ages of 45 and 65 are limited in their daily functioning by at least one chronic condition (U.S. Department of Commerce, 1980). One outcome of improvements in medical technology has been the transformation of acute, life-threatening diseases into chronic illnesses that must be addressed over an ever-lengthening portion of the individual and family life cycle. Chronically ill patients are cared for primarily by families. Family members "are the ones who help most with the physical demands of an illness, ranging from preparing special meals for a family member with heart disease, . . . to running a home dialysis machine" (McDaniel, Campbell, & Seaburn, 1990, p. 229).

Family members provide the emotional support that an ill member needs and shoulder the stress that often accompanies illness in the family. At the heart of the culture of collaboration are the needs of patients living in the context of families. Families shape their members in a variety of critical ways: they provide a primary social context, a rich source of history and rootedness, and a context for the development of personal meaning.

The Family as Social Context

Our first and most important social context is the family. And just as "no organism" can be understood "apart from the social context in which it is shaped" (Berger & Luckmann, 1966, p. 50), no person can be adequately understood apart from the family in which he or she has been shaped. For some, family is parents and siblings; for others it is extended family, aunts, uncles, grandparents, cousins; for still others it is a close circle of friends with whom they live or work. And for some it may include professional helpers who have played an important role in their lives over a long period of time. In its first meaning, then, family can be understood as a relationship context (Ransom, 1993). It is "any group of people related biologically, emotionally, or legally" (McDaniel et al., 1990, p. 4).

The Family as History

The "family as history" (Ransom, 1993) refers to the transgenerational flow of families across time, the mix of legacies, loyalties, blessings, and curses passed down from one generation to the next. Families, like individuals, develop and evolve (family life cycle). A person does not live his or her whole life in just one family. At any given age, the family may present itself in different ways, depending on the configuration of its members and the events that shape its history. The family that includes an 8-year-old and his grandparent is not the same family that child lives in when he is 15 and the grandparent has died. The family changes continuously.

The family as history also implies continuity and stability over time. Each generation is connected to the next by what often seem to be invisible strands of loyalty (Boszormenyi-Nagy & Spark, 1973). Patterns of interaction, roles, expectations, and beliefs are passed on to each generation through various rituals and interpersonal processes. In a sense, the family as history refers to the family we carry within us (Ransom, 1993). The family we carry within us provides a foundation for who we are and how we are. The power of family can play a significant role in a patient's health or mental health beliefs and practices (Doherty & Campbell, 1988).

A physician, frustrated with an obese patient who had uncontrolled hypertension, explained in detail the importance of eating an appropriate diet, losing weight, and taking medication. She was concerned about the patient's risk for a stroke. The patient appeared to understand his situation and the need for the recommended treatment but did not comply. The physician suspected that family issues were influencing her patient's behavior. She consulted with a therapist colleague, and with the agreement of the patient they convened a family meeting. The meeting was attended by the patient's parents and the patient's two adult brothers, each of whom was also obese and had hypertension.

During the interview, the physician and therapist learned that the family was well aware of the health risk they all faced. They talked openly about relatives who had died or been incapacitated by strokes in the past. When asked what they believed would happen to them, each family member said he or she would face the same fate. The physician and therapist worked slowly with the family to understand and respect them better, without agreeing with their view of what the future held. They also introduced the idea that things could be different for the patient, if not for themselves. They appealed to the family's concern about the patient. Eventually, family members gave the patient permission to accept help, a new experience in the life history of the family.

The Family as Context of Meaning

This case also illustrates the family as "access to meaning" (Ransom, 1993). Meaning is created in a context of dialogue that occurs over time, sometimes over many generations (Berger & Luckmann, 1966; Rolland, 1994a; Seaburn, Lorenz, & Kaplan, 1992). The family provides the context of meaning in which dialogue takes place.

In a sense, children inherit their reality as it is filtered through the family, especially their parents. This reality is passed on to them through the stories, rules, blessings, and admonitions of family members. In the family the child learns "I am good" and "I am bad"; about relationships and hope and fear and joy; acceptable and unacceptable ways of being a family member; and which problems can be solved and which must be endured. All of these experiences create the ground of meaning upon which a person stands.

This inherited world is not static. Over time it evolves and expands. Each person develops greater opportunities for dialogue with others. As one's context for living grows, one's perspective on reality changes and evolves. We revisit what was and alter it to fit what is and what will be. Nevertheless, the family remains a vital presence within and around us throughout our lives. Without access to the family, no provider can fully understand a patient. Family provides the history that shapes a person's being. The family is the initial and often most lasting source of a person's Weltenschauung (Wittgenstein, 1953), or "meaning scheme for living."

In Linda's case, the family was involved in a variety of ways. At a symbolic level, they were invited into the room at the first visit when the therapist did an initial family genogram (Bowen, 1978; McGoldrick & Gerson, 1985). They were also involved in family meetings to discuss Linda's health and problematic family patterns. Family members were contacted by phone and letter when they were reluctant or unable to attend. At each treatment stage, the physician and the therapist took the family into consideration as the primary relational context of the patient. And at each stage, family members made shifts in their behavior to show Linda they cared. Without the family's inclusion, Linda would have remained an even more complicated puzzle, one with many of the most important pieces missing.

Mental Health and Health Care Providers

The health and mental health care providers involved in Linda's care could have felt they had enough pieces of the puzzle to effectively address her problems from their own areas of expertise. Linda's long history of abuse, depression, and family conflict provided ample material for any therapist to deal with. And her history of diabetes, back pain, chest pain, and the like provided a full agenda for any health care provider.

The difficulty and the challenge lies in the interconnectedness of all these problems. Many patients' experience cannot be easily divided into psychosocial and biomedical domains. Efforts to do so may be not only ineffectual but in some cases harmful. Linda's therapist realized that if he moved forward independently of Linda's family physician, he could precipitate a health crisis. By focusing exclusively on Linda's history of abuse without being sensitive to her need for insulin treatment, the therapist could have inadvertently encouraged Linda to resist taking injections because of its painful connection to her past. In like manner, had the family physician pushed Linda to comply with the insulin treatment without being aware of her background of abuse, she might have withdrawn further from medical care because of the flashbacks the treatment precipitated.

In the meantime, Linda, feeling caught in the middle, might have complained to her physician about problems she was having with her therapist, and to her therapist about problems she was having with her physician. Without communication between them, the physician and therapist could have misunderstood each other's approach to treatment and become frustrated with each other.

Effective collaboration without regular communication among providers is impossible (see chapter 3). One of the authors was consulting to primary care physicians and nurse-practitioners in a community health center who complained that they never heard back from the therapists to whom they had made referrals. When the primary care providers tried to call these therapists, they could never be interrupted, and when they did get through to the therapists, they were often blocked from further communication by the latter's concerns about confidentiality.

The health center took the bold step of inviting a few community therapists to a monthly case consultation group. At the first meeting, they learned of the frustrations that therapists experienced trying to work with primary care providers. The therapists complained that patients were ill prepared for referrals, that it was impossible to get referring primary care providers to return therapists' calls, and that too often the referring professional expected a quick fix. This unique group of health and mental health care providers recognized that despite these problems, collaboration would be valuable to the patients they shared. They also quickly learned that many of the hurdles that stood between them disappeared through conversation. The more they talked, the more possible collaboration seemed.

Effective collaboration involves communication between differing cultures (McDaniel, Hepworth, & Doherty, 1992; Seaburn, Gawinski, Harp, McDaniel, Waxman, & Shields, 1993). Each culture has its own way of thinking, its own language, and its own rules of communication. The bridge across these differences is dialogue. Through dialogue each culture expands to make room for the other. Through dialogue both cultures are informed and changed. Over time they may develop a culture together with a common language and a shared perspective.

BASIC TENETS OF COLLABORATION

In this section, we focus on the conceptual basis for collaboration. What are the underlying tenets that make it possible to create a culture of collaboration in which professionals, patients, and families can "work closely together, trying to offer more comprehensive care than is usually available" (Glenn, 1987b, p. viii)? In our view, the basic tenets of collaboration are:

1. An integrative paradigm regarding health and mental health problems
2. An ecological perspective on the interaction between professionals who collaborate
3. The treatment of patients and families as partners in care

These tenets cannot be found in pure form in any one collaboration, but they are present in some form in all collaborations.

An Integrative Paradigm

George Engel developed the biopsychosocial model as an antidote to what he perceived as the reductionistic tendencies of the prevailing biomedical model in medicine (Engel, 1977, 1980). The biomedical model assumes that disease can be reduced to "measurable biological variables" (Engel, 1977). The chief task of medicine under the biomedical model is to analyze and eliminate all possible disease-causing factors until the most basic biological elements of a disease can be identified. These disease-producing elements are then treated as the primary cause of the problem.

The biomedical model has achieved much success in treating disease. The main difficulty with the biomedical model, however, as Engel points out, is that it excludes psychological, interpersonal, and social factors and assumes that complex situations can be explained entirely by biology. The biopsychosocial model places illness into this larger framework of multiple systems interacting with each other. These systems include cells and organ systems as well as the person, the provider-person relationship, the family, and the social context.

The relationship between these systems or levels of experience is continuous and reciprocal (Dym, 1987; Medalie, 1978). For example, Linda's diabetes cannot be adequately understood and treated by considering only a single level of her problem. Not only do her blood sugar levels need to be assessed, but her levels of personal and interpersonal stress must be understood as well. Each level of experience interacts with other levels and contributes to the development of symptoms. The biopsychosocial model is a common approach for training health care professionals, particularly family physicians (Christie-Seely, 1984; Crouch & Roberts, 1987; Doherty & Baird, 1983; McDaniel et al., 1990).

The biopsychosocial model challenges health care professionals to broaden their perspective on illness. It challenges mental health professionals to broaden their perspective as well. Just as the biomedical model may focus too exclusively on the micro level in the development of problems, mental health professionals may overlook these factors and their influence on individuals and their interpersonal difficulties. One of the authors was reminded of this possibility by the following experience in his own practice:

A patient presented with slurred speech, difficulty maintaining his balance, and exhaustion to the point of falling asleep in session. These symptoms coincided with a recent financial crisis in the patient's life. Since the patient had a history of depression and a prior suicide attempt, the therapist assumed that he was overdosing on his antidepressant medication. At a home visit with the patient and his family, the patient's father and aunt expressed concern that the patient was secretly trying to kill himself. The patient admitted he was depressed but denied any attempts at suicide.

The therapist discussed these issues with the patient's primary care physician. Since the patient strongly denied any suicidal behavior, his symptoms became more confusing. The physician suggested that some routine blood tests be done to see whether anything could be learned. Test results revealed that the patient was suffering from hypothyroidism, which was causing the symptoms. The physician treated the patient's illness by prescribing thyroid medication, and within a week the symptoms dissipated.

This case was a valuable reminder that patients have bodies and that within their bodies are systems just as influential as the systems outside of their bodies.

The biopsychosocial model integrates these multiple systems in a way that respects and enlarges the domains of both health and mental health professionals. But this integration does not come without change. Though the biopsychosocial model has been criticized for being more conceptual than practical (Griffith & Griffith, 1994), physicians and other health care professionals trained in the model learn many new skills, such as constructing genograms, conducting family conferences, and providing brief forms of counseling. In addition to developing a broader perspective on the influence of organ systems, circulatory systems, and electrochemical interactions on behavior, mental health care providers who accept the biopsychosocial model as an integrative paradigm must make other changes as well. This is particularly true for family-oriented mental health professionals, whose training often leaves them unfamiliar with or hostile to the medical illness itself.

Lyman Wynne, Cleveland Shields, and Mark Sirkin (1992) have identified several reasons mental health professionals may have a "jaundiced" view of illness as a concept. They note that the concept of illness is seen by many therapists as "reductionistic," "pathologizing," "disempowering," and "stigmatizing" (p. 4). Wynne, Shields, and Sirkin go on to argue for a broader understanding of illness among mental health professionals. From their grounding in the biopsychosocial model, they suggest that illness is a complex dialogic and interactional process. They describe, for instance, how a headache moves from being a "nuisance" to an "illness." That transformation occurs when the headache affects a person's daily functioning. Impaired daily functioning may be related to how family members and others respond to the headache sufferer; they may suggest that he or she is sick or needs rest. As the person's functioning decreases, other family members often take over his or her responsibilities, altering the functioning of the family as a whole. By common agreement, the person with the headache has an "illness."

Treatment usually begins in the family with home remedies and suggestions by loved ones. If the illness does not abate, the person may seek the input of a professional health care provider. The professional health care provider will listen to the patient's illness account and translate it into the "disease" language of diagnosis, prognosis, and treatment (Hunter, 1991). This language, in turn, will influence the patient's and family's response to the illness. The diagnosis of a disease such as cancer will have a different impact on the patient and family than a report of "no findings." One diagnosis may elicit anxiety and increased support of the patient by the family; the other may stimulate doubt and even resentment about the patient's illness.

While disease refers to "an alteration in biological structure and functioning" (e.g., the multiplication of cells that characterizes cancer), illness is the "experience of symptoms and suffering. Illness refers to how the sick person and the members of the family or wider social network perceive, live with, and respond to symptoms and disability" (Kleinman, 1988, pp. 3, 5–6). The concept of illness is not reductionistic. Illness is inherently transactional and systemic in how it is defined and how it is experienced. Understanding illness in this way makes it entirely relevant to the nosology of any mental health theory.

The biopsychosocial model enables health and mental health care providers to conceptualize problems in an integrative manner. When systems theory is applied to the biopsychosocial model, the levels of the biopsychosocial hierarchy come alive with interaction and the health and mental health professionals become more than observers of the process—they become an integral part of the interaction, contributing to it and being influenced by it. Such a dynamic model stimulates dialogue and encourages professional care providers to work together. This cross-fertilization helps each professional understand the illness and disease experience of patients and families better.

An Ecological Perspective

Collaboration is characterized by efforts to resolve problems by bringing professionals from different disciplines together. This interdisciplinary approach has been called a "putting together of heads" by Edgar Auerswald (1968). Auerswald suggests, though, that an interdisciplinary approach may not foster the very thing it is intended to create—a clearer vision of problems and solutions.

In his classic paper "Interdisciplinary versus Ecological Approach" (1968), Auerswald begins with a discussion of how knowledge is accumulated when addressing a problem. The steps in the process are familiar; they include

the collection of information or data, the ordering of that data within a selected framework, analysis of the data, synthesis of the results of analysis into hypotheses, the formulation of strategies and techniques . . . to test the hypotheses, the construction of a delivery plan . . . the implementation of the plan, and the collection of data from the arena of implementation to test its impact. (p. 203)

For the purposes of collaboration, the most important step is "the ordering of data into a selected framework." What information is deemed important or unimportant will be determined by the conceptual framework of the person collecting the data. How professionals select and prioritize data or information guides all the remaining steps in the process. Auerswald argues that in an interdisciplinary approach, each professional maintains the vantage point of his or her discipline. Each professional uses his or her framework of origin to look at a problem and uses only that framework when addressing the problem. The family therapist stays within a family systems perspective, the psychologist within a psychological perspective, the nurse within a health care perspective, the physician within a biomedical perspective, and so on. Like the characters in the Japanese play *In the Grove,* each looks at the same event but sees different things. The problem is not that each discipline has a different perspective; the problem is that each professional remains married to his or her perspective and does not communicate adequately with those from other disciplines. As a result, we remain perspective-bound, unaware of what our perspective and its language keep us from seeing (Griffith & Griffith, 1994). In Auerswald's words, each discipline borrows "only those concepts which pose no serious challenge or language difficulties" (1968, p. 204). Sometimes this tendency may encourage professionals to believe that part of their mission is to "convert" other professionals to their point of view.

An ecological approach does not require professionals from different disciplines to abandon their perspectives. It does, however, invite professionals involved in collaboration to focus on the process of interaction between the professionals, the patient, and the family. By focusing on the process of communication among the parties involved, each collaborator minimizes the risk of maintaining too narrow a vision of the problem. Instead, each is invited to see with the eyes of the other participants in a given problem. The collective viewpoint is thus enriched.

Put simply, the ecological approach proposes that the process of communication is just as important as the content of communication in determining how a problem will be understood and addressed. By focusing attention on the process of professional interactions, the ecological approach builds bridges between conceptual frameworks by creating connections between people. In the case of the patient with hypothyroidism, the ecological approach makes communication among the participants (a form of data collection) central to analyzing the problem. Had the therapist focused exclusively on how his discipline's framework of origin (family systems) conceptualized the problem, he would not have learned from the physician's framework of origin (biomedicine). The collaborative process not only encourages an interface between different disciplines but recognizes that such an interface provides the best means for gathering the most comprehensive information needed to address complex problems.

An ecological approach is to professional interaction what the biopsychosocial model is to illness. The biopsychosocial model focuses on the interface of different systems in the development of illness. The ecological approach emphasizes the interface of professional disciplines with varying degrees of expertise in the treatment of illness. The ecological approach reminds us that the content of that expertise, while very important, is no more important than the capacity to "give and take" that expertise across disciplines.

Partners in Care

William Doherty and Macaran Baird (1983) developed the "triangular model for medicine" in an effort to break the "illusion of the dyad" in health care. The "dyad" referred to is the physician-patient relationship. The emphasis on the quality of the health care provider–patient relationship has been a positive step in the humanization of medicine; it calls attention to the curative elements inherent in that relationship. However, as Doherty and Baird point out, an exclusive focus on the physician-patient dyad overlooks the impact that families have on health, illness, and how the patient relates to health care providers. They argue for the inclusion of the family in the treatment, thus creating a treatment triangle.

In our view, a similar process has prevailed in collaborative efforts between health care and mental health professionals, who have focused on how they can work together. As we have just argued, this focus is a crucial part of the collaborative process that needs care and attention. But just as a narrow focus on the physician-patient dyad may perpetuate an illusion, an exclusive focus on the mental health–health care professional dyad may create a similar illusion—that effective professional interaction is all that is needed for effective collaboration.

Because patients and families are the ones facing illness or distress, and because they are the experts on their own experience and the source of many of their own solutions, they must be included in the conceptualization of collaboration. Wynne and his colleagues (1992) remind us of the dual nature of the illness experience. On the one hand, illness affords a legitimized reduction in functioning; on the other hand, illness requires that the patient and family take responsibility for doing whatever is necessary to facilitate health, healing, or adjustment. An exclusive focus on professional interaction as the key to collaboration may overlook the important role that patients and families play in the treatment of illness. In many cultures, such as China, the patient and family are active partners in health care. Kleinman (1988) suggests that patients and families be seen as "colleagues" and that "the act of training patients and families as caregivers is a message of empowerment that is of symbolic and practical significance" (p. 261).

Family strength and competence is a major focus in contemporary family therapy (Sprenkle & Bischof, 1994). Froma Walsh (1993) notes a shift in the field from "limitations, deficits, and pathology to a competency-based, health-oriented paradigm" that changes the emphasis of treatment from "what went wrong to what can be done for enhancing functioning" (p. 53). Successful therapy depends as much on the resources of the patient and family as it does on the resources of the therapist (Karpel, 1986). Utilization of family strengths and resources is common in many approaches to family therapy, including solution-focused therapy (DeShazer, 1982), narrative therapy (White & Epston, 1990), transitional family therapy (Landau-Stanton & Clements, 1993; Seaburn, Landau-Stanton, & Horwitz, 1995), larger systems approaches (Imber-Black, 1988), and family therapy of children and adolescents (Combrinck-Graham, 1990).

Patient and family strength and competence is also reflected in the training of many health care professionals (McDaniel et al., 1990) and in the development of the medical family therapy field. McDaniel, Hepworth, and Doherty (1992) put patient and family "agency" at the center of their medical family therapy model. Agency refers to "a sense of making personal choices" (p. 9). To facilitate agency, health and mental health care providers must actively elicit the patient's and family's goals, identify their strengths, and involve them in decisions related to care. In essence, professionals must treat patients and families as partners in the collaborative process.

Later in the course of Linda's treatment, she informed her physician and therapist that she did not feel they were giving adequate attention to her problems. The therapist was tempted to see this complaint primarily as a reflection of Linda's frustration with the lack of attention she was feeling from her family. The therapist and Linda explored family issues and talked with family members, who responded by staying in more regular contact with her.

Linda reminded the therapist, though, that her complaint was that the therapist and physician were not attending adequately to her. As a consequence, Linda, her therapist, and her physician met. At that meeting, Linda taught her providers how to structure a medical/psychotherapeutic interview so that her needs could be fully addressed. She did an excellent job of training the professionals as she clarified what her concerns were and set an agenda at each visit. For her part, Linda agreed to write down her agenda before each visit so that she could more clearly state her concerns.

As this vignette indicates, collaborative dialogue facilitates changes not only among patients and families but among professional providers as well. Dialogue and openness are keys to any collaboration. They facilitate the creation of an atmosphere of respect and inclusion in which more effective decisions can be made.

CONCLUSION

A culture of collaboration does not just happen. It must be formed and fashioned by many hands, all of which are influenced by many factors, including professional training, theoretical paradigms, and the prevailing health care delivery systems. Leading the way for collaboration are professionals who share common beliefs about human problems (an integrative paradigm) and how best to address them (an ecological perspective). These professionals are only as effective in their work together, however, as their capacity to develop partnerships with patients and families allows them to be. Creating effective partnerships among professionals, patients, and families is both the challenge and reward of collaboration.

In the next chapter, we discuss the historical factors that have made collaboration the exception rather than the rule among health and mental health professionals.

CHAPTER 2

Collaboration in Historical Perspective

TO HELP US UNDERSTAND collaboration and what it means today, we can look back through the past and trace the development of predominant themes. Collaboration has not evolved in a nice, smooth, easily understood, linear way. Rather, its course through history more closely resembles the path of a tumbling gymnast: It has leaped and bounded, started and stopped, twisted and turned. In part, this is a quality of collaboration because it is a group effort, and each member of a group has a unique background. Their backgrounds may differ enormously: For example, some professions have been around since antiquity, and others for less than one hundred years. Each profession has its own focus, strengths, and idiosyncrasies. This diversity allows the health care system to accommodate and respond to the diversity of human suffering, but it can also lead to many interprofessional misunderstandings.

Collaboration can be viewed as the latest adaptation to a changing health care environment. The purpose of this chapter is to describe this complex evolution so as to illuminate our current situation and professional behavior. It is not intended to be a complete review of each profession; that is already the work of many other books. We will touch on the fields of medicine, nursing, psychiatry, psychology, social work, and family therapy. Limiting our discussion in this chapter to collaboration in the health care setting and to Western society, we will focus on collaboration between mental health and health care providers and on their attitudes about collaboration with patients and their families.

To organize the discussion, we trace three influential themes: mind/body dualism, dyadic and systems orientations, and paternalism versus empowerment. These three themes culminate in the basic tenets of collaboration noted in chapter 1. An "integrative paradigm" responds to the challenge of mind/body dualism. An "ecological approach" incorporates the healing power of a dyadic orientation with systems theory. And an attitude of "partners in care" speaks to the debate about paternalism versus empowerment. For conceptual ease, we divide our discussion of each theme into three time periods: antiquity to the Industrial Revolution, the Industrial Revolution to World War II, and World War II to the present. We view history with an eye on the role these themes have played in forming our current health care system, and on the way the basic tenets of collaboration represent a logical and necessary evolution of health care delivery.

MIND/BODY DUALISM

Mind/body dualism, which dates back to at least Plato, is a dichotomy that cleaves our experience into two disparate entities. One could argue that the single conceptual element that most characterizes Western culture is mind/body dualism. Likewise, our health care has been divided into care for the mind and care for the body. An integrative paradigm links mind and body with a language that can be understood in both cultures. An integrative paradigm allows health care providers to work together while accommodating our intellectual inheritance of .mind/body dualism. Creating a culture of collaboration bridges the conceptual chasm created by splitting mind and body.

Roots of Western Culture: Antiquity to the Industrial Revolution

> The medical art heals diseases of the body, whereas wisdom relieves the soul of passions.
>
> Democritus (1922)

Western culture dates back to the time of the Greeks, roughly 500 B.C. The foundations of our current culture were laid by Plato, Aristotle, Hippocrates, and others. Their ideas permeate every aspect of Western civilization. Ancient Greece witnessed great revolutions in thinking. Health and illness, along with just about all aspects of life, had previously been considered a reflection of the individual's relationship with the gods. It was a time of pagan beliefs; incurring the disfavor of the gods was thought to wreak illness, pestilence, and drought. In his efforts to secure a place in society for the profession of medicine, Hippocrates nurtured mind/body dualism. Rather than try to explain all of human suffering, Hippocrates focused narrowly on the body. The philosophers of his time were happy to reinforce his view so that they could become undisputed experts in the realm of the mind.

Hippocrates' contribution was to "make medicine rational" (Temkin, 1991). He took medicine out of the realm of magic and the domain of the gods. By focusing medicine on the patient's body, he distinguished the body as the exclusive province of the physician. Skilled in dissection, Hippocrates relied heavily on anatomy as a way to both describe and treat illness. His curriculum begins with anatomy as a map for understanding pathophysiologic processes. To this day, most medical school curricula begin with anatomy and dissection.

The focus on anatomy is also significant in that it fosters a way of thinking, a kind of cognitive attitude. Physicians are trained to think visually and to see problems as mechanical perturbations. This thinking has led to many current-day misunderstandings. When one who is trained to think mechanically tries to communicate with one who is trained to think organically, their cognitive styles can clash. Hippocrates' biomechanical orientation wrought many such problems, but it also led to a great many positive advances in surgery and orthopedics. Today simple fractures are set in the exact same way they were during the time of the Greeks. Over the years Hippocrates and his followers became quite proficient at all the manual skills of healing.

While Hippocrates established the body as the domain of illness, and the physician as the expert on treating illness, he left the mind to the philosophers. Both medicine and philosophy flourished once their separate domains were defined. In Western culture, following the time of Christ, religion took up much of the work of philosophy. The soul became part of the mind, and clergy became healers of the soul's ailments.

After Hippocrates, the perception of the body went through several transformations. The Greeks saw the body as glorious and worshiped its accomplishments (hence the Olympics). With the spread of Christianity, however, the body came to be seen as a source of sin, and the impulses of the body as something to be resisted (Magner, 1992). Following the Renaissance, during the Age of Reason, and beginning with Descartes, mind/body dualism was extended metaphysically and became a part of the Truth. The mind was part of the soul, and the body merely an earthly machine, or deus ex machina (god in the machine) (Brown, 1989).

The Modern Age: The Industrial Revolution to World War II

The Industrial Revolution marks the beginning of the modern age. The period 1800–1941 was characterized by diversity, complexity, and new growth. Men, along with some women and children, left their families, homes, and fields to work in factories. These changes had a profound effect on families and gender roles (Bly, 1990), and capitalism had a tremendous effect on communities; Karl Marx and Friedrich Engels hypothesized that the resulting alienation would lead to massive social revolution. Society became increasingly mobile, and the world became a smaller place. The expansion of technology led to more diversification and specialization in every field.

The well-established mind/body split became even more entrenched during this period. Professions were spawned that specialized in various aspects of either the mind or the body. With the goal of studying mind and body objectively, these new professionals made many new insights into the condition of humankind and developed new treatments for illness. Both professionals and the general public became quite enamored with the successes of the new specialties. However, professional specialization increased the need for communication between different health care disciplines.

Many important advances in medicine were made. The discovery of anesthesia (1811) radically transformed surgery. Now the body really could be reduced to a "machine" and be repaired. Internal fractures could be fixed. People no longer died of appendicitis. Cesarean sections could be performed on women and babies who might otherwise have died during childbirth. Germ theory gave physicians a model for disease (though some resented its reductionism). Many contagious diseases could at least be explained, if not treated. The incidence of waterborne diseases, especially cholera, was dramatically reduced as a result of the sanitation measures inspired by germ theory. Such a reduction was an enormous success for public health. Penicillin was discovered. The use of X-rays was initiated. Nursing emerged as a profession devoted to caring for the sick and injured. These innovations and others brought physicians greater success in treating illness and raised the public's opinion of medicine in general.

Florence Nightingale, the founder of professional nursing, presaged some of the gender issues, and related power issues, between nursing and medicine when she began her seminal 1860 work *Notes on Nursing* with the phrase, "Every woman is a nurse." Certainly nursing was done prior to Nightingale's time (Reverby & Rosner, 1979; Shryrock, 1959), but she established it forever as a profession. Born in 1820 to affluent English parents, Nightingale was raised to be freethinking, egalitarian, and assertive. She was interested in helping the sick and injured from the beginning and as a young woman dreamed of turning her family's large estate into a hospital. She sought training the only way she could get it— through the Catholic Church. During the Crimean War, she led a group of women to care for the sick and wounded. In the military hospital she found chaos, filth, and very high mortality rates. Patients were housed in close and drafty quarters amid rats and vermin. Bandages were reused, and surgical instruments were not cleaned between patients. Her reform efforts were vigorously opposed by military medical officers, who took her ideas as personal criticism. Nightingale had powerful friends in London, however, and succeeded in carrying out her reforms. As it turned out, she was immensely successful and eventually became a hero.

On her return to England, and shortly thereafter in the United States, support grew for the Nightingale System, a training program for nurses. Some of the training took place in universities but for the most part was provided in hospitals. The discovery by hospitals that nurses-in-training were an inexpensive source of valuable labor expedited the growth of the profession.

Nursing's position relative to medicine in the hierarchy of health care has always mirrored the power differential between women and men in Western society. Barbara Melosh, in explaining the title of her book *The Physician's Hand* (1982), nicely captures the spirit of nursing:

> The title evokes three central aspects. It calls attention, first, to the relationship that defines nurses' position in the medical hierarchy.

By law and custom, nurses are subordinate to physicians. At the same time, it captures the nurse's critical role in executing the physician's work. Second in the line of command, nurses are closely associated with the power and prestige of medicine. In the intricate hospital hierarchy, they reign over practical nurses and aides, orderlies, and a plethora of other auxiliary workers. Second, interpreted in a rather different way, "the physician's hand" suggests the strength of character of nurses' occupational culture, a tradition of pride in manual skills, of direct involvement with the sick, of respect for experience and often a concomitant mistrust for theory. Finally, "the physician's hand" is a phrase that symbolizes years of struggle, for nurses have never been content to define their work solely in relation to doctors. Both in professional associations and on the job, nurses have sought to claim and defend their own sphere of legitimate authority. Leaders called it professional autonomy; nurses on the job might well have named it workers' control. (pp. 6–7)

Nursing made an enormous contribution to the care of patients in the medical setting. Besides their biologic training and their work with physicians, nurses were also trained to emphasize family, social, and psychological well-being (Baggs, 1994; Baggs & Schmitt, 1988).

On the mind side of mind/body dualism, the rise of science and technology during and after the Industrial Revolution brought an accompanying decline in the religious life of the general population. In earlier times, religion had answered some of the basic questions of life: What is the meaning of life? How do you explain the problem of suffering, or the problem of evil? What happens after you die? During the modern age, the task of addressing these core life questions was taken up in part by two new professions and colored by new developments in philosophy. The fields of psychology and psychiatry sought to provide insight into the human condition and, if not address, at least help reformulate these questions. The establishment of the "mind" professions, partly replacing and partly supplementing religion, embellished the mind/body split, making collaboration among those attempting to alleviate human suffering ever more complex.

Following Friedrich Nietzsche and his well-known meditation "God is dead," the dean of Harvard was so terrified that the decline of religious life would lead to rampant nihilism and suicide among educated youth that he hired William James to put meaning back into the lives of Harvard students. James conducted a number of experiments in perception, and these studies, especially of visual perception, eventually helped legitimize psychology as a way to study the mind when they were applied to examinations of how people think (James, 1890, 1961, 1970, 1971, 1974).

By the late nineteenth century, the scientific method was accepted and could be applied to a study of the mind, further embuing the mind with a life of its own apart from the body. James continued the task set for him by the dean of Harvard, blending metaphysics with science in an attempt to come up with a more "scientific" response to the meaning of life. His followers, however, would place more emphasis on the scientific aspects of the study of the mind and abandon the attempt to answer the larger questions.

The writings of Sigmund Freud, a physician and the founder of psychoanalysis, further increased the number and breadth of professionals devoted to the mind. He hypothesized that dreams are a major route to revealing the unconscious. He did his own dream analysis and published his findings in the well-known *Interpretation of Dreams* (1900/1965). He wrote that a part of the self of every person is invisible to his or her mind's eye. This unconscious part includes unacceptable aspects—such as sexual and aggressive urges or memories of specific life events—that would cause anxiety if the individual were consciously aware of them. These unconscious forces and memories affect health and can play a role in illness. For example, an inability to perform a certain task could relate to unconscious, irrational fears about its meaning and consequences. Bringing those fears to light allows a person to rethink his or her response, decide whether the previous fears and avoidance remain necessary, and hence obtain greater freedom to pursue life satisfactions. Through the process of psychoanalysis, and the help of a trained professional, the unseen is brought into awareness, thus promoting in the patient greater autonomy and improved health (Freud, 1990/1887–1938).

There was some struggle in the 1930s over the question of which profession would continue Freud's work, but since he was trained as a physician, medicine won out and psychiatry became a medical specialty. Since that time psychiatry has garnered particular expertise in prescribing psychoactive medications.

There were also major new movements in philosophy during the modern period. The existential philosophers, most notably Jean-Paul Sartre, presaged postmodern thought by expanding the idea that there is no absolute truth and life has no ultimate meaning beyond what the individual mind attributes to it. The heuristic philosophers, most notably Martin Heidegger, went further by saying that since reality is merely a linguistically defined concept, and language is a social process, reality is only a socially defined entity.

Griffith and Griffith (1994) note the relation between this formulation and the medical context: "Philosophical hermeneutics showed the division between mind and body on which modern medicine is built to be a socially negotiated interpretation imposed on life as humans experience it, rather than a reflection of an objective reality that stands outside human experience" (p. 35). Mind and body are constructs and as such can be rethought (or deconstructed) and in the process reconnected. Their book offers an excellent review of this philosophical movement, which has evolved into the social constructionism of today. This philosophical idea was ahead of its time and has had considerable impact on the theory of psychotherapy today, though at the time of its development it had little actual effect on health care.

These three threads—psychology, psychoanalysis, and the precursors of postmodern philosophical ideas—wove a fabric that established the mind as a field of scientific study as well as a source of illness, suffering, and meaning and established mental health as an integral part of health care (Anderson & Goolishian, 1988; Berger & Luckmann, 1966; Gergen, 1985; Howard, 1991; Rorty, 1979; Seaburn et al., 1992; White & Epston, 1990).

The Age of Technology: World War II to the Present

The explosion of technology and information since World War II, in all fields, has come at a considerable price. Many parts of our experience are now broken into very different pieces. There are specialists for every conceivable aspect of our daily lives. Machines separate us from even the simplest tasks, and telecommunications has made the world an extremely small place. In health care, specialization and diversification have only increased. There has been a backlash to the resulting alienation. More and more people cry out for holistic health. Collaboration is the natural solution to the problems created by diversification.

Before World War II there were few medical specialists; after World War II (in the late 1940s and 1950s) 30% of all physicians were specialists; now more than 60% of all physicians are specialists. Why are there so many? The myriad reasons include but are not limited to: Specialists make more money and often have a nicer lifestyle than most generalists; specialty medicine produces more income for hospitals; specialization offers a different intellectual appeal (depth instead of breadth); focusing on a specialty presents less ambiguity; and perhaps most important, the public thirsts for medical miracles. Mind-boggling feats of heroic medicine are played out every day: Antibiotics treat life-threatening infections; cancer is detected earlier and often cured; coronary arteries are bypassed; critical organs are transplanted. The list of achievements goes on and on. What were once life-threatening or terminal illnesses are now chronic illnesses, and people are living for considerably longer periods of time. Meanwhile, the care of patients has become splintered among specialty groups, with one doctor taking care of the heart, one the lungs, one the joints, and one the psyche.

The mental health fields have seen a similar burgeoning of specialties, among them, clinical psychology, psychiatry, social work, and family therapy. Within each field are many different perspectives and clinical interventions: behavioral, solution-focused, Bowenian, Jungian, transpersonal, insight-oriented, biologic, family/contextual, and more. Approaches, and the corresponding training, can be divided up by age or by problem. People can be seen as individuals, couples, families, with other families, or in groups. The diversity is enormous. It is fitting that, as the biomechanical orientation of medicine divides the body into anatomical parts, the organic orientation of mental health divides the field by approaches.

The 1960s saw the rise of primary care specialties in response to the fragmentation of medical care. The purpose of family medicine, also born against this backdrop of superspecialization, was to integrate health care provision and "to not discriminate on the basis of age, sex, race, or problem" (Stephens, 1982, p. 75). Family medicine incorporated many of the ideas of the time. Patients were seen in the broader context of the family, which was the focus of care. Ninety percent of all health problems could be cared for by a family physician.

General internal medicine and pediatrics sought to incorporate many of these same ideals. Greater emphasis was placed on preventive care, and psychosocial and socioeconomic factors were again considered integral to health. Nursing, which had always paid attention to these factors, expanded into the field of primary care during the 1960s with the development of nurse-practitioners. At about the same time the number of certified nurse-midwives (CNMs), who had been providing care for several decades, began to increase substantially. Today there are now physician's assistants (PAs) who can provide primary care, though both nurse-practitioners and physician's assistants may work with specialty physicians as well.

There have been several attempts to construct an overarching paradigm to resolve mind/body dualism. The biopsychosocial model postulated by George Engel (described in chapter 1) enables providers to recognize the different levels of a patient's experience. We have found this model to be the most appealing and the best at accounting for the diversity of human experience. Perhaps more important, this model is best able to accommodate and link the diversity of preexisting explanatory models. Systems theory embellishes the biopsychosocial model by stressing the importance of focusing on the interaction between different systemic levels. Also, with the increasingly cosmopolitan nature of the world, other cultures and ways of thinking have influenced our own. Mind/body dualism is not present in many other cultures. A cultural cross-fertilization of ideas has taken place, and some of our new ways of thinking are hybrids of this interaction (Kleinman, 1988).

DYADIC AND SYSTEMS ORIENTATIONS

Since the Greeks, healing has focused on three critical aspects of health: modification of external factors, modification of internal factors, and cultivating a healing dyadic relationship. The next section on empowerment elucidates the issues related to modification of internal factors. In this section, we concentrate on the role of the dyadic relationship and the evolution of our thinking about the role of external factors. An ecosystemic approach respects the power of the dyadic relationship while using systemic thinking to determine the influence of external factors.

The dyadic relationship between healers and patients has a long and prestigious place in the history of healing. According to ancient Greek legend, the healer took illness out of the afflicted person's body and brought it into his or her own, where it could be combated and destroyed. It was through this close contact between healer and patient that healing occurred. This idea of the special healing powers between two people has been perpetuated throughout history in all the healing professions.

A variety of external factors have been thought to play a role in health. Since Hippocrates, who espoused a naturalistic approach, nutrition has been thought to be important. Air and water quality has always been emphasized. The Greeks believed that exercise was integral to good health, but this notion fell into disfavor when attitudes about the body changed with Christianity. Being in a state of war was also thought to be deleterious (especially to the soldiers). Although the Greeks seldom mentioned the family, both the Greeks and Christians often spoke of community. People continued to take systemic factors into account as they searched for a way to explain health and illness. As Glenn (1987b) notes, "For centuries, physicians sought for the fit between people's illnesses and their way of living. The Hippocratic tradition reigned, especially through the writings of his follower Galen, and his influence was still strong in nineteenth century Europe before the germ theory of disease took hold" (p. 58). The biopsychosocial model, systems thinking, and an ecological perspective all look at the patient in this broader, more complex context that stresses interrelatedness and the power of context.

Mental health and health care providers are also located within a larger context. Every health care professional works amid other professionals, and every professional needs to be aware of his or her own role and the contributions of others. For example, social work has long understood the value of working with various agencies and creating care-providing networks. Doctors have collaborated with professional nurses since Florence Nightingale. More recently, the health care team has expanded from nurses, social workers, mental health care providers, and others to include dietitians, physical therapists, and occupational therapists. All health care providers need to be aware of their own issues as well as their strengths and skills. Thus, an awareness not only of the context of the patient but of the context of the mental health and health care providers is critical to understanding the ecosystem in which care is provided.

Antiquity to the Industrial Revolution

One of Hippocrates' greatest contributions was in the area of the doctor-patient relationship. Hippocrates valued the healing dyad. The confidentiality that protected the discourse between healer and afflicted allowed a more accurate illness history to emerge. He also observed that this protected intimacy was in itself healing. Humans are social beings who need a protected relationship for healing.

With the advent of Christianity, this dyadic healing focus was perpetuated in the practice of confession. Priests carried on the role of the philosophers in their counsel about spiritual and metaphysical matters and learned from physicians about the power of confidentiality. The same rule of confidentiality was applied to confession, and the confessional booth became a place of psychological as well as spiritual healing. This carryover into religion reinforced the norm of confidentiality in the world of medicine. With the Reformation, confession was dropped from the practice of Protestant faiths, but the notion of confidentiality between clergy and members of their faith remained. This norm also characterized the relationship between the rabbi and his congregation.

Healers rarely collaborated. In Greek and Roman antiquity, there is some evidence of consultation between physicians, dietitians, and gymnasts and cooperation with water specialists. (The Roman aqueducts were well-known public health projects.) Greek philosophers and physicians had little contact and did not collaborate on individual patients; each outlined his own "turf." Likewise, there would be little contact later between physicians and priests or rabbis, except during the Middle Ages, when the church took over much of the education of physicians until the emergence of the university system.

The Industrial Revolution to World War II

The social tension and suffering that resulted from the early industrial age sensitized many of the great thinkers to systemic issues. It became more and more difficult to focus on the individual without accounting for the family, social, and political contexts. For example, Marx and Engels noted the influence of capitalism on the social alienation of families and communities. Their analysis of the whole community, including its economic status, as a function of health was a major contribution (Navarro, 1976). These ideas were some of the early seeds of the public health movement that was trying to influence medicine. Glenn (1987b) points out that Virchow, a pathologist at the turn of the century, "like Engels linked workers' illnesses to the effects of the Industrial Revolution" (p. 60). But organized medicine was threatened by this kind of political analysis, and such notions quickly faded from the medical literature.

The field of social work focused on the impact of poverty on families and the neighborhoods they lived in. With the initial goal of providing places for families to come together and guaranteeing them food and shelter, social workers created recreation centers, soup kitchens, and shelters and developed various outreach activities. Social workers also coordinated and facilitated access to available services. Social work's family orientation is summarized by Axinn and Levin (1975).

> Amazingly rapid development occurred in social work during the period 1900–1929. The organization and professionalization of social work was carried out by the Charity Organization and Settlement House movements. Both movements claimed a concern with the family as the core unit of society, and each, to its own lights, developed its program so as to bring stability and fulfillment to family living. While the economy appeared to prosper, social work turned to family dynamics and individual personality development. Therapy had become the door to social well-being. (p. 143)

As physicians grew more enamored of medical technological advances, their interest waned in the psychological and social well-being of hospitalized patients. Thus, starting in 1905, medical providers and administrators brought medical social workers into hospitals to help in these areas. Caring for the psychological well-being of patients was seen as more menial work, while medicine maintained its position atop the health care hierarchy.

During this period, Michael M. Davis, one of the early proponents of collaboration, helped organize the Committee on the Cost of Medical Care (Board of Trustees, AMA, 1932a). The committee's main thesis was that collaboration between providers of different aspects of a patient's care ensured more complete and more cost-effective care. Presumably threatened by this apparent attempt to decrease its power, the American Medical Association (AMA) lambasted the committee's report, calling it "communistic," in a series of 1932 editorials in the *Journal of the American Medical Association* (Board of Trustees, AMA, 1932b).

In the 1920s and 1930s, there were several health demonstration projects that focused on family health and collaboration with health care professionals. The most notable of these was the Peckham Project in England (Pearse & Crocker, 1943). It was cooperatively set up and run by a group of social scientists, with consultation from physicians, nurses, midwives, and dietitians. The Peckham Project was designed to foster the health of a small community of neighborhoods and to combat the alienation associated with poverty, especially for young families. It was housed in a large structure in which health care services were not directly delivered (no prescriptions were written) but many social and recreational opportunities were provided. Prenatal care was provided as well, but all deliveries were done at a nearby hospital by other personnel. The many educational and support efforts focused on parenting and on the struggles of young families. Besides activities for parents, children, and whole families, classes in nutrition, housekeeping, and health were offered, and job skills assessment and retraining opportunities were also available. The Peckham Project was quite successful in health promotion but was not financially self-sustaining. Lack of funding and the strain of the depression brought it to an end.

World War II to the Present

As the world has grown more complex, so has the understanding of individual systems. Systems theory grew out of an appreciation for the interdependence of living organisms and their environments. One event ripples out, like waves in the water after a stone is thrown in a pond, and affects everything to which it is related. These effects ripple back, and so on, as the relationships keep evolving. Cybernetics, originally a communications field, further defined these effects and relationships systemically. The notion quickly caught on, and systems theory was widely applied to many different disciplines.

Family therapy was started in the 1950s by psychiatrists such as Lyman Wynne, Murray Bowen, Nathan Ackerman, and Don Jackson who were interested in schizophrenia. Initially, they took the traditional medical approach of looking for the systemic cause (or "germ") of the problem. As interaction systems came to the forefront of thought, the body and biology were eventually left behind. Thus, family therapy developed away from the medical model and away from the physical body. Family systems approaches have expanded over the years to include the extended family, transgenerational processes, culture, gender, and the person of the therapist.

Systems theory also had an effect on medical health care delivery systems. During the 1960s, there was a tremendous resurgence of community health centers. This trend was not unlike the progressive movements of the early 1900s, when it was thought that health care needed to be delivered in the neighborhoods where people lived. The community health centers of the 1960s emphasized complete care, ranging from dental, medical, social, and mental health care to social work (see Montefiore experiment in Levenson, 1984). These centers were popular and apparently effective, though largely unstudied.

Many of these efforts were experiments in the participation movement, a grassroots effort that emphasized nonprofessional involvement. In fact, professionals were often purposefully left off of planning committees and administrative boards. During the era of the Great Society, money was available to provide for the poor and carry out these experiments in health care delivery. However, keeping track of which interventions were most cost-effective was not given priority, and these clinics were not self-supporting. When the stripped-down budgets of the late 1970s and 1980s came along, the great majority of community health centers closed. However, collaborative clinics have once again begun to appear, especially ones that foster a collaboration between agencies (Huebel, 1993). In fact, in the field of social work the term "collaboration" primarily refers to collaboration at a larger systemic level—between agencies, not between individuals.

A truly ecosystemic approach also respects the role and power of the healing dyad. In mental health there has always been room for individual therapy, and most therapists are willing to see individuals. In medicine, partly as a result of the distance created by technology, there has been renewed interest, mainly among primary care internists, in focusing on the special doctor-patient relationship. Numerous seminars and conferences that focus on this one-to-one relationship are now offered. Some of this renewed interest is centered on the physician's own person and family of origin and how they affect the doctor-patient relationship. New national groups dedicated to fostering this interest have arisen, in particular the Society of General Internal Medicine and the American Academy on Physician and Patient. New journals that chronicle this fascinating chapter in medicine—for example, *Second Opinion*—have also been started.

In a recent survey, as many as 60% of all physicians said that if they had to do it all over again, they would not choose medicine as their career. There has been tremendous burnout and job dissatisfaction among physicians. For the many physicians who have embraced this renewed emphasis on the doctor-patient relationship, like a long-lost traveler savoring a home-cooked meal, it is a return to what initially attracted them to medicine.

PATERNALISM VERSUS EMPOWERMENT

The third theme, paternalism versus empowerment, has to do with the locus of control and influence—who has the power and the responsibility for health and healing. Paternalism assumes that the healer is in charge, and that the healer is embued with many god-like qualities: all-seeing, all-knowing, and all-powerful. To get well, the patient must do what the provider says. There have always been political implications to paternalism—since it designates an artificial hierarchy—as well as gender implications: In Western society men have more power, and their role as healers may increase this power.

The goal of empowerment is to make the patient an integral participant in health care decisions. In fact, outside the biomedical world the term "client" or even "consumer" is used in place of "patient," since "patient" often connotes a passive, one-down position. The healer's role is to help patients become more active in their own health care and to empower them to take more responsibility for their overall health (Brickman, 1982). On the provider side, empowerment fosters certain attitudes about power distribution among health care providers and attitudes about spheres of influence ("turf") and working together. A philosophy of empowerment replaces rigid hierarchy with differential expertise, directives with consensus, and compliance with cooperation, and it relies on trust, respect, and a spirit of working together. Since power is a key ingredient in any relationship, the locus of control is a central feature in any collaborative relationship, be it between health care providers or between health care providers and patients and their families.

Antiquity to the Industrial Revolution

> The art [of medicine] has three factors: the disease, the patient, and the physician. The physician is the servant of the art; the patient must cooperate with the physician in combating the disease.
>
> Hippocrates, *Epidemics I* (1988)

This quote summarizes physician attitudes from the time of Hippocrates to the Industrial Revolution and beyond. The Hippocratic tradition made giant strides in improving the efficacy of medicine in treating the ailments of antiquity. Physicians also became very good at predicting the outcome of diseases (making prognoses) and knowing their limitations. If the physician did decide to do something, then it was the responsibility of the patient to follow the doctor's orders. If no cure resulted, it was either because the patient did not follow the treatment properly or the patient was beyond treatment.

Sometimes the physician elected to do nothing and allow the illness to take its natural course. As implied by the famous dictum *primum non nocere* ("first do no harm"), this decision reflected a faith in and respect for the body's natural healing powers. If the physician could do nothing to promote healing, then his or her job was simply to comfort the patient. Thus arose a paternalistic attitude in many physicians, and a neutral (nonpaternalistic, but non-empowering) attitude in others.

Industrial Revolution to World War II

Paternalism was reinforced during the modern age by its emphasis on objectivity. Not only did physicians know what was best for their patients, but now they had scientific "truth," not just theories, to support their claims. Psychoanalysts knew the right interpretation of dreams. Physicians knew that germs cause disease. In some ways, such certainty was an even more pernicious form of paternalism. How could one argue with science?

The evolution of obstetrical care illustrates how medicine succeeded in expanding its territory and promoting its methodology. Prior to the turn of the century, most babies were delivered at home by midwives. Midwives knew their patients and the patients' families well, often living in the same neighborhoods. Physicians wanted more deliveries to be made in hospitals, partly as a source of income and partly to provide training opportunities for medical students and interns. Dr. Joseph Price wrote in 1894, "The rich have to take care of the poor, and I feel the pauper element of society should be wisely and humanely used for educational purposes that we may have more finished doctors" (p. 41). Then, in the landmark case Commonwealth (of Massachusetts) v. Porn (1905), a lay midwife was successfully prosecuted for illegally practicing medicine. Subsequently, midwifery went underground. The medical profession, with science on its side, had persuaded the public, and the courts, that it was superior, though in fact the morbidity and mortality associated with hospital deliveries far exceeded that of home deliveries. Before the turn of the century, 90% of deliveries were done at home; by 1938 the number had dropped to 50%; by 1955 the medicalization of obstetrics was almost complete, with only 5% of deliveries done at home. Only recently has midwifery regained any status as a health care discipline.

The evolution of social work, which was built on the notion of empowerment, was quite different. George Bellamy of Cleveland's Hiram House nicely summarized this orientation in 1914 when speaking about the role of recreational programs: "It is far better for the city to throw the responsibility of self-support and self-improvement upon the people themselves than to hire at great expense . . . others to entertain the community. We need a recreation by the people, not, for the people" (Axinn & Levin, 1975, p. 73).

There is little in the medical literature of the Progressive Era—which peaked during the term of Theodore Roosevelt in 1912 but ended with World War I—on empowerment, but it is clear that most medical providers became increasingly threatened by health care providers who advocated this approach. For example, following the Progressive Era, the Sheppard-Towner Act of 1923 promoted the rapid expansion of health conferences, the development of centers for prenatal care, and an increase in the scope of visiting nurse services. During the 1920s patients were increasingly able to pay for more and more expensive services. Physicians saw these new providers as competing for health care dollars. Organized medicine (the AMA) was soundly against the Sheppard-Towner Act.

World War II to the Present

As noted at the beginning of the chapter, any discussion of paternalism naturally involves a discussion of power. Likewise, any discussion of power entails a description of hierarchy. The health care hierarchy has gone through several convolutions in the past five decades, especially recently. Through the establishment and enormous growth of the Medicaid and Medicare programs, the federal government has taken a greater role in controlling the provision of health care. The insurance industry, especially in the form of managed care, has garnered tremendous power in the provision of health care. In general, physicians have seen their power steadily eroded.

Not only has the total power allotted to health care providers decreased, but physicians have had to share their power with an expanding group of professionals. Power is being transferred from the specialists to the primary care physicians. Increasing numbers of nurse-practitioners and physician's assistants provide both primary and specialty care; new, and newly recognized, allied professionals and paraprofessionals are now on the scene. Lawyers and the threat of malpractice suits have also transformed the way care is delivered. All in all, physicians, particularly specialists, remain at the top of the health care hierarchy. That may change, however, as health care reform proceeds.

The change in the relative power of patients and their families in health care has been a bit less dramatic. The consumer movement has promoted education and informed consent among patients. For the most part, however, patients are still supposed to do what the doctor says, and if they don't, they are labeled "noncompliant," or "bad," patients. Some physicians have changed that attitude recently as they have come to a greater understanding of why patients don't do what their doctor tells them and of the role families play in taking care of ill members. But in general, the doctor, armed with all the latest technology, continues to know "what is best."

One problem with the physician's aura of power is that it engenders false hope in medicine; many patients are bound to be disappointed. As doctors recognize the problem of false hope, they are more and more willing to step down off their pedestals. Moreover, as doctors treat patients more as partners in care, they are finding that they get better histories and better cooperation with treatment plans from their patients, their patients appreciate them more (and consequently sue them less), and perhaps most important, they enjoy medicine more.

As noted in chapter 1, the notion of empowerment is central to many schools of family therapy. Historically, family therapy has taken one of two approaches to empowerment. The cybernetic model has emphasized symptoms in families as if they were from homeostatic systems. Therapists practicing with this perspective from the early 1970s to the early 1980s used the interventions of unbalancing, restructuring, and redefining boundaries (Minuchin, 1974; Minuchin & Fishman, 1981) and emphasizing hierarchies, giving directives, and prescribing tasks (Haley, 1973, 1976; Madanes, 1981). These therapists saw the direction the family needed to take and pointed them toward it.

Those taking the second approach view families as evolutionary, as living and evolving rather than as homeostatic systems. From this view, families are capable of making transformations on their own. Therapists with this perspective take the posture of "standing behind" (White & Epston, 1990) individuals to support them through their change rather than directing them into it. Particularly in working with black families, Nancy Boyd-Franklin (1982, 1989) sees empowerment as the central goal of therapy. Today family therapy has moved toward this second vision of empowerment as a basic goal in therapy and, more important, as a critical component of continuing health beyond therapy.

CONCLUSION

The mind/body dualism nurtured since Hippocrates is deeply embedded in our culture and in our health care delivery system. Part of the success of the Hippocratic method, and of medicine, has been attributable to its focus on the body. Over the centuries tremendous technical expertise has evolved with the elaboration of numerous specialties. Now medical miracles are performed every day. In the past century, the study of the mind and the provision of mental health services have burgeoned at a similarly breakneck pace. Our understanding of illness, health, and the provision of mental health and health care services has grown increasingly complex. Meanwhile, the public cries out for an appreciation of the whole person. Only an integrative paradigm will be able to take into account the wide range of perspectives between mental health and health care providers.

History recognizes that mental health and health care providers and patients and their families exist in their own contexts, and that these contexts (or ecosystems) are related and connected. Mental health and health care providers operate in the contexts of their own life history, their clinical setting, their unique training, and in their relationship with other providers. These relationships take place in the context of the health care environment, which encompasses prevailing social norms and the myriad facets of health insurance and economics. Patient contexts include family, genetic heritage, community, culture, job, and all the other external factors that affect an individual's health. Simultaneously, it is critical not to lose sight of the special and time-honored healing role of the primary dyadic relationship between the professional and the patient. Effective collaboration takes a balanced position that recognizes the power of the healing dyadic relationship within a larger ecosystem.

Finally, effective collaboration begets certain norms about power distribution. Paternalistic attitudes can no longer predominate. In the pluralistic world of health care today, there must be a recognition of the expertise of all concerned, including all providers and patients and their families. To become partners in care, patients and their families need to be empowered to take control of certain aspects of their own health and well-being. They also need to accept the responsibility that goes with this power.

Mental health and health care providers need not abdicate all power and responsibility and become passive. The sharing of power among providers and patients and families should reflect each one's unique expertise and responsibility for health. Given the evolution to our current setting of diversification of professional disciplines, technological advances, intellectual inheritance, and the need for individual and family involvement, it is clear that the basic tenets of collaboration represent the most meaningful elaboration of health care at this time.

CHAPTER 3

Key Ingredients for Effective Collaboration

COLLABORATION BETWEEN mental health and health care providers is co-evolving with collaborative approaches in every area of society. From the arts and sciences to business, manufacturing, and architecture, one hears repeatedly of the need to collaborate. With the information explosion and the complexity of today's world, it has become increasingly difficult for one person to grasp and steer an entire enterprise. The days of Ford and Carnegie are gone. No longer can one person direct while others follow blindly, not understanding how their individual parts fit into the larger whole.

This new thinking challenges some long-cherished approaches. Collaboration questions the modern tendency to divide complex tasks into smaller, more specialized components to increase efficiency. Collaboration disputes the assumption that rigid hierarchy is essential to organizational functioning. Collaboration may even challenge us to confront our cultural roots in rugged individualism. As a society, we are developing work and home environments that respect each individual's need to learn and contribute. We now recognize that one person's contribution may complement and strengthen the contributions of others. Shared decision-making and a common purpose enhance everyone's commitment to a common goal. From total quality management (TQM) approaches in health care, business, and education to multiracial children addressing the issue of prejudice through theater, the trend toward working together for a common goal is sweeping through every sector of our society.

As collaborative approaches to health and mental health diversify and multiply, several key ingredients can be identified within the multitude of final applications. These key ingredients are essential to all cultures of collaboration, no matter what the particular ecosystem. The exact "recipe" within each ecosystem may vary. Like recipes for chocolate chip cookies, some may be more labor-intensive; some may call for more expensive ingredients; and sometimes a shortfall of ingredients may call for more creativity on the part of the baker. The same is true for collaboration—the key ingredients may be mixed in a variety of different ways depending on the context, what is available, and individual preferences. Competing demands will undoubtedly shape and change the ultimate form of future collaboration in health care, though certain fundamental ingredients should remain the same.

The key ingredients for health and mental health collaboration are: relationship, common purpose, paradigm, communication, location of service, and business arrangement (Figure 3.1). We illustrate the conceptual material with real cases of mental health and health care providers working together, though some details may have been changed to protect anonymity. A short list of practical suggestions closes each key ingredient section. The chapter ends with a summary that offers our ideal blend of the key ingredients.

RELATIONSHIP

Relationship is the most important ingredient in any recipe for collaboration. The quality of the collaboration often reflects the quality of the relationship between the collaborators. Sharing the same geographic space, and even optimizing all the other variables, means nothing if the individuals trying to collaborate cannot develop a working relationship. Effective collaboration can take place between people of widely divergent backgrounds, experience, and viewpoint if they have a good relationship. In this section, we focus primarily on collaborative relationships between mental health and health care providers, and only secondarily on collaborative relationships with patients and families. We note that

FIGURE 3.1

KEY INGREDIENTS FOR EFFECTIVE COLLABORATION

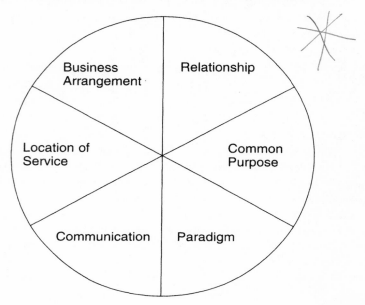

building relationships takes time and occurs on a developmental continuum, and we highlight the principles of mutual respect, good manners, influence, and flexible hierarchy.

The concept of development is critical. There are, of course, the occasional relationships in which everything "clicks" from the beginning; however, such relationships are rare, and most of them take time to build. Collaborative relationships go through all the familiar stages of other relationships. There is an initial period of self-disclosure, checking each other out, and building trust. Most of the self-disclosure is indirect and communicated through discussions of cases. Many collaborative relationships work effectively at this stage.

Over time, though, the relationship may mature, trust may deepen, and the discussions may turn more often toward what is happening for the providers. This quantum leap in development brings collaboration to a new level, beyond the pure, case-focused work relationship, and produces a kind of second-order collaboration. The collaborators become vulnerable to each other, care for each other, and grow together.

At the far end of this developmental continuum may be peak collaborative moments when the goals of the patient, family, mental health care provider, and health care provider are all united. It becomes crystal clear to everyone how things need to change and what role everyone needs to play to move toward health. Of course, these rare moments are not necessary for collaboration to occur; rather, they are insightful endpoints on the continuum of collaborative relationships.

Mutual respect is the cornerstone upon which a good working relationship between any group of individuals is built. Virtually all forms of therapy emphasize an effective relationship and respect for the validity of each person's perspective as essential parts of mental health care. Likewise, since every mental health and health care provider has his or her own area of special interest and knowledge (framework of origin), each collaborator must value the perspective and expertise of the others in order to work effectively together. These areas can be diverse and wide-ranging, but they must be acknowledged if effective collaboration is to take place. While recognizing the expertise of others, we must also recognize our own limitations; doing so not only makes us open to the other's expertise but promotes mutual respect.

The good manners most of us learned are essential to a respectful relationship with another professional. By offering simple politeness and consideration, we create an open space for another person to be himself or herself. My courteous behavior in a professional relationship is an invitation to enter safely into "my culture." Once this has occurred, the professional collaborators have the opportunity to discover what each has to offer and how each is incomplete in the task of patient and family care without the other. Promoting mutual respect and making room for one another, professional care providers greatly reduce the chances of misunderstandings and inadvertent sabotage. For example, when a patient feels that the health care provider is held in high regard by the mental health care provider, she may listen more attentively to what the health care provider says. And conversely, when she feels the health care provider holds the mental health care provider in high regard, she may then attentively hear everything the mental health care provider says and fully engage in therapy.

Directly related to the issue of respect is the dynamic of influence. Collaboration implies recognizing and sharing influence as a function of mutual respect. Respect is the ethical counterpart of influence. Influence should vary with the situation and each professional's expertise. There should be no preconceived notions of who should make all the decisions.

In the middle of a therapy session, Mike, a 63-year-old executive, was relating the story of physical abuse he suffered at the hands of his alcoholic father when he experienced chest pain and broke out into a sweat. He was seen by a physician in the same office, evaluated, and transported to a hospital, where he was admitted to the intensive care unit for a heart attack. Multiple high-technology interventions saved his life.

Mary came in to see her doctor ostensibly for a sprained ankle. When asked generally how she was doing, she broke into tears and described her suicidal feelings. A therapist working in the same office was able to see her promptly and arrange a family safety watch. Mary's life was saved.

These two examples illustrate the same point. In each situation, the professional with the most expertise in the problem at hand exerts the most influence. In these extreme examples it is easy to see how that should be the case. Situations in which influence needs to be shared are more challenging, as in the case in the first chapter. These extreme examples do show, however, that a flexible hierarchy provides the optimal care for the patient.

The logical outcome of mutual respect, the trust that goes with it, and a sharing of influence is a flexible hierarchy. Every situation presents a hierarchy, either implicit or explicit. If collaboration is to take place, the hierarchy must be flexible. This element of relationship-building depends on a differential sharing of power. After the relationship has matured and evolved, the hierarchy becomes fluid, continually changing with the needs of the system. Of course, relationships do not get to this point overnight; it takes time to build an integrated, mature relationship with a flexible hierarchy. This pace can be significantly accelerated, however, by modeling.

The principle of flexible hierarchy also applies to relationships with patients and their families. If patients are more involved and more responsible for their own health care, they are more willing to take greater responsibility for their health. Changes in health behavior cannot be forced upon people. Patients need to be empowered to make changes themselves. What better expert on patients' situations than the patients themselves?

Mental health care providers have particular expertise in the realm of relationships. They are both blessed and cursed with more extensive training in interpersonal skills. The blessing is that this training enables them to facilitate collaborative relationships; the curse is that they may at times feel that they are doing all the work to make such relationships happen. In our experience, the mental health care provider usually has to take the initiative in building a collaborative relationship. Once the initiative is taken, though, modeling of collaborative behavior often leads to health care providers responding more collaboratively in return. It is important for the mental health care provider to be inclusive in his or her approach to collaboration. By remaining inclusive, he or she can facilitate dialogue that can help all voices be heard and point everyone toward the common purpose.

Though there are many similarities between the collaborative relationships mental health care providers have with other health care providers and those they have with patients and their families, there are some differences as well. The relationship between providers is at minimum a working relationship, with a focus on the patient's goals. The relationship with the patient is a healing relationship. The relationship with the patient's family is somewhere in between, combining elements of both a working relationship and a healing one. However, as these relationships evolve, they all become both working and healing relationships focused on mutual goals.

Suggestions:

- Contact the health care provider of a shared patient; ask for his or her perspective, impressions, and any goals for the patient. Be brief and practical.
- Start slow and be patient. It takes time to build good collaborative relationships.
- Model respect and good manners.
- Recognize spheres of influence.

COMMON PURPOSE

The central purpose of health care delivery is to effectively manage or treat each patient's concerns and to promote health in all members of the community. When working together, professionals, patients, and their families may unite around this common goal. Schrage (1990) describes this process: "At the very heart of collaboration is a desire or need to solve a problem, create, or discover something" (p. 36). The common goal keeps the group together until the task is completed or the product is made. Senge (1990) identifies the process as the development of "shared visions." He describes collaborative efforts at an organizational level where shared visions "create a sense of commonalty that permeates the organization and gives coherence to diverse activities" (p. 206). Susan McDaniel suggests that the glue of collaboration is "shared mission" (personal communication, 1994). Whether called the "heart," "shared vision," or "shared mission," a common purpose draws people together like a campfire on a cool evening.

Although effective collaboration is augmented by a common purpose, at times collaboration can take place when the parties involved have very different short-term goals—as long as these goals are not mutually exclusive and can be blended in an overarching common purpose. Making the general purpose of any collaboration clear often dramatically facilitates the process of weaving short-term goals together. Also, making explicit the specific short-term goals of each party augers effective progress toward those goals. This strategy can be very helpful when conflict arises. It would be unrealistic to expect all parties to have identical goals. When the different goals appear to be the source of conflict, a review of each party's specific short-term goals and the overall common purpose often helps to resolve the conflict by putting each party's needs in perspective and bringing everyone together around a common purpose.

Michelle had a long history of both psychiatric and medical problems. She had struggled with life-threatening anorexia for years. She also had multiple orthopedic problems, and recently her carpal tunnel syndrome had become extremely painful and disabling. She was terrified of surgery, especially the loss of control associated with general anesthesia. After several phone calls between surgeon, therapist, and anesthesiologist, the team elected to go with regional anesthesia. The surgery went off without complication, and the patient recovered well.

This case demonstrates short-term collaboration. The exact goals of all participants are quite different, but the common purpose is to get the patient through surgery with a minimum of complications. The anesthesiologist knows well that anxiety and its concomitant adrenaline can cause life-threatening heart rhythm irregularities during surgery. The orthopedic surgeon knows that not all carpal tunnel surgeries are effective, and that minimizing the patient's psychological trauma will enhance her rehabilitative efforts and her recovery (as well as minimize the likelihood of a lawsuit). The mental health care provider knows that if surgery does not go well, the patient's eating disorder and general well-being will be affected. All collaborators have their own specific short-term goals, but they all have a common, uniting goal: Get the patient through surgery with as little psychological trauma as possible. In this case, a few phone calls probably saved them all an enormous amount of time and facilitated effective patient care.

Collaboration can take place in short-term situations or at a more global level. Like the community health centers and health demonstration projects of the 1950s and 1960s—most notably the Peckham and Macy's projects (see chapter 2 for the Peckham Project)—an entire health care facility can be organized around a common purpose. More recently, and at an even larger level, some health maintenance organizations (HMOs), such as Group Health Cooperative (Seattle), Kaiser Permanente (the West Coast), and Sharpe (San Diego), have tried to organize their entire plans around a common purpose (see chapter 13).

Suggestions:

When mental health care providers collaborate with health care professionals, each participant's purpose and goals should be clarified. These are some questions to keep in mind:

- What is the general purpose of the collaboration?
- What is the health care provider's goal for the patient?
- What is my goal for the patient?
- What is the patient's/family's desired outcome?
- How are these goals different?
- What goals are held in common?

PARADIGM

It is not necessary for all collaborators to share the same paradigm for collaboration to take place. Just as many different routes can often be taken to get to the same place, many different paradigms can be used in collaboration as long as they are not mutually exclusive. In the example of Mary, it is likely that neither the surgeon nor the anesthesiologist was very familiar with the biopsychosocial model. Even so, they were able to collaborate effectively. This would not have been possible if the surgeon or anesthesiologist had ignored the psychosocial aspects of the case. Likewise, if the therapist had believed that all participants in professional collaboration had to be systems thinkers, the collaboration and successful outcome would not have taken place. It should be noted, however, that the person who initiates collaboration is often a systems thinker (either by nature or by training) and is often the one who fosters relationships.

The importance of forgoing any requirement that collaborators share the same paradigm should not be underestimated. In attempts at professional collaboration, differing views about what is actually happening may give rise to conflict. These arguments are usually unresolvable since they are rooted in differing paradigms. As long as there is mutual respect, a good relationship, and a common purpose, even widely divergent paradigms can be managed. Nevertheless, if you have a similar paradigm in addition to all of the above, collaboration is a lot easier.

Implicit in every paradigm is a theory of change. Identifying your own and your collaborators' theories of change augments effective collaboration. The important question is: Who is responsible for change? Each participant must be aware of his or her own theory, and of where the locus of control over change lies. Broadly speaking, in health care the physician takes greater responsibility for change, and in mental health care the patient (or family) is expected to take greater responsibility. These issues are important for patients and their families. If the health care provider thinks it is his or her job to be responsible for change, the mental health care provider thinks it is the family's job, the family thinks it is the patient's job, and the patient thinks it is the mental health care provider's job, there will be no end to the confusion and chaos. Making explicit who is responsible for what change, and recognizing differences of perspective, will influence how collaborators negotiate treatment with each other and with patients and families.

Paradigms and theories of change are linked in another way. Both delineate a field of focus, or where each provider looks for information he or she considers important. For example, physicians tend to focus on the microsystems level. Therefore, physicians tend to heal by attempting to manipulate the microsystem within the patient by way of medications. On the other hand, many mental health care providers focus on what Robert Like and his colleagues (1993) described as the "meso" level or mesosystem. The focus, and the locus of responsibility for change, is on patients and their families. Social workers and public health providers (even politicians) focus on the macrosystem and tend to see change, and work for change, within very large systems. These notions are all connected: One's descriptive system (paradigm) is tied to where one looks for information and to how one sees the system change. A paradigm becomes what Thomas Kuhn (1970) described as a model of and a model for reality. Having different paradigms, and all that accompanies such differences, is not a problem as long as they are not mutually exclusive.

Suggestions:

- Elicit and respect the perspectives and paradigms of others.
- Do not take differences personally.
- Identify and utilize the strengths of each paradigm.

COMMUNICATION

Clear, concise, direct communication is essential for effective collaboration, especially early in the process. The cultures of mental health and health care can be quite different. It takes time to learn the language and rules of each field. At first, collaboration can feel like doing family therapy with a family from a faraway land, or even like doing family therapy with a family from a faraway land *in* a faraway land. Mental health and health care providers need to understand and respect the cultural norms regarding rules for and forms of communication that are unique to each field. The same is true for communicating with patients and families.

This section is divided into five aspects of communication: language, frequency and duration, form, content, and confidentiality.

Language

In the beginning, dialogue between cultures can be fraught with confusion and misunderstanding, as this excerpt from a tongue-in-cheek video on medical family therapy indicates:

> FAMILY THERAPIST (*talking about working in an outpatient medical clinic*): It is important to have an understanding of . . . medical

stuff. For instance, the language, you know, medical jargon. Medical education is a laborious process of changing the alphabet into a series of acronyms and words that are designed to mystify patients and confuse other professionals. So, you have to know about CA, and HTN. You have to understand about COPD. Another good example is MI, which means "heart attack." Why they don't call it HA I'll never know.

Luckily, we in the family therapy field don't have problems with unclear language, although health care people act like we do. Just the other day a family physician conferred with me about a case he wanted to refer. It was clear to me early in his presentation that he had made a common epistemological error by overlooking the dynamics of cybernetics in the case. But when I told him this he looked at me like I had two heads. When I told him we were dealing with an undifferentiated ego mass in this case, he wondered if we should refer the patient to a surgeon or just order a CT scan. (Seaburn, 1988)

Language differences can be humorous, but they can also be intimidating, making us hesitant to enter a new culture. Language differences are meaningful. They often reflect shorthand ways of summarizing important information that is valuable to others in the same culture: "Undifferentiated ego mass" and "MI" are condensed ways of talking about more complicated processes. Language symbols can be easily deciphered by those who are initiated into a particular culture but remain puzzles to the uninitiated.

Learning the meaning of language symbols is extremely valuable to collaboration. Doing so teaches us what people say, the content of their language, in different cultures. It can also teach us how people in different cultures talk, the style of their communication. For example, we find that the style of health care communication is more concrete and instrumental than the language of family therapy (Seaburn et al., 1993). Often the concerns of referring health care providers about their patients and their expectations of family therapists are also concrete and instrumental. They want something to be done more than they want something to be explained. This can pose a challenge to those family therapists whose language tends to be broad and theoretical—an appropriate vehicle for their desire to give insightful explanations of interpersonal processes.

Learning each other's language can also help us understand the rules for how communication should take place in a given culture. For instance, when a primary care provider refers a patient to a cardiologist, it is understood that the cardiologist will send a written summary of the consultation back to the primary care provider. Therapists may not have a standard protocol for follow-up communication. They may be more likely to call a referring provider to discuss a patient than to write a letter of report. Clarifying the expected mode of communication can greatly facilitate relationship-building and collaborative work.

Frequency and Duration

In addition to the language differences, the pace is different in the two cultures. Most health care providers see patients for 6 to 15 minutes, whereas the standard psychotherapy visit is 50 minutes. In general, primary care providers believe they will see their patients for the rest of their lives; pediatricians expect to see their patients until they become adults. For mental health care providers, the time course is shaped by the severity of the illness and often is measured in weeks or months. Primary care providers, as well as specialists, are routinely interrupted by phone calls, emergencies, and urgent messages. Mental health professionals generally have much more control over their time and are subject to fewer interruptions. Thus, in general, primary care providers measure time with patients and families in short "bits" over an extended period, whereas mental health care providers measure time in extended bits over a shorter period. Health care providers are interested in prompt, brief conversations, whereas mental health care providers encourage more extended and in-depth discussion. Obviously, neither way is "right"; each simply reflects a different orientation to time.

Nevertheless, even given these different orientations to time, there are accepted norms around the minimum frequency of contact. At the very least, mental health care providers need to contact health care providers at the time of referral and at the time of termination. The frequency of communication needs to be flexible and will vary from provider to provider, patient to patient, and situation to situation.

Pam, diagnosed with multiple personality disorder, was seen in an office that had physicians, nurse-practitioners, and a psychologist. She was seen weekly by the psychologist, every four to six weeks by one of the physicians (who was male), and periodically by one of the nurse-practitioners (who was female) for women's health concerns. Some of her alternate personalities were occasionally suicidal. The physician and psychologist met on a biweekly basis to discuss her care. The nurse-practitioner joined this meeting on an as-needed basis. In addition, one chart was maintained on the patient so that all her providers routinely read each other's notes.

This is an example of high-intensity collaboration based on the needs of the patient. The frequency of communication here is high as a result of regular scheduled meetings. Sharing space is extremely useful in such a case and often makes the communication needs less intense.

Marjorie was 47 years old and well known to her physician, who had cared for her since she was 12. Her mother had recently died, her youngest child had gone off to college, and she had changed jobs. She maintained internal and external resources but was having trouble adjusting to so many changes. Her physician wrote a brief note to a therapist and made the referral. The therapist followed up with a phone call about every six weeks, simply saying that Marjorie's therapy seemed to be coming along.

This more common and considerably less intense scenario requires only occasional brief contact. It is all that was really expected by everyone involved.

Form

There are a variety of methods of communication between collaborative providers. We feel that face-to-face communication, which allows for questions and immediate feedback, is best. Face-to-face encounters are certainly facilitated by sharing a service location or being very close by (e.g., in the office next door). Face-to-face encounters occur in a variety of forms. Scheduled meetings—biweekly lunchtime meetings, for example—to discuss mutual patients is a common scenario. Making joint appointments and scheduling time to meet before or after an appointment are other ways to arrange face-to-face meetings. Of course, there is also the "bump in the hall" interaction in which brief updates are given spontaneously.

Same-site providers must make decisions about charting. Clearly, there are many advantages to sharing charts. Sometimes locating a chart is more of a challenge, but that is the only real disadvantage. When providers share a chart, it can be forwarded to the collaborative partners for review after the patient has been seen, thus keeping everyone up-to-date. Mental health notes can either be kept in a different section of the chart from the medical progress notes or included with the medical progress notes when appropriate.

Phone calls, probably the next-best option, also provide opportunities to exchange information. It is best for a mental health care provider to make it known when he or she can be reached (e.g., 10 minutes before every hour) and to let the health care provider's secretary know which patient the phone call is about so that the chart can be pulled.

Letters are also extremely helpful and can be filed for future reference and as part of the permanent record. (For this reason, be sure to write about only one patient per letter.) Letters have the advantage of permanence and lend themselves to thoughtful consideration. They are also the most familiar form of communication between primary care providers and specialists.

Electronic communication is a new and increasingly popular form of interchange. E-mail has the advantage of quick turnaround time but raises serious concerns about confidentiality. Nevertheless, as the paper chart disappears and we move toward electronic medical records, this form of communication will undoubtedly become more widespread.

Content

Certain basic pieces of information should be exchanged between collaborators. Most referrals are made by a health care provider to a mental health care provider, and most are made by a primary care physician. (Although sometimes mental health care providers do make referrals to health care providers.) The referring health care provider should include the reason for referral, pertinent background information, and goals for treatment in a letter. Many new managed-care plans also require that the number of visits be specified. Following the initial evaluation by the mental health care provider, a response that includes initial assessment, diagnosis, and treatment strategy should be communicated to the referring party.

In addition to these basic pieces of information, any content that helps the provider receiving the referral accomplish his or her goals is appropriate to communicate. Since the goals for each patient and family are unique, this information will vary.

Michael and Deborah were referred to a multifamily group for chronic pain. Michael suffered from severe back pain caused by degenerative disk disease. In the multifamily group, Michael shared the story of his father's struggle with back pain, inability to hold a job, long-term disability, and coming to terms with his limitations. In contrast, Deborah shared a family story of her mother's struggle with rheumatoid arthritis and virtual cure with the medicine methotrexate. Sharing these stories from the multifamily group with Michael's physician helped explain both Michael's attitude of resignation and Deborah's continual search for a "magic bullet" at every visit.

Sharing these kinds of goal-specific stories, and their implications, often provides helpful information for further care. Sticking to goal-oriented guidelines helps to clarify exactly which details to share.

Confidentiality

Protecting the norm and the oath of confidentiality is absolutely critical to nurturing a healing relationship. However, the norms around confidentiality are very different for health and mental health professionals. For physicians (psychiatrists are often an exception), nurses, physical therapists, and other traditional biomedical health care providers, the envelope of confidentiality is generally thought to contain all health care providers and the patient. Information is freely exchanged between nurses and physicians in the hospital about the most intimate details of the patient's life. In fact, most patients expect that such exchanges will and should take place. Likewise, physicians are very forthcoming about a patient's life history with a mental health professional. In general, the mental health professional shares fewer details with the biomedical team.

The much stronger prohibition against disclosure of patient confidences enforced by mental health professionals is often a major bone of contention between them and health care providers. Physicians frequently complain, "I referred this patient for mental health services, and I never heard back." Protecting the particularly private nature of therapy conversations is essential to cultivating a trusting relationship between therapist and patient. There are also strong legal ramifications to any disclosure of confidential information. However, some kind of disclosure is necessary if communication is to take place. Only rarely is the barrier of confidentiality invoked to cover feelings of inferiority or a fear of scrutiny. Negotiating issues around confidentiality is a tricky balancing act that needs to be constantly and individually monitored.

These reflections and guidelines on communication between providers also apply to communication between providers and patients' families. Similar rules of confidentiality obtain in this area, although they can be very complicated at times, especially when minors or potentially life-threatening illnesses are involved. Families can be our most important allies in providing health care, yet nothing is more damaging than violating a patient's confidence with a family member. Therapists need to obtain the same permission from a patient to speak with family members as they seek to speak with health care providers.

The guidelines about the form and frequency of communication apply to patients and families as well. It is important to establish explicit and reasonable expectations about availability and about the intensity of the communication. Once the ground rules are laid out, everyone can work together more effectively within a mutually agreed upon framework.

Suggestions:

- Discuss confidentiality issues as soon as possible—ideally at the outset, or at the first relevant point.
- Clarify which issues you want to discuss with the patient's health care provider.
- Have release-of-information forms handy.
- Contact the health care providers of patients you are currently seeing as soon as possible.
- Discuss common goals for the patient/family, diagnosis, and treatment.
- Clarify frequency and form of communication.
- Ask about any specific content requests.

LOCATION OF SERVICE

In his seminal work *Collaborative Health Care* (1987b), Michael Glenn organizes his description of collaborative practices around the issue of geography. Simply put, the ease of collaboration is related to the proximity of the providers. Collaboration is more difficult for providers who do not share an office. For those who share an office, share charts, think alike, and see patients together, collaboration is a natural way of working together. Close proximity usually makes collaboration easier but is not an absolute necessity. We condense Glenn's categories into three: service locations that are separate, together but separate, and together.

The Separate Model

Glenn (1987b) writes that the "traditional model" of mental health care provider interaction is "separate" locations. "The physician refers to a therapist who is not in the same practice" (p. 106). The geographical separation between the physician and the therapist often defines and symbolizes the nature of their communication. While being respectful of each other's roles, these professionals may not discuss the patient beyond the initial referral letter and perhaps a letter on completion of treatment. Their relationship, characterized by low frequency and low content of communication, is a minimal form of collaboration. The patient is the key link—in fact, the only link—between their two worlds.

Sheila had been diagnosed with irritable bowel syndrome for the past six years. Recent stressors had exacerbated her symptoms to the extent that she only felt comfortable if she knew the exact location of the nearest bathroom. This need had isolated her by limiting her activities outside of home and work. Sheila's physician suggested that it might be helpful for her to see a counselor to improve her stress management skills. Sheila agreed, and the physician wrote a referral on the encounter form. When Sheila gave the encounter form to the physician's secretary, she was given the counselor's phone number. She called to make an appointment, and a letter of referral preceded her first visit. As therapy progressed, a series of childhood traumas were unveiled, and Sheila eventually worked through them. During this time, the only communication between physician and therapist was a brief letter from the therapist outlining Sheila's diagnosis and anticipated treatment. After nearly a year, it made sense for therapy to terminate, at least for the time being. The therapist sent a brief summary of treatment to the physician. At the next visit with the physician, Sheila was very grateful for having been referred, and the physician was very pleased that her irritable bowel symptoms were quiescent and satisfied with her overall care. A few months later the physician ran into the therapist at the store and complimented her for the "nice work."

This example from one extreme of the separate but respectful continuum shows how good health care can be delivered with even minimal explicit collaboration.

In another extreme example, a partner of one of the authors moved across the country. He had been collaborating with a psychologist in his office on the case of a severely disturbed patient. The patient had become quite attached to her physician and occasionally but regularly needed to make contact with him. Periodically, the psychologist and the patient would together call the patient's former physician as part of therapy. This is but one example of how even a distance of 2,000 miles does not necessarily get in the way of collaboration; if there is a will, there is a way. One could say this is an example of separate in location, but together in mission.

Under special circumstances, it may be better for a patient to see providers in different offices. One of the authors recalls a patient who did not want to be seen for mental health services in the same location where he received medical care. He was afraid that family members who also received care there might inadvertently be exposed to his mental health records. This scenario is an argument for different entrances to mental health offices, even in shared-space situations, where confidentiality may be more of a problem, for example, in a small town.

The Together-but-Separate Model

Glenn (1987b) refers to "together but separate" work as "collaborative, but traditional: Physicians have therapist colleagues in their practice, but are clearly the leaders of the working group" (p. 108). Health maintenance organizations, hospital settings with social workers, and consultation-liaison psychiatry fit this category. This model is organized hierarchically with the physician at the top. The physician takes the lead and directs recommendations for services provided by other professionals. When providers are in separate locations, each has greater autonomy; no one has to be subsumed under the direction of another. Such autonomy is probably the greatest appeal of the separate model for the therapist. However, the rigid hierarchy that often underlies the together-but-separate model is virtually always led by the physician. Sharing space is not equivalent to collaboration.

Caplan and Caplan's (1993) description of their work in a pediatric hospital setting demonstrates this more hierarchical arrangement. Treatment teams are run by pediatricians. Members of the team include social workers, nutritionists, mental health care providers, teachers, and recreational therapists. The team leader solicits the opinions of team members but is responsible for making final treatment plans. The mental health professionals accept responsibility for the mental health of the patient and play the important role of assessing, diagnosing, and recommending treatment. Separation in this model is based less on geography than on hierarchy. Responsibilities and decision-making are hierarchically based. However, co-location does enhance regular communication through both the medical record and face-to-face contact.

The Together Model

In the together model, health and mental health professionals work closely together in the same office to provide comprehensive mental health and health care services, offering the opportunity for "one-stop shopping." The key here is that providers are colocated in a setting in which differential expertise is respected. This is not to say that the model is nonhierarchical, but that the hierarchy is flexible and the person with the most expertise sits at the top. This person could be the professional, the patient, or a family member. Partly as a function of geographic proximity and the discussion that inevitably ensues, a common purpose and a comprehensive paradigm eventually evolve. A wide range of options may develop even within this practice style.

Glenn (1987b) describes one variation as "together in location and learning." In this arrangement, "physicians not only work with a therapist in their practice, they also learn counseling skills themselves" (p. 110). It should be noted that mental health professionals learn a lot of medicine in the process too. The health care provider maintains a central role in this practice style, since patients attend the practice for the health care provided by the physician. The physician hires a colleague to supplement what he or she is unable to provide because of limited time, training, or interest. As necessary to meet the needs of the patients, the physician or health care team recruits nurse educators, social workers, or family therapists. The resulting teams of health care professionals demonstrate the various ways physicians develop collaborative practices initially to care for patients but ultimately to provide professionals with ongoing development of their skills and competencies.

Glenn (1987b) describes a primary care collaborative practice style that he and one other family practitioner developed. Glenn and his partner actively sought out and secured the services of two family therapists. These therapists were free agents and billed separately for their services. About 10% of the patients in the total active practice were referred for problems that involved other family members or needed special psychological expertise to be resolved. The patients' medical and family therapy notes were maintained in the same charts. Weekly meetings were held with the provider teams. The families for whom they shared care were discussed, observations reported, and issues researched. Of course, the luxury of informal hallway discussions assisted in keeping each professional up-to-date on changes. Over time their collaborative style evolved and was modified to fit their style and the needs of their patients.

Another example of the "together in location of service" model has been described by some of the authors (Seaburn et al., 1993). This model is situated in a family medicine residency training program in Rochester, New York. The physician/therapist is seen as the center of the "primary health care network" (p. 187). The goal is to determine what can be done together when working with the patient and family. The model encourages therapists and health care providers to find a way to proceed with treatment so that the goals of each professional and those of the patient and family are respected. In addition, the model recognizes the "clinical family" (Stein & Apprey, 1990, p. 187) as a community of care providers that includes both "the community of health care providers and patient families" (Seaburn et al., 1993, p. 186). From this perspective, the practice of health care collaboration follows Schrage's view that "the issue isn't communication or teamwork—it's the creation of value. Collaboration describes a process of value creation that our traditional structures of communication and teamwork can't achieve" (1990, p. 39).

The practice of Dym and Berman (Dym, 1986) supported the

notion that each primary care medical appointment can be viewed as an opportunity for health and mental health care collaboration. Each presenting patient is met by the colleague team, which conducts the interview together for the initial appointment and makes interventions at a biopsychosocial level each time. No opportunities are lost for successful engagement in the family system. The members of this "primary health care team" (p. 9) mutually share all patients and consult with each other before any decision in health care change is made. Dym describes the new role for the therapist who becomes a working partner of the primary care physician as the "primary care therapist." The therapist in this role requires different skills, as most of his or her time is spent in the medical interview. The mental health care providers actually make interventions during the physician-patient-family health care encounter. The relationship of this team with patients and families is modified over time as the needs of the professionals, the patients, and the families change. The length of the relationship is not determined by the patient's needs of service but rather by the decision to apply the model to the clinical practice at large. All notes on the patient and family are maintained in the family chart by all professionals and staff who encounter the patient and family during visits.

This concept has been further elaborated by the physician Don Bloch as the "generic health care team" (1993a, p. 119), which he sees as "an equal partnership between biomedical and psychosocial providers in the clinic and at the patient's bedside" (1988, p. 2). He proposes the "primary care provider as a team" (p. 2), which sees all patients for all visits as a team, not just at the initial visit, as Dym and Berman do. The recognition of the magnitude of psychosocial issues in clinical care is the basis for his position that a mental health care provider should be present at all health care visits. Bloch calls for a change in the current health care system, which he would redesign so that the biomedical model "include[s] psychosocial medicine as a full clinical partner" (1993a, p. 119). So far this concept is only theoretical and has yet to be tried in practice. It does serve to illustrate complete togetherness on a collaborative continuum.

Suggestion:

- Share office space, at least part-time, with, or adjacent to, a health care provider.

BUSINESS ARRANGEMENT

A culture of collaboration recognizes all aspects of the relationships between all participants in the health care system—including the financial relationship between the parties, the way the relationship is described publicly, and the design of the larger organization. Gone are the days of care at any price and the blank checks written to providers. Patients, hospitals, health maintenance organizations, and insurance companies, along with federal, state, and local governments, have all become acutely focused on the cost of providing health and mental health care. Now cost-effective care is trumpeted by reformers, enforced by insurance companies and health maintenance organizations, and studied by researchers. In this section, we focus on the importance of the business arrangement between providers and between providers and patients. For many of us, money, power, and hierarchy are all linked. The business arrangement between providers may reflect each provider's relative power and place in an implicit hierarchy. The effects of this arrangement must be explicitly recognized and accommodated if effective collaboration is to occur.

Currently there are several models of financial arrangements: employer/employee, parallel, and colleague.

Employer/Employee

When one provider is the employee of another, most commonly it is the mental health care provider who is an employee of the physician, and the traditional hierarchy with the physician on top is recapitulated. Providers in this scenario must have a very mature relationship if this business arrangement is not to impede collaboration, especially if conflict arises. It would take an extra bit of boldness on the part of any mental health care provider to challenge and confront a physician cocollaborator who is also his or her employer. This situation also motivates the physician to ensure that the mental health care provider has a full schedule; this priority may reduce flexibility and even be a conflict of interest. Such employer/employee situations are rare.

Parallel

It is common for mental health and health care professionals to have parallel financial arrangements—for example, when each professional is in a private practice, or when one provider is a hospital employee and the other is in a community mental health setting. Each provider bills separately and maintains separate accounts and possibly separate offices, secretaries, and so forth. They may be close collaborators but have separate financial arrangements. Sometimes the providers may be colocated and share charts, secretaries, billing, and so forth, but be financially independent in terms of income. In another variation, each provider is self-employed, but one of them (usually the mental health care provider) rents space from the other.

This has been a popular model, but as health care in this country moves toward managed care, it is becoming less common.

Colleague

Today it is becoming increasingly common for both providers to be employees of a larger organization, such as an HMO, hospital, or government-funded clinic. There still may not be financial parity between them, but neither is their relationship characterized by the tremendous mismatch of power in an employer/employee relationship. Nor do they have the equality and autonomy of parallel private practices. In this situation, there may be closer collaboration between the providers and the administrators of the organizations than with each other.

With the movement in this country toward managed care and capitation, the link between the cost of care, the patient, and the provider is shortened. In the past, the payer was a distant company to which one sent bills and from which one received payments. With the focus on the cost of care, the financial arrangement between provider and patient has changed. Now the providers must focus on providing cost-effective care. Any excessive costs are indirectly passed on to the patients and eventually passed on to the providers in the form of declining reimbursements.

Insurance companies are just now realizing that the provision of mental health services can save them money in the long run (see chapter 4). Insurance companies need to make mental health services affordable and focus on the long-term health of the patient (see chapter 15). The current debate over the provision of mental health services centers on the notions of "carving in" and "carving out." In carving in, mental health services are purchased in a block and provided with other health care services. In carving out, mental health services are sold to the outside service that makes the lowest bid. Collaboration can work in either of these scenarios but is greatly facilitated by an integrated system. Even carved-in mental health services run the risk of being separate if they are conceived of as separated by a carving line—that is, if they are not integrated with primary care and other medical specialties. Totally shared risk creates an incentive to work together. With the financial arrangement of totally carving out, placing as much responsibility for care as possible on the other providers is financially advantageous.

Grasping the intricacies of the business arrangements between providers is essential to collaboration between providers. Likewise, the arrangements between providers and their patients are important in the modern era of cost containment. Providers must share some responsibility for the cost of care and the so-called risk pool. Health care reform raises possibilities for radical changes in how health and mental health care providers work with patients and their families. We hope the change will be for the better.

Suggestions:

- Identify and acknowledge the implications of various business arrangements.
- Consider what arrangement best suits your personality, style, means, and environment.

CONCLUSION: A RECIPE FOR EFFECTIVE COLLABORATION

Much of the success of any recipe for effective collaboration depends on the available ingredients: What is an ideal mix in one situation may not be ideal in another. This fact notwithstanding, some universal principles and concepts do apply to every situation. Successful collaboration arises from success in each of these areas.

Building good working and healing *relationships* is the most important ingredient in any collaboration. Doing so takes time and is facilitated by mutual respect, good manners, and a flexible hierarchy. Having a *common purpose*, especially one that is clear and explicit, is essential to working together. This purpose may evolve over time and may encompass the different short-term goals of providers, patients, and their families. A comprehensive *paradigm*, including ideas about change, health, and illness, helps provide a language and a framework within which providers, patients, and families can communicate. Timely, understandable, and mutually agreed upon *communication* is also essential. A shared *location*, with frequent informal exchanges of information, shared charts, and joint meetings, is an ideal arrangement. Having a shared responsibility for the cost of care, with a view to the long-term health and well-being of the patient, is crucial to providing cost-effective care. A *business arrangement* based on a flexible hierarchy also makes for an ideal collaborative recipe. Partners in such an arrangement can be in mutual private practice or employed by the same large organization.

Successful collaboration blends these ingredients in the manner best suited to the palate, growth, and health of all parties involved.

CHAPTER 4

The Efficacy of a Collaborative Approach

THE FIRST THREE CHAPTERS describe the foundations, history, and models of collaboration in health care and other settings. In this chapter, we outline prior efforts, both in this country and abroad, to test the efficacy of mental health interventions in medical settings. For integrated health/mental health systems to gain acceptance, they must be scrutinized for their efficacy in creating better outcomes for patients, their families, and the health care system. We describe the results of studies conducted in medical settings using various populations and different medical and psychosocial outcome measures. We highlight models in primary care practice that have been developed and are being evaluated. Finally, we make recommendations for studying these models in the future.

To date there has been no comprehensive, well-controlled study that looks specifically at collaboration. However, a variety of processes have been studied and outcomes measured. They more clearly demonstrate the effectiveness of collaboration in health care when considered as a whole. We describe four of these outcomes, each of which addresses collaboration from a different angle. The first is *patient/family outcome*. What are the medical and/or psychosocial outcomes for patients or family members when mental health interventions happen in medical settings or are used to address the psychosocial aspects of disease processes? The second area is *employer satisfaction*. Employee assistance programs (EAPs) have been widely utilized for the past 30 years. When there is a collaborative relationship between the employer, the employee, and the EAP, what outcomes are achieved? The third area is the *cost-offset effect*, that is, the decreased use of medical services as a result of mental health interventions. To what extent does providing mental health services in close proximity to medical services decrease current and future utilization of direct medical services as well as indirect ancillary services such as laboratory, physical therapy, X-ray, and so forth? The fourth, and least studied, area is *provider effects*. In what ways and to what extent does working closely with a mental health care provider affect a medical care provider's attitudes, skills, and effectiveness? How does working in a primarily medical environment affect the attitudes, skills, and effectiveness of a mental health care provider? Does increased effectiveness translate into better patient/family outcomes or greater cost-offset effect for the system?

EVALUATING SERVICE DELIVERY SYSTEMS OUTCOMES

The inherent difficulties in evaluating service delivery systems have been detailed elsewhere (Von Korff, Katon, Lin, & Wagner, 1987). First, the available studies often have different definitions of a mental health intervention and the dependent variables that should be measured. Does a one-time psychiatric consultation compare to a six-session educational program or a ten-week brief therapy by a clinical social worker? Should the outcomes be measured in physical recovery, psychosocial adjustment of the patient, effective cost utilization to the system, or enhancement of provider skills and satisfaction? A second problem is the generalizability of methods. If treatments are tailored to the unique needs of individual patients, how does one describe a collaborative approach that can be replicated? Third, the rigor of scientific inquiry must be considered. How does one get a large enough population, create random groups, and compare an intervention/collaborative practice to a control group? A fourth problem is the way in which psychiatric problems have been diagnosed. Criteria based on the Diagnostic Interview Schedule (Robins, Helzer, Croughan, & Ratcliffe, 1981) or the Schedule for Affective Disorders and Schizophrenia (Endicott & Spitzer, 1978) have been used to describe psychiatric clinic patients in diagnostic terms. These instruments may not be suited to the issues seen in primary care because they pay little attention to anxiety disorders, adjustment disorders, and, most important, disorders presented in somatic language. Do new structured interviews need to be created and applied to collaborative models? Fifth, there has been some discussion about the most appropriate length of time to study the effect of an intervention. Should effects be judged after three months, five years, or both?

All of the studies and reviews described in this section have methodologic limitations, a common problem in clinical research exploring multivariant, multisystem issues (Shemo, 1985). Some of them did not use control groups but looked at the change of a particular group naturalistically on a pre-post comparison. Although results can be significant, attribution of the causes of those results without comparison groups is difficult. The studies that used matched comparison groups also face questions about the differences between groups when the members of one of them did not seek or accept psychiatric treatment. Many of the studies used small samples and lacked specific information on the nature of the psychotherapy provided. Since many of the studies were done in prepaid plans, differences in outcome between them and fee-for-service situations have not been determined, although some initial studies suggest no difference (Schlesinger, Mumford, Glass, Patrick, & Sharfstein, 1983). Despite these limitations in design, the sheer number of studies addressing collaboration directly or indirectly, combined with the face validity of an integrated approach to care, provides a convincing argument for further development and usage of these models.

Patient/Family Outcomes

This section looks at the effects of psychosocial interventions on physical illness using patient and family variables as the outcomes of interest. Although there have been efforts to look at the effects of psychosocial factors within individual disease processes (e.g., hypertension and diabetes), there have been relatively few attempts to review studies across illnesses. A notable exception is a review of the effect that family interventions have in the treatment of physical illness (Campbell & Patterson, 1995).

In this section, we review studies conducted in four related areas of health care delivery: patient recovery from serious acute illness such as heart attack or surgery; preventive medicine and health promotion efforts such as smoking cessation, weight loss, or hypertension management; dealing with chronic physical illness; and symptoms of depression. Work in these four areas, while not directly addressing the effects of collaboration, demonstrates that consumers of health care benefit from treatment approaches that emphasize medical and psychosocial factors.

Recovery from Acute Illness

Mumford, Schlesinger, and Glass (1982) provide a review of controlled studies that tested the effects of providing psychosocial support as an adjunct to traditional medical treatment for patients going into surgery or recovering from a heart attack. Thirty-four studies in which the treatment group received some type of therapeutic or educational program were examined. The interventions provided included brief supportive counseling, group therapy, and relaxation training. The type of provider was not controlled in the studies; psychiatrists, surgeons, psychologists, and nurses were among those included.

Mumford and her colleagues (1982) found that, on the average, surgical and coronary patients who are provided psychosocial services to help them deal with their medical crisis do better than patients who receive only the routine medical care. This careful analysis concludes:

> It is often argued that the medical care system cannot afford to take on the emotional status of the patient as its responsibility. Time is short and costs are high. However, it may be that medicine cannot afford to ignore the patient's emotional status assuming that it will take care of itself. Anxiety and depression do not go away by being ignored. The psychological and physiological expressions of emotional upheaval may be themselves disastrous for the delicately balanced patient or may lead to behavior that needlessly impedes recovery when surgery or medical treatment was otherwise successful. (p. 144)

Health Promotion and Disease Prevention

A second area receiving increased attention is health promotion and disease prevention. What are the effects of psychosocial interventions that encourage patients to stop smoking, eat better, exercise regularly, and effectively manage high blood pressure? Two examples described in the literature on families and health follow (Doherty & Campbell, 1988).

In the complex area of weight reduction, four controlled studies examined the effect of involving the partner in treatment (Brownell, Hecherman, Westlake, Hayes, & Monti, 1978; Pearce, Lebow, & Orchard, 1981; Saccone & Israel, 1978; Wilson & Brownell, 1978). All of these studies used a structured program in which the spouse gave positive reinforcement for weight loss. Three of the four studies demonstrated that with spouse involvement, more weight was lost and the loss was maintained longer than in the non-spouse-involved group. This study is interesting both for the beneficial effect of the intervention and the notion that increased collaboration, in this case between the spouses, has a positive effect.

Morisky, Levine, Green, Shapiro, Russell, and Smith (1983) compared three different educational interventions in improving appointment attendance, weight control, and medication compliance in patients with severe hypertension. The interventions were brief individual counseling, group sessions, and instruction of the spouse or significant other during a home visit. All groups showed significant positive effects on the variables described. The group that improved the most was the spouse education group, again suggesting the beneficial effects of collaboration between spouses.

Management of Chronic Illness

Chronic physical illness is an area in which psychosocial consultations and interventions are often recommended and utilized. As the population ages and services become more outpatient-based, effective treatment of chronic illness will become even more critical. One area often addressed in chronic illness research is the role of social support. This variable has been extensively studied to determine the morbidity and mortality of chronic illnesses (Cohen & Syme, 1985; House, Landis, & Umberson, 1988). It is one's social support network, most importantly the family, that has the greatest influence on health risk behavior. House, Landis, and Umberson state:

> The evidence regarding social relationships and health increasingly approximates the evidence in the 1964 Surgeon General's report that established cigarette smoking as a cause or risk factor of morbidity and mortality for a range of disease. The age

adjusted relative risk ratios are stronger than the relative risks for all causes of mortality reported for cigarette smoking. (p. 543)

The strength of this statement supports the idea of a partnership with patients and families, which is one of the core principles of collaboration.

Rinaldi (1985) reports on two studies that looked at the effects of psychotherapy on specific chronic illnesses. The first (Svedlund, 1983) focused on patients with irritable bowel syndrome, a difficult disorder to define and treat. Its symptoms are often exacerbated by stress, and thus collaboration with mental health professionals is frequently utilized. In the study, those patients who received psychotherapy along with standard medical treatment showed significantly more improvement than a comparison group in somatic symptoms, including abdominal pain and bowel dysfunction. The patients receiving psychotherapy were also less depressed and showed better overall psychosocial adjustment, at both a 3-month and a 15-month follow-up to the treatment. The second study was designed in the same way but focused on the chronic condition of peptic ulcer disease (Sjodin, 1983). At both 3- and 15-month follow-ups, significant positive differences were noted for the treatment groups in number of somatic symptoms, coping ability, self-confidence, and belief in "their own capacity to resolve problems."

Asthma is another chronic condition that often has significant biological, psychological, and relational components. Approaches that employ cognitive-behavioral therapy, education, relaxation training, biofeedback, and family therapy have been successfully utilized. Teaching self-management strategies to the asthma patient may be a critical component in controlling symptoms (Lehrer, Sargunaraj, & Hochron, 1992). Creation of a collaborative partnership between the patient, the family as often as possible, and the health care provider is an essential element of this approach.

Group therapy for cancer patients has been the focus of two studies (Fawzy, Cousins, & Fawzy, 1990; Spiegel, Bloom, & Kramer, 1989). In the Fawzy study, immediately after the group stopped and six months later, patients who received group therapy were less anxious and depressed and considered themselves more active and satisfied. They also had increased immune system activity.

Spiegel worked with 83 women who had metastatic breast cancer. The women met weekly for one year and then were followed and compared to a control group. Remarkably, the therapy group lived on the average twice as long as those in the control group. Several members of the treatment group were alive 12 years post-treatment, compared to none from the control group. While oncology teams are responsible for setting up support groups for cancer patients, these studies may reflect the collaborative influence of group members sharing a similar problem and working together to maintain a focused attitude.

Depression

There is an extensive literature on the treatment of depression with both medication and psychotherapy. Some combination of these two treatment modalities seems to be most effective. Most efforts to research effective treatment for depression have been made in clinical trials in psychological or psychiatric settings. However, a majority of patients with depressive symptoms, such as headaches, chronic fatigue, and other somatic difficulties, present in a general medical setting. Most such medical patients do not find their way to specialty mental health services but continue to need help.

Wayne Katon and his research colleagues at the Group Health Cooperative of Puget Sound in Seattle are conducting research on the collaborative treatment of depression in primary care settings. They state:

> Major depression is one of the most common illnesses among primary care patients and is associated with high medical utilization, multiple unexplained symptoms such as pain and fatigue, and substantial decrements in vocational functioning. Specific psychopharmacologic and psychotherapeutic interventions have demonstrated efficacy in randomized trials among patients with major depression treated in specialty settings. (Katon & Gonzales, 1994, p. 269)

The Group Health Cooperative began by providing limited information about high-utilizing patients' functioning to primary care physicians. They found that when primary care physicians were given screening data on a patient's mental and emotional state, there was little effect in terms of more adequate treatment by the physician or adherence by the patient. In the next study, they increased the collaborative potency of the intervention. They focused on depression syndromes and utilized psychiatrist-consultants collaborating with primary care physicians. Each provider met separately with a depressed patient twice. This treatment, combined with psychoeducational material on depression, was given to one group and the results compared to those for a control group of depressed patients who received the usual care. Results showed relative improvement in the experimental group in adherence to adequate dosage of antidepressants, a reduction in depressive symptoms for the patients with major depression, and higher ratings by patients on the quality of care they received. In addition, patients were more likely to rate the antidepressants as helpful (Katon et al., 1995). This well-designed study is one of the few efforts that have looked directly at the effects of collaboration on patient outcome. The research team is continuing to investigate collaborative interventions in depression. A study of the use of psychologists as collaborators with the primary care physicians in treating depression will be published later this year.

Employer Satisfaction

Employee assistance programs were originally developed to enhance the accurate detection of alcohol-dependent employees and provide for their care. Currently, most EAPs have expanded to not only treat troubled employees and their families but also to help supervisors and the overall workforce recognize potential problems early and be proactive about designing strategies to address them. The primary concept behind EAP work is that troubled employees cause excess absenteeism, turnover, and poor productivity. The link between mental illnes or emotional difficulties and physical disability/overall health at work has been established (Wells, Stewart, et al., 1989). Early detection is the key to improved productivity and increased morale. EAPs are examples of collaboration between the employer/supervisor, the employee, and the mental health professional but are not often linked to occupational health services. They do keep accurate data about employee productivity, providing yet another way to measure the efficacy of a collaborative approach.

Nearly two-thirds of Fortune 500 companies employ EAPs. Firestone Tire and Rubber, for instance, estimated savings due to its EAP of $1.7 million, or $2,350 per person involved, after one year of operation. United Airlines reported a return of $16.35 for each dollar invested in EAP costs. Corporate executives often associate EAPs with improved employee morale and job satisfaction (Jansen, 1986).

One of the most rigorous studies of an EAP was the one conducted at McDonnell Douglas by the Alexander and Alexander consulting group (Smith & Mahoney, 1990). The study involved 25,000 employees from 1985 through 1989. A crucial component of the McDonnell Douglas EAP was insisting that the whole family be included in treatment. That requirement resulted in higher first-year costs, but "it seems to be a very important aspect of long-term recovery and long-term health care management" (Winslow, 1989, p. 8).

Over four years, employees who used the McDonnell Douglas EAP for chemical dependency treatment missed 44% fewer workdays, had 81% lower attrition, and filed $7,300 less in health care claims than those who used an HMO mental health plan instead of the EAP. Savings were somewhat smaller in all categories for psychiatric care. Employees who used the EAP were four to five times more likely to stay with the company than those who sought mental health care outside. Absenteeism and productivity were significantly improved over the four-year period. The company estimated that it would save $5.1 million over the next three years as a result of reduced employee medical claims, reduced dependent medical claims, and reduced absenteeism.

Quirk, Rubenstein, Strosahl, and Todd (1993) state that even though the EAP is a limited service, employers and employees see it as value-added because of its joint advocacy role for the patient and employer. In the future we need better linkages between occupational health services—located on-site in large companies—and EAPs. This kind of collaboration arrangement is currently in place in some locations, for example, at Duke Medical Center in North Carolina. In the Department of Community and Family Medicine's Division of Occupational Health, a team of occupational health physicians and mental health care providers offer integrated services to 30,000 employees at local as well as national locations. Studies documenting successful outcomes of these kinds of partnerships are needed.

Cost-Offset Effect

The cost-offset effect refers to the savings, both financial and in terms of improved quality of care, when mental health services are provided to high utilizers of the health care system who have mental health issues. A direct cost savings will result in fewer visits to medical providers as well as indirect savings in fewer ancillary costs such as laboratory and X-ray fees. The cost-offset effect has been studied over the last 20 years with considerable interest. If true, it could provide a convincing rationale for saving overall health care dollars and providing more comprehensive services. However, the best rationale for including mental health services in medical settings should combine cost savings with other important values:

> It is important to acknowledge the primary rationale for the provision of mental health services, which includes alleviation of the individual pain of mental illness, provision of help in leading more productive lives by increasing the patient's repertoire of available behaviors, and curtailment of the rippling effect of mental illness in families and larger social units. Thus, the offset effect is not presented as the primary rationale for the inclusion of mental health benefits as much as the demonstration that the values described above can, in fact, be provided at reasonable cost, with part of the expense being defrayed by the savings incurred in other segments of the health care system. (Shemo, 1985, p. 21)

Nearly all reviews of the cost-offset effect find that it does exist. Jones and Vischi (1979) described the combined results of 25 studies of alcohol, drug abuse, and mental health treatment. In the mental health area, they found both outpatient and inpatient utilization reductions in 12 of 13 studies analyzed, with a median reduction of 20%. The one study that did not show the effect was done in a poor Mexican American neighborhood. Since there was no health care center of any kind in this setting, it is not surprising that inclusion of a mental health component actually encouraged more overall health care utilization.

The combined results of these studies are convincing. The admission rate per 1,000 for chemical dependency decreased from 2.02 to 0.77, and the hospitalization rate for mental illness decreased from 1.57 to 0.43. In addition to this decrease in hospitalization rates, average bed days per admission were also decreased. One of the studies found that the prepaid plan was able to decrease the percentage of its mental health budget that went to providing inpatient treatment from 71% in 1975 to 20–25% in 1979 by integrating the mental health services.

One of the studies reviewed by Jones and Vischi deserves a more complete description. Follette and Cummings (1967) at Kaiser Permanente in California designed a study 20 years ago that remains one of the seminal works in this area. Their study group consisted of 152 adult patients drawn from the psychiatric population at Kaiser. This study group comprised every fifth initial psychiatric interview. Fifty-three percent received only the initial session, 27% received brief therapy consisting of two to eight sessions, and 20% were engaged in long-term therapy comprising more than eight sessions. The researchers developed a comparison group matched on a variety of variables, including level of psychological distress, age, sex, and prior medical care utilization. For all three experimental groups, utilization of nonpsychiatric medical services dropped significantly. Outpatient utilization declined each year for five years. Inpatient hospital utilization fell for each of the first two years and then began to level off. Medical care utilization by the comparison group, however, underwent no statistically significant changes.

In an interesting follow-up to this study, those patients who received brief therapy (85%) were contacted eight years after the intervention. All but one remembered seeing a psychotherapist, although most thought of the time lapse as being only two or three years instead of eight. The critical finding was that the great majority remembered their problem as a psychosocial one identified by the therapist, not as the somatic one that originally brought them to the physician. In other words, in the typical patient's understanding, the mental health problem was more real than the biologic symptom. However, the great majority felt that the visit to the therapist had not been of much benefit and that they had worked out the problem on their own. In any event, this study supported the hypothesis that an individual's insight into his or her underlying problem reduces the somatisizing of emotions and the resultant need for medical visits.

Since leaving Kaiser to form Biodyne, a mental health specialty model, Cummings has continued to research the cost benefits from providing mental health services in medical settings. With the support of the Health Care Finance Administration (HCFA) and Senator Daniel Inouye, a longtime champion of mental health care issues, Cummings conducted a six-year investigation of the cost-offset effect in Hawaii (Pallak, Cummings, Dorken, & Henke, 1994). The goal of this project was to examine the effect of mental health treatment on medical costs in both a Medicaid population and a comparison population of federal employees. The project was also designed to study two additional variables. The first was the differential cost savings when "brief targeted interventions" were used compared to "traditional" mental health treatment. The second was the differential cost savings when patients also had chronic medical conditions. This large study reviewed over 40,000 patients' medical utilization records over six years.

Results from the Hawaii study showed a decrease in medical costs with the provision of mental health treatment (particularly the targeted, focused type) ranging from 18% to 38%. However, these encouraging results need to be considered in the context of the methodology of the study. Despite extensive outreach efforts, only a small proportion of the experimental group actually utilized the mental health intervention. As a result, the research team made the comparison between those in the experimental group who received mental health intervention and those in the control group who did not. This strategy makes it more difficult to conclude that it was the intervention and not some other difference between the groups that determined the outcome.

In another frequently referenced review, Mumford, Schlesinger, Glass, Patrick, and Cuerdon (1984) did a meta-analysis of 58 controlled studies and an analysis of the claims file for the Blue Cross and Blue Shield Federal Employees Plan for 1974–78. Decreases in medical use following psychological intervention were reported in 85% of these studies. The subset of studies in this group using naturalistic (unrandomized) experimental designs yielded an average cost-offset effect size of 33.1%. The studies using randomization yielded a lower percentage change, but cost reductions were still significant. Approximately three-quarters of this effect is due to the subsequent decrease in need for medical hospitalization (versus outpatient visits to the physician). Savings for patients 55 years of age and older tend to be maximized by psychotherapeutic interventions. These results have been replicated by other research teams (e.g., Sloan & Chamel, 1991).

Somatization disorder is a good target for collaborative interventions because it falls in the middle of the psychosocial and medical domains. A team of researchers in Little Rock, Arkansas, has conducted two studies involving brief psychiatric interventions for patients with this disorder. Smith, Monson, and Ray (1986) report on both the cost of providing health care and the overall functioning of 38 patients randomly assigned to a treatment or control group. The treatment group received standard care from their physician as well as psychiatric consultation and suggestions on patient management from a consultant. The nature of the interaction between the psychiatrist and the physician was not described. The control group received standard care (no psychiatric consultation). After nine months, the control group received the same psychiatric consultation as the treatment group. After the psychiatric consultation, the quarterly health care costs in the treatment group declined by 53%. In contrast, the cost in the control group showed wide variations but no overall change. The quarterly costs in the control group were significantly higher than those in the treatment group. After the control group was crossed over to receive treatment, its quarterly costs declined by 49%. The reductions in expenditures in both groups were due largely to decreases in hospitalization. There were no differences in functional health status of the patients in the two groups, or in the satisfaction they described.

The same design was used by this research team in a recent study of somatization syndrome. This syndrome is defined as a less severe form of somatization disorder, which is understood to be a history of seeking help for 6 to 12 unexplained physical symptoms. Patients meeting criteria for somatization syndrome were divided into two groups. One group received a consultation letter immediately. The letter outlined steps for treating the syndrome. The control group received a letter after one year. In the year following this brief intervention, positive physical outcomes were noted for the first group of patients, and as in the first study, significant cost savings were obtained (Smith, Rost, & Kashner, 1995). Although this study is encouraging because of the crossover aspect of the design, as well as its dramatic effect with a relatively small intervention, caution should be used in interpreting the results. The small number of patients and physicians in the study makes generalization difficult. In addition, the cost savings are reported using pre-post intervention comparisons rather than experimental-control comparisons. Replications are needed with other populations to more fully support the conclusions.

Finney, Riley, and Cataldo (1991) evaluated the impact of psychological treatment on 93 children, ages one to fifteen, with common behavior, toilet, school, and psychosomatic problems. The children and their parents, who were members of an HMO, made one to six visits to a primary care–based psychological consultation service. Individualized treatment was guided by problem-specific behavioral protocols. Parent outcome and behavior checklist ratings indicated improvement or resolution for 74% of the children and high satisfaction with the psychological service. However, one primary variable of interest in the study was the impact on the family's use of medical services, especially acute primary care visits following the consultation. The treatment group was compared to a matched comparison group. There was a significant reduction in medical utilization for the treatment group, reflecting, according to the authors, possibly excessive visits before treatment. The comparison group did not show the same decrease. Despite methodological problems, this study does lend support to the effectiveness, from a cost-offset standpoint, of psychological treatment for children's behavioral problems.

From these studies of the cost-offset effect several conclusions can be made:

1. *When mental health services are provided for appropriate patients, such as high utilizers of medical care, there is a reduction in nonpsychiatric medical utilization.*
2. *The most significant cost reductions can be seen in the lowered use of hospitalization.* This is the case both for those with chronic physical illness and for those suffering from psychiatric illness.
3. *The most significant cost reductions in outpatient care occur with those patients who receive brief to moderate treatment.* The cost-offset effect is seen less in outpatient care for those with severe or chronic mental illness or with comorbid medical and psychiatric illness.

Provider Effects

Sherri Muchnick, former director of family therapy training at Nova Southeastern University, recently described the experience of two family therapy interns who were incorporated into specialty physician practices. One intern, working in an oncology setting, reported that the physician with whom she worked felt strongly about the positive effect she had discussing affective issues with families as well as resolving treatment decisions. The physician decided to incorporate a medical family therapist into his staff as a result of the experience. Another intern from the same program described her experience in a rheumatology/immunology clinic. The physician in this case described increased personal satisfaction from the decrease in anxious patient phone calls she was noticing as a result of the intern's interventions (Muchnick, Davis, Getzinger, Rosenberg, & Weiss, 1993). These family therapy interns also reported high personal satisfaction from working in a more ecosystemic manner.

Health and mental health care providers commonly have a small number of cases at any one time that pose particular personal challenges. Therapists typically use supervision to address issues that arise when working with challenging patients and to find direction for effective treatment. Although the medical culture has not incorporated this kind of peer supervision, working collaboratively allows conversations about challenging clinical encounters to occur more often. Health and mental health care providers meeting together to discuss difficult patient care situations can provide mutual support.

Macaran Baird, former chairman of the Department of Family Medicine at Syracuse University, tells of his entry into a small family practice in Minnesota. He hired a consulting therapist on a part-time basis but found after six months that instead of filling the consultation time with patients, he would use the time for himself. He reports that the conversations with the therapist about his challenging cases, and his part in making them challenging, provided new ideas to try in practice. Although clearly not therapy, Dr. Baird found these meetings energizing and helpful in his care of patients.

In England, Strathdee, a psychiatrist, studied a liaison-attachment model. Underlying this approach is the belief that "administrative and medical logic alike suggest that the cardinal requirement of the mental health services in this country is not a large expansion and proliferation of the psychiatric agencies but rather a strengthening of the family doctor in his therapeutic role" (Shepherd, Cooper, Brown, & Kalton, 1966, p. 26). In the liaison-attachment model, the mental health specialist closely collaborates with the general practitioner (GP). Strathdee polled a sample of providers (70 psychiatrists and 58 GPs) to understand their experience with and perceptions of this model. The majority of the psychiatrists were extremely enthusiastic about their role and felt strongly that the standard of clinical care improved. "The ability to have a close liaison with the GP appeared to be the fountainhead from which this improved clinical care stemmed" (1987, p. 104). Further, the psychiatrists described the ease of access for patients, the reduction in stigma, and the educational benefits to providers as significant advantages. Administrative and logistical problems, such as space and secretarial support, were described as disadvantages.

The perceptions of the GPs were also overwhelmingly positive. Most of them felt that communication improved as a result of having regular discussions about clinical cases. They also noted the positive effect of removing the anonymity that had existed between local GPs and hospital specialists. There was increased understanding of training, interests, and mutual limitations.

Provider satisfaction, and its effects on patient satisfaction and outcomes, is a relatively unexplored area. In the changing health care scene, with the increasing demands on primary care physicians and nurses, the impact of collaboration on provider satisfaction will be a valuable area of research.

COLLABORATION IN PRIMARY CARE

In the 1970s, a fascinating primary care project looking at collaboration between family therapy and family medicine was undertaken in a Dutch family practice. Subjective and objective outcome measures were used to evaluate this effort. In 1978 Dr. F. J. A. Huygen published the results in *Family Medicine: The Medical Life History of Families.* Physicians from the primary care practice referred patients for brief (four sessions) family therapy. When the book was written, some 300 families had been seen in therapy. Dr. Huygen reported on both the level of family physician satisfaction and the new skills physicians learned. He also reported on patient care from a cost-offset perspective. Physicians in the project learned a number of skills basic to good family therapy or psychotherapy, including assessment of family structure and function, the possible relationship meaning of physical symptoms, circular causality, and the best ways and times to address mental health issues. Following is Huygen's summary of subjective outcomes.

> Taking all things into consideration, our experiences with family therapy have been very favorable. The way of thinking and acting of family therapists and family doctors are in certain respects much alike. We are glad to have found one another and we have learned that by cooperation in a short time changes for the better can sometimes be brought about, even in families which we regarded as hopeless and where other helping professionals had failed. Family therapy proved to be a kind of adventure for us general practitioners. I often held my breath and was impressed by the risks that were taken. The family therapist challenged and rated our patients higher then we were used to doing as their general practitioners. (p. 138)

The design for the objective analysis of outcomes involved selecting 30 families at random, obtaining a matched comparison group, and looking at medical utilization and prescription data. The therapists also collected perceptions of outcome from both the families and the general practitioners. It should be remembered that the numbers are small, so generalizations must be made with caution. However, the differences in utilization between the 12-month period before referral and the period leading to the completion of family therapy were significant for lowered number of contacts and lowered number of diagnoses. Huygen concludes that the families were made more self-reliant by the intervention.

Further analysis showed that the number of contacts with the primary care physician diminished significantly not only for the identified patient but also for the family members! The same was true for the total number of prescriptions for psychoactive drugs. More than half the families said that their problems had disappeared or improved, while one-quarter of the families said their problems remained the same. The physicians reported that the presenting problems improved in 56% of the families. Also of importance, the physicians said that medical requests were reduced in 45% of the cases. The numbers of prescriptions decreased in 42%, remained the same in 57%, and increased in 1%.

In this country for the past 16 years, the National Institute for Mental Health (NIMH) has sponsored research looking at mental health consultation/intervention in primary care. One example of the kind of project supported by NIMH is described by Barbara Burns, former director of the Division for Primary Care Research (Jacobsen, Regier, & Burns, 1978). In Boston the Bunker Hill Neighborhood Health Center has always had a comprehensive mental health program that provides active interaction between medical and mental health care providers. Due to this collaboration, medical providers were better able to recognize and treat psychosocial difficulties. As a result of increased collaboration, morale also improved among the staff. Improved morale seemed to be associated with the increase in information shared about patients served and services provided. One additional result of the Bunker Hill project was being able to identify specific practice needs, such as increased services to the elderly. The Bunker Hill project and others in the early 1980s were successful but did not endure because of funding difficulties. They continue to serve as a model for working collaboratively.

Gonzales and Norquist (1994) provide a review of the few controlled studies done using consultation-liaison interventions. Of the 13 studies that met their stringent research requirements, almost all showed modest to strong positive outcomes in the areas of mental health symptoms, patient satisfaction, social functioning, primary care visits, and/or prescription usage. They also reflected the complexity of practice and research in primary care. The mental health professionals involved in these interventions were from various disciplines—social work, psychology, nursing, and psychiatry—and research protocols ranged from 2 to 36 months. The interventions included consultation (Katon et al., 1990; Ross & Scott, 1985), time-limited focused therapy (Klerman, Weissman, Rounsaville, & Chevron, 1984), and an internist liaison program (Thompson, Stoudmire, & Mitchell, 1982). Each study included some measure of psychological distress; however, definitions of distress varied, from nonspecific (as measured by general screening instruments) to more symptom-specific (as measured by disorder screening instruments) to frank mental disorder (as measured by structured interviews). The studies were carried out in diverse settings both here and in Great Britain, making generalizations difficult. The fact that all of these studies showed positive effects in their stated outcomes is impressive given the diversity of situations investigated and methodologies used.

In 1977 the President's Commission on Mental Health was charged with the responsibility of identifying how the mentally ill were being served, to what extent they were underserved, and who was affected by underservice. Regier, Goldberg, and Taube (1978) estimated that 15% of patients in the primary care/outpatient population were affected by a diagnosable mental disorder for a period of one month to one year. Of that group, only 3% were seen in the specialty mental health setting, while fully 9% were treated in the generalist office. Their article called for further integration of general health and specialist mental health services, as well as more training for generalists working in this area.

Since this seminal article, there have been a number of replications. Schurman, Kramer, and Mitchell (1985), who examined the 1980 and 1981 National Ambulatory Medical Care (NAMC) surveys, reported that close to one-half of the mental illness visits made to office-based practitioners were made to nonpsychiatrist physicians. A large percentage of mildly or moderately troubled patients were seen by primary care physicians for mental health services.

The Mauksch and Leahy (1993) report on data from the Group Health Cooperative of Puget Sound confirms the NAMC data that roughly half of the mental health patients in that practice are managed by their primary care physician (Von Korff, 1990). This latter study indicated that mental health patients going to physicians perceive themselves as having poorer health; they also present more frequently with somatic complaints and often refuse referrals to mental health professionals.

There are a number of good reasons patients and families may receive mental health treatment only in a primary care setting. First, access to quality mental health care may be difficult owing to an unavailability of specialized providers. In most areas of the country, general health care is more accessible. Second, on a more affective level, patients may trust and feel a connection with their primary care provider and fear losing that relationship. Third, their psychosocial distress may be so intertwined with their somatic symptoms that they are not open to their physician's suggestion that psychotherapy may be warranted (Bridges & Goldberg, 1985; Katon, Kleinman, & Rosen, 1982). Fourth, mental health consultations continue to bear a societal stigma. Frequently, patients would rather have something "medical" wrong with them, even if life-threatening, than something "emotional" related to life events or family stress. Finally, significant financial issues are involved. Often medical care is reimbursed at higher rates, either fully after a deductible is met or at least at 80%. Mental heath services typically are reimbursed at 50%.

In 1994 a task force was developed by the Commission on Health Care Services of the American Academy of Family Physicians (AAFP). Its assignment was to review the literature and make recommendations on the provision of mental health services by family physicians. AAFP's concern was the trend in public and private insurance to manage the cost of mental health care by eliminating or limiting benefits to the insured population.

This task force reviewed much of the literature on the prevalence, utilization, and cost of mental health services in general medical settings. In coming to many of its conclusions, it referenced many of the studies cited in this chapter, as well as a recent demonstration project at United Behavioral Health Systems, a behavioral managed-care organization in Wauwtosa, Wisconsin. This organization initiated an overall restructuring that included an integration of medical and mental health services. In a large health care delivery system, they were able to reduce by 33% their overall costs, while retaining high consumer and provider satisfaction. They credit integration of services as the key factor in the changes in cost and satisfaction (German, 1994).

This task force concluded:

A uniform benefits package must include coverage of mental health care services. The prevalence of mental health disorders, the health care needs of our patients, together with the high societal cost of failure to provide treament, make such an inclusion mandatory. A collaborative model, which integrates both primary care and specialty mental health services, can best meet the needs of our patients and introduce substantial cost savings into a benefits package. Third party payment policies should encourage the provision of mental health services through a primary care based collaborative model. (American Academy of Family Physicians, Commission on Health Care Services, 1994, p. 4)

As health care systems change, primary care settings will be viewed with even more interest, particularly the ability of physicians to provide for the mental health needs of their patients and families. It is clear that a significant percentage of patients presenting in primary care practices have psychosocial problems in need of assessment and treatment. However, these problems are not presented directly, as they would be in a mental health setting. They are confused and complicated by co-occurring medical conditions and vague presentions of aches and pains.

Efforts to describe and evaluate services that address the complicated interactions between the biological and psychosocial domains have looked increasingly to collaborative teams rather than individual practitioners. Such teams seem particularly effective at increasing confidence and competence while reducing anxiety throughout the treatment system. Patients and families are more satisfied and less anxious in these settings because it is clear that mind, emotions, and body are addressed in an integrated way. Medical care providers are less anxious because they do not feel responsible for the entire solution and can trust themselves to set reasonable goals. Mental health care providers are less anxious because they know more about medical conditions and can address their impact directly. The natural (but unproductive) blaming of others that occurs in stressful situations is diminished. Finally, because of the emphasis on prevention and lifestyle changes in primary care settings, problems and solutions can be addressed earlier, before they reach a high anxiety level. Reductions in anxiety in patients, families, and professionals have contributed to care that costs less (e.g., more unnecessary testing is eliminated), is more satisfying (less burnout, higher patient adherence), and leads to better medical and psychosocial outcomes.

FUTURE RESEARCH QUESTIONS IN
COLLABORATIVE CARE

There are compelling commonsense and anecdotal arguments for establishing collaborative relationships between mental health and medical care providers. There is also evidence of its efficacy. However, more well-designed research into the value and effectiveness of collaborative approaches to health care needs is critical. Efforts are currently being made to study these approaches. Frank DeGruy (1995) highlights some of them in the most recent newsletter from the Collaborative Family Health Care Coalition.

The following general questions should be considered.

1: *What groups of patients are most likely to benefit from a collaborative approach?* Research needs to identify these groups to be able to clearly monitor outcomes. Some examples are:

- Patients for whom clear biologic and psychosocial issues are present (e.g., hypertension, depression, marital distress)
- The top 10–15% of high utilizers of medical services
- Undiagnosed, poorly differentiated problems that may or may not achieve a clinical diagnosis owing to their transitory or subthreshold nature (e.g., minor depressive symptoms presenting with fatigue)
- Chronic pediatric conditions such as diabetes, asthma, or ADHD
- Work-related injury or disability

The general approach and methods of each practice need to be well defined, and a full documentation of treatments administered provided. After identification, such patients would be randomized and different interventions made, using various degrees and types of collaboration—structured referral, assessment versus informal consultation, brief treatment provided by primary physician, family-oriented versus individual focus, and so forth.

2: *What mental health interventions provided by a collaborative team for specifically designated populations are most care-effective and most cost-effective?* The study described earlier in the section on mental health diagnoses (Katon et al., 1995) addresses this question as it affects one designated population, those suffering from depression. We believe this study points in the right direction by highlighting the care-effectiveness of providing brief, intensive exposure to different perspectives on the same problem, thereby increasing patient options. The approach outlined in this study will also be indirectly cost-effective as a result of the informal education, training, and support involved.

3: *What are more efficient and effective ways of training providers and delivering care?* Studies need to be prospective, looking at effects two to four years after initiation of a model. Outcomes need to be measured in at least the following categories and measured for the interaction between the categories:

- Patient outcomes—psychiatric, illness behavior, social dysfunction, illness outcome
- Service utilization—utilization of direct service and ancillary costs
- Physician outcomes—diagnostic skills, psychopharmacologic and psychotherapeutic skills, orientation to psychosocial factors, job satisfaction
- Mental health care provider outcomes—diagnostic skills, consultative skills, orientation to biology as a contributing factor

4: *What are the core components of a collaborative relationship between health and mental health care providers that make a difference in patient/family outcomes? How can they be developed?* This book describes the best current thinking on these questions. Explorations of possible answers through experimentation with rigorous designs, both qualitative and quantitative, need to continue.

An important arena for these studies is primary care medicine, which includes occupational medicine. All efforts at health care change have a strong primary care component. It is clear that physicians and health care practitioners from family medicine, general internal medicine, and pediatrics will be critical collaborators with employers as well as mental health professionals in the future. Further, it will be important to set up these studies using existing practices to gather data about existing collaborative relationships and interventions. Fortunately, there are some preexisting structures around which to design such studies. It is certainly the mission of managed-care companies to design cost-effective care, and much of the literature cited in this chapter comes from those settings. However, their efforts to be maximally efficient may not make them the best settings in which to experiment with new collaborative models of practice. Networks such as ASPN (Ambulatory Sentinel Practice Network) and PROS (Pediatric Research Organization Services) could be utilized. For example, these two networks are currently participating in a collaborative study to determine the kinds of psychosocial problems in children that present in a family practitioner's or pediatrician's office. As part of this ongoing study, physicians are being asked questions about the nature of their relationships with mental health practitioners. Results should lead to a better understanding of current collaborative efforts.

5: *How does working together affect the skills, confidence, and satisfaction of health and mental health professionals?* The provider effects of collaboration have not been looked at closely, but with increased pressure and job dissatisfaction, doing so seems critical if burnout and general provider stress are to be prevented or alleviated. "Working together" refers not only to accomplishing the task—providing quality patient care and achieving the best possible outcomes—but also to creating the culture of collaboration described in chapter 1. The questions are: Does collaboration enhance both medical and mental health care providers' confidence, skills, and excitement about their role? Does this enhancement of confidence and skills then translate into better patient outcomes, more cost-effective processes, and more satisfied consumers?

CONCLUSION

This chapter has provided an overview of previous efforts to describe the demonstrated costs and benefits of mental health interventions in health care environments. It is a standard conclusion that "more work is needed in this area"; however, it certainly holds true in the study of health care collaboration. We are in a time of great crisis in which cost-effectiveness has become the rallying cry for any new model. The Japanese character for "crisis" means both danger and opportunity. The danger is that in emerging models of health care, mental health consultation will be devalued or go completely unsupported. The opportunity is to use this time of transition to create and systematically study collaborative models of health care that increase rather than decrease our joint capacity to be healers.

PART II

Perspectives on Collaboration

The first part of this book laid the foundation for a collaborative approach to health care. We presented the fundamental tenets of collaboration, the historical trends that have contributed to a division of disciplines, the key ingredients for collaborative practice, and the research support for the efficacy of a collaborative model. In this part, we build on this foundation by focusing on the practical aspects of collaboration, drawing on the experience and wisdom of professionals whose work has shaped the collaborative movement in the last two decades. We regret that we could not interview all of the prime movers in this rich period of collaboration, but we are pleased with the number of leaders who did share their work and ideas with us. We want to thank them for their invaluable contribution to the field: Macaran Baird, M.D., associate medical director for Primary Care, Health Partners, Minneapolis, Minnesota; Donald Bloch, M.D., former director of Ackerman Institute, editor of *Family Systems Medicine*; Thomas L. Campbell, M.D., associate professor of family medicine and psychiatry, University of Rochester, School of Medicine and Dentistry and Highland Hospital; William J. Doherty, Ph.D., professor of family social science, University of Minnesota; Barry Dym, Ph.D., private practice, Cambridge, Massachusetts; Michael Glenn, M.D., private practice, Cambridge, Massachusetts; Jeri Hepworth, Ph.D., associate professor and associate residency director, Department of Family Medicine, University of Connecticut and St. Francis Hospital; Larry Mauksch, M.Ed., clinical associate professor, Department of Family Medicine, University of Washington; Susan H. McDaniel, Ph.D., associate professor of psychiatry and family medicine, University of Rochester, School of Medicine and Dentistry and Highland Hospital; John S. Rolland, M.D., codirector of Center for Family Health and clinical associate professor of psychiatry, Pritzker School of Medicine, University of Chicago; Lorraine Wright, R.N., Ph.D., professor, Faculty of Nursing, and director of Family Nursing Unit, University of Calgary.

To their perspectives we add our own, offering a practical guide to collaboration applicable in any clinical setting. In "The Role of Personal Experience in the Decision to Collaborate" (chapter 5), we explore the factors that influence a professional's choice to pursue such a different model of practice; we also provide a guide for the reader's "self-assessment." "Wrong Turns, Blind Alleys, and Paths to Follow" (chapter 6) gleans from the experiences of leaders in the field some of the most common mistakes made by those new to collaboration; it also provides a map for those getting started. "The Influence of Collaboration on the Mental Health Professional's Identity and Practice" (chapter 7) takes a detailed look at the role of context in shaping what the mental health collaborator does; it delineates the central practice issues facing mental health professionals working in medical settings and makes concrete suggestions for handling them.

CHAPTER 5

The Role of Personal Experience in the Decision to Collaborate

MANY COMPLEX FACTORS shape how patients and families respond to an illness. Among those factors is their personal experience with illness and other adversities prior to the onset of the current problem. Such experiences can have a lasting effect on the life of a family. One elderly husband whose wife had a terminal cancer worried more about her suffering than her death because as a boy he had watched his mother die in pain from a similar cancer. Another man explained his capacity to adjust to his wife's multiple chronic illnesses by recalling how his family dealt with oppression in eastern Europe two generations before. A mother of a three-year-old with cystic fibrosis explained her tenacious parenting as a way to ensure that her daughter would live longer than the mother's sister, who died of cystic fibrosis at age 15.

Personal experience has a similar impact on professionals who collaborate. Professionals are shaped as much by their own personal experiences as they are by their training and expertise. Many schools of psychotherapy encourage students to enter therapy during their training or require a family-of-origin course as part of their program. Many medical residency programs offer Balint groups, which focus on the complex elements of the doctor-patient relationship. The Society of General Internal Medicine's Task Force on Doctor-Patient Relationships provides intensive training that focuses exclusively on the value of self-awareness in doctoring. Courses for medical and mental health professionals interested in collaboration taught at the University of Rochester and at that city's Highland Hospital also emphasize the role of personal and family-of-origin factors in the development of effective treatment and collaboration skills.

In this chapter, we look at the personal experiences of health and mental health professionals and at the influence of those experiences on their decision to work in a collaborative model. Our discussion will not be exhaustive. However, it will remind health and mental health professionals to examine the reasons they are willing to venture off the traditional professional paths into the still foreign land of collaboration.

A commitment to collaboration often evolves for serendipitous reasons. For example, William Doherty notes that working with physicians was not a career track he originally intended to follow. His interest emerged after being invited to give a talk to family physicians. They were so interested in what he had to offer that they eventually invited him to join the family medicine faculty at the University of Iowa.

While circumstance and serendipity may have ignited the fire of collaboration for many health and mental health professionals, we found that the fire is sustained by other life experiences that have shaped their identities and how they think about their work. We focus on the four primary influences that health and mental health professionals discussed most often with us: family-of-origin experiences, social currents, critical life events, and professional socialization. We also provide readers with a guide for assessing the influence of their own personal experiences on how and why they collaborate.

FAMILY OF ORIGIN

One of the authors was cofacilitating a group of therapists discussing their interest in working with health care providers and families dealing with illness. The therapists in the group felt frustrated by how difficult it was to work with physicians, whom they characterized as professionals who did not care adequately about their patients and who were inaccessible to therapists who genuinely wanted to collaborate. Furthermore, physicians seemed resistant to the obvious benefits of systemic thinking. As part of the group process, each participant was asked to share an illness experience from his or her own family of origin. To a person, the therapists told stories of seriously ill family members who, in the eyes of their families, had not been taken care of appropriately by their physician. Further discussion helped these therapists recognize the connection between their family-of-origin experience and their later professional struggles with physicians.

The power of our families of origin is with us always. As Boszormenyi-Nagy and Spark (1973) indicate, we are bound by invisible strands of loyalty that connect us to previous generations and influence how we enter into any new relationships. For professionals interested in medical family therapy and collaboration, these strands may be even more powerful because they are often connected to matters of life and death. Entering into new relationships with professionals and families around issues of illness without an awareness of personal family-of-origin influences can greatly diminish a therapist's effectiveness (Mengel, 1987).

A family physician consulted with a family therapist colleague about the difficult case of a patient who was dying of cancer. The physician found it difficult to stay connected with the patient despite his genuine concern and sadness. Upon further exploration, the physician recognized that when his own mother was dying, he had felt unable to help her, even though he was a medical student at the time. The physician realized that he was pulling back from his patient because he was afraid of not being able to "cure" someone again.

Awareness of the impact of family of origin on one's professional life can be a potent resource. Macaran Baird discusses the role of his family in his development as a physician:

> My family of origin has shaped my interests in a powerful way. My sister, who died four years ago, was diagnosed with schizophrenia. I grew up in the late 1950s. I was about five and she was fifteen when she had a break. She was disturbed and intermittently violent. I remember days when it seemed like she understood reality and the days she couldn't. It taught me the tragedy of incomprehensible behavior. When I went to college, I remember sitting in the science library thinking there must be a solution. Having grown up in a culture so influenced by science, I thought it must be a biochemical problem. It never dawned on me until

halfway through medical school that while genetics is important, there may be other actions that may be helpful, if not curative. I'm sure this helped create my interest in mental health. Actually, part of the reason I'm a family doctor and not a psychiatrist is that I don't want to deal daily with people that have such a hard time getting better.

The role of illness in the families of health and mental health care providers is an important and recurring theme in our conversations with professionals (Rolland, 1994b). It often contributes to the individual's choice of profession and his or her areas of special interest. Baird insightfully discusses an illness that was a powerful "member" of his family. The strengths that enabled him to become an effective and innovative physician were born in his family's effort to deal effectively with this problem. He experienced first-hand the impact of serious illness on a family, as well as the influence that a family can have on the course of an illness.

A more subtle yet equally powerful influence derives from the worldview of one's family of origin. Families commonly develop a family Weltanschauung, or "meaning scheme," regarding life (Seaburn, Lorenz, & Kaplan, 1992; Wittgenstein, 1953). The amalgamation of viewpoints that represents the family's overall perspective is of great importance. For example, a family's capacity to attribute meaning to a chronic genetic disease such as cystic fibrosis is often a key indicator of how well they will adapt and function (Patterson, McCubbin, & Warwick, 1990; Rolland, 1994a; Venters, 1981).

The capacity to value differences is a key indicator of how well professionals will collaborate. This quality of openness to multiple viewpoints and respectful curiosity often finds its roots in the family Weltanschauung. John Rolland, a family psychiatrist, and Larry Mauksch, a family therapist, both come from refugee families who survived the Holocaust. For Rolland, this experience made him sensitive to issues of "difference"—to how, for example, being seen as different may contribute to being oppressed. "Since I grew up in a family that had experienced oppression, I've always been sensitive to patient advocacy and consumer groups. Collaboration is not just professional to professional; it must include patient involvement and decision-making as well."

Mauksch's parents always fought for the underdog in any situation. His mother's decision to enter nursing was motivated in part by her feelings of "survivor guilt." His parents always tried to approach the worlds of others with an open mind, and their experience shaped Mauksch's openness to working with different disciplines and perspectives: "Both of my parents were always very interdisciplinary in their understanding of the world and their understanding of health care. So that was a normal way of thinking for me. I didn't have to make a paradigm shift when I became interested in professional collaboration. Before I graduated from college, I knew I wanted to work in an interdisciplinary setting." Family-of-origin factors enabled both Rolland and Mauksch to be sensitive and open to viewpoints that differ from their own and to appreciate the intrinsic value of dialogue about those differences. Fundamental to their commitment to collaboration is the inclusion of voices that are often excluded from dialogue and decision-making—in particular, patients and families.

These stories are a reminder that each time the professional enters a therapy office or an exam room to work with a patient, it is a very crowded place. The patient may be accompanied by invisible yet influential family members from past generations. In the ways they interact with patients and families and with each other, health and mental health care providers may also bring significant and vocal members of their own families of origin into the room. It is important for mental health professionals, physicians, nurses, and other health professionals to listen to those voices and track their impact on why and how they collaborate.

SOCIAL CURRENTS

Rolland's and Mauksch's stories also illustrate that families do not evolve in cocoons; they are constantly interacting with the social context. Among the many other legacies we inherit, besides the ones our families pass on to us, are cultural shifts and historical events. These influences, reflecting and at times challenging the dominant values of the larger culture, also shape the values of health and mental health professionals.

Many of the professionals who have played an important role in the development of contemporary approaches to collaboration either reached maturity or began their professional work during the foment of the 1960s and early 1970s. This era was characterized by trends that can generate collaboration: challenging hierarchical forms of organization, questioning authority and the misuse of power, advocating for civil and human rights, struggling for gender equality, and fostering a spirit of experimentation. It is no coincidence that this turbulent period saw the emergence of the Peace

Corps, Vista, community mental health, and family medicine—
each focused on grassroots efforts to work together to address the
needs of the human family. A lasting concern with power and its
use in relationships also emerged from this cauldron of social
forces.

These values are easily transferred to the arena of collaboration.
Susan H. McDaniel, a family psychologist, was strongly influenced
by the women's movement in college. She sees a clear relationship
between that movement and collaboration: "I think professional
collaboration is about the same issues. If you don't have some con-
ception about sexism or racism or equality, then you'll have a hard
time understanding what collaboration is all about."

Seeing how those values can transform even a small system can
permanently transform one's sense of what working together is all
about. John Rolland was a young medical student in a traditional
medical school when he had the opportunity to volunteer in a free
clinic:

> Medical school is very hierarchical. You are taught to exercise
> authority over people. You say, "I am Dr. Rolland," even when
> you are a second-year medical student. That's where it begins.
> Even when I was working with nurses who knew more than I did,
> I was to call myself "Doctor." I remember it felt awkward to me,
> like I was the Wizard of Oz behind the screen. At the free clinic
> where I did volunteer work, faculty physicians who were also
> there behaved in a much more nonhierarchical way. We worked
> more as a team. And we were working out a lot of issues, such as
> gender. I was impressed with that.

Medicine has traditionally been dominated by males, who
occupy most positions of power. Mental health care providers who
do not have an "M.D." after their name enter the medical world at
a disadvantage. Women are at an even greater disadvantage,
owing to the gender inequity that pervades not only medicine but
our culture.

A collaborative perspective is both a response to social currents
and an attempt to change the flow of those currents. The values
that underlie collaboration often challenge hierarchical forms of
organization. These values—better conceptualized as circles than
as pyramids—emphasize negotiation and the respectful give-and-
take that leads to compromise. By their very nature, they pose a
challenge and provide an opportunity not only to deliver health
care differently but to organize it differently as well.

CRITICAL LIFE EVENTS

Lorraine Wright, a nursing professor and family therapist, recalls an event in her early nursing education that transformed the direction her work would take:

> You have to grow up fast being trained in a hospital. One of the experiences that shaped me occurred on a Christmas Eve. A patient for whom I had been caring died in my arms. I went out into the hall to be with the family. I remember the family weeping and coming into the room to be with the family member who died and my having to be with them. I wondered, "What do I do? What can I say to this family?" I was only 19 years old. When you watch a patient you've cared for die in front of you, and you are just 19, you develop a very different perspective about health care and life.

Almost 50 years ago, the philosophical theologian Paul Tillich (1948) wrote about personal, social, and cultural changes of such significance that they can only be called a "shaking of the foundations." This idea approximates the personal experience of many professionals engaged in collaboration: Critical life events have shaken their foundations and transformed how they think about themselves, about families, about illness, and about how they practice. These critical events often fuel the passion and the purpose that enable them to pursue collaborative approaches even when support from other quarters is not forthcoming. Wright was in graduate school before she was introduced to the significance of and the competencies for the family work she had started doing with the death of that patient. Now she is the director of a family nursing unit that educates nurses to work with families dealing with the trauma of illness and loss. She has also written extensively about collaborating with families, including the coauthored text *Nurses and Families: A Guide to Family Assessment and Intervention* (1994) (see also Wright & Leahey, 1987a, 1987b, 1987c).

For Wright, a critical life event refashioned her understanding of her role as a nurse. For others, a critical incident may have taken them out of their professional role so they could experience an illness or loss from an entirely different perspective, one that might have been inaccessible to them while wearing professional garb. John Rolland came to a family systems viewpoint through just such an experience. His first wife died of cancer: "She was ill four years before she died. I felt what it was like to be a family member with an ill loved one. The need to be involved with her care and decisions about treatment was strong. My wife and I worked hard to be included." This loss contributed to his pursuit of advanced training in family systems theory and therapy. Rolland subsequently developed the ideas about families and illness conveyed in his book *Families, Illness, and Disability* (1994a). "I felt very strongly that around illness, in particular, it was important for the family to be involved and included in the collaborative process."

Wright's experience as a nurse helped her think differently about her role with families. Rolland's experience as a family member helped him think differently about the same thing. Barry Dym, a family therapist, had an experience that enabled him to rethink how health and mental health professionals should work together when helping families.

When Dym's son was three months old, he developed conjunctivitis. It spread to his ears, and the boy developed fevers of up to 106°. Dym and his wife began to panic as their son got progressively worse. When they saw their physician, though, they felt he minimized their concerns and did not heed their anxiety. They felt dismissed but also wondered if they were overreacting. The situation went on for several days. They were hesitant to go to their physician again because they did not feel he would take them seriously. Finally, as their son's condition worsened, they made another appointment. This time their physician told them to go immediately to the hospital or their son might die. At the hospital, they were told that their son might not have made it through the night had they not brought him in.

Dym's son did make it. From that experience, Dym developed a belief that "it is impossible to treat a child, no matter what the illness, if you do not treat the family, the parents, in particular." Shortly after that incident, Dym started the Boston Center for Family Health. The professionals at the center worked in teams that included a few therapists and a physician-consultant. There were a variety of teams, including oncology, cardiology, and neurology. Dym felt that this model would make it easier to bridge the gap between the medical model and a family systems model, a gap in which many patients and families get lost.

Many health and mental health professionals drawn to collaboration with families and other professionals have had critical life experiences that helped define them personally and professionally. From these often disorienting experiences emerges a new vantage point that, not merely cognitive or intellectual, includes a certain resolve or commitment that shapes the direction of the professional's work.

PROFESSIONAL SOCIALIZATION

The development of one's professional identity is often a subtle process. Through exposure to a professional group over time, one learns how to be a nurse, physician, psychologist, family therapist, social worker, or other health professional. This almost invisible process is similar to what occurs within families. The younger generation learns from the elder generation not only necessary skills but traditional ways of being and interacting.

The injunction to call oneself "Doctor" teaches the medical student more about his or her place in relationship to others than about any particular skill and fosters a sense of loyalty to the group, a loyalty similar to that felt by children toward parents and grandparents. In this manner, the professional internalizes the ways and means of those who have gone before.

The obvious value of this socialization process is that it creates a sense of belonging and identity, a "home world" (Berger & Luckmann, 1966) for the professional that may be essential to functioning competently. Professional socialization also ensures the survival of the profession from one generation to the next. The socialization process may make it difficult, however, to take a different path within one's profession. Professional novitiates may be encouraged to conform rather than experiment with different ways of being. When he was trying to decide whether to enter medical school, Macaran Baird went to his college chaplain for advice: "I told him I wanted to be a 'regular' doctor who talked to people as well as did medical things. The chaplain looked me straight in the eye and said, 'Doctors don't do that.'"

The pressure to conform and conserve that characterizes much professional socialization may discourage collaboration with professionals who come from other "home worlds." When Susan McDaniel first told colleagues that she was working in family medicine, many of them responded by asking, "Why would you want to work with a bunch of doctors?" McDaniel wryly notes that another definition of collaboration is "to cooperate with the enemy."

Collaboration with patients and families or with professionals often involves pioneering, venturing out from traditional definitions and carving out narrow paths into foreign lands. One may sometimes feel disloyal to one's own professional identity. Traveling in foreign lands can teach us customs and practices that may contradict what we feel is "true." Imagine the shock of a well-socialized family systems therapist working in a medical setting who learns that antidepressant medication can be a valid and effective intervention. Collaboration requires an openness and flexibility that may at times leave us feeling very far from "home."

A common lament of psychotherapists working in health care settings is the isolation. They feel that full citizenship may be denied them and that, at best, they have a "green card" that allows them to travel in a foreign culture. An unfamiliar setting can indeed engender a nagging sense of homelessness. While it is important to be open to the richness of any new culture, it is equally important to remain connected with one's home world. A child psychology colleague working in a primary care medical clinic joined an outside group of psychologists who had similar research interests. After a few meetings, she reported how good it felt to speak the same language and share common assumptions.

With the emergence of medical family therapy as a professional entity, new forms of professional socialization are developing that support collaboration as a basic ingredient of professional identity. The Joint Task Force on Collaboration of the American Association for Marriage and Family Therapy and the Society of Teachers of Family Medicine worked for several years to promote the cross-fertilization of disciplines. Division 43 of the American Psychological Association (APA), the Academy of Psychosomatic Medicine (representing consultation-liaison [C/L] psychiatry), the Working Group for Family Therapists Practicing in Medical Settings, and, more recently, the Collaborative Family Health Care Coalition (40 W. 12th St. New York, NY 10011–8604) support collaborative approaches to practice. The Working Group and the Coalition advocate for collaboration as central to professional identity.

As the field develops, an emerging critical mass of professionals and structures will socialize the next generation of health and mental health professionals interested in collaboration. While this is a promising perspective, a cautionary note is warranted. The warnings made by Shields, Wynne, McDaniel, and Gawinski (1994) to the family therapy field not to become "marginalized" must be heeded by all mental health disciplines and psychiatry. Mental health care must not become an outpost on the periphery of health care but must remain in constant dialogue with medical disciplines so that an integrative approach to health care can be fostered. Only in this way can we maintain truly collaborative relationships.

A GUIDE FOR SELF-ASSESSMENT

The family therapy pioneer Harold Goolishian was fond of saying that the best resource a therapist has is his or her own self. We hope this guide for self-assessment will help health and mental health care providers explore that resource in greater depth. We do not predict that the reader will come to claps of thunderous awareness or lightning bolts of insight. Some parts of the guide may not be as relevant as other parts. Pick and choose what seems most interesting or challenging. The exercises and questions are intended to be used as tools for looking more closely at the role life experience plays in how and why one collaborates with patients, families, and other professionals around issues of health and illness. While personal reflection on these exercises is valuable, dialogue with others about them is even more valuable. We encourage the reader to talk to colleagues about the issues raised by these questions.

Family-of-Origin Factors

Construct your family genogram using the conventions established by McGoldrick and Gerson (1985). Include a minimum of three generations, talking with parents, siblings, aunts, uncles, cousins, or grandparents if necessary. The more detail one has about dates (births, deaths, marriages, other significant events), relationships, and illnesses, the better. Once you have gathered this information, choose a family experience with illness and write a brief account of it.

- How do members of your family respond to physical symptoms? Are they discussed? Denied? Do family members "keep going" or "stop"?
- Who in your family defined when someone was sick or gave permission for family members to be sick?
- How were family members treated by others when they were sick?
- What illnesses or conditions have been a part of your family? Were these illnesses acute, chronic, progressive, remitting, disabling, terminal?

- How would you characterize your family's style of coping with illness? Is the coping style of some family members different from the family norm?
- What does illness mean in your family (e.g., bad luck, sinfulness, genetics)?
- How does your family relate to health care providers? What positive experiences has your family had with health care providers? What negative experiences?
- How has your family experience influenced how you respond to your own or others' illnesses?
- What kind of patients are most difficult to care for? How is your experience with them similar to or different from your experience in your family of origin?
- How do you interact with health care professionals? What do you expect of them? How are your expectations influenced by your family's experience with health care providers?

Social Currents

Write a brief narrative about a major social or political event or trend that has influenced your personal or professional development.

- How has this experience shaped your worldview?
- What values underlie that worldview?
- How has this experience influenced your beliefs and attitudes about power, hierarchy, and collaboration?

Critical Life Events

Write a brief story about a critical incident that you feel has contributed to your interest in collaborating with patients, families, and other professionals around illness. How did this incident "shake the foundations" of how you approach your work?

Professional Socialization

Write a profile of the behaviors and beliefs that best characterize someone in your profession.

- What theoretical framework best characterizes your professional discipline? How does that framework either enhance or hinder your capacity to collaborate?

- How does your profession socialize members? How does that socialization influence the way you work with professionals from other disciplines?
- How do you remain connected to your professional "home world"?
- Do you have a "sponsor" in the medical or health care system in which you work? Are you a part of structures that help socialize you into collaborative ways of practice?

CONCLUSION

Typically, professionals who collaborate have either departed from or expanded their traditional professional pathways to accommodate a different perspective about families, mind and body, and the ways in which professionals work together. Some of their motivation to work collaboratively, to be sure, can be attributed to training. Until recently, though, formal training in collaboration has not been available. Those pursuing collaborative approaches to health and mental health care have been guided and shaped by personal experience as much as by anything else, and much of the training now available acknowledges the influence of such experience.

Understanding the role that personal experience plays in one's desire to work collaboratively can be useful in a variety of ways. First, it can help the beginning collaborator assess the degree to which personal experience has contributed to his or her professional choices—that is, when and how he or she is working out personal concerns through professional avenues. Second, understanding personal experience can help the professional identify areas of strength that he or she brings to collaborative work; a person who has dealt with family or personal illness, for instance, brings a wisdom to his or her work that can be a tremendous advantage. Third, much of collaborative work brings professionals and families face to face with illness, uncertainty, and loss. Being able to draw upon and utilize personal experience helps the professional struggle creatively with the questions of meaning that often arise under these conditions.

CHAPTER 6

Wrong Turns, Blind Alleys, and Paths to Follow

GETTING STARTED in collaboration is much like preparing to visit a foreign land. It stimulates excitement as well as a degree of anxiety. And it calls for preparation. This chapter is for anyone planning a trip into the culture of collaboration. It may also provide a helping hand to those who feel lost in this new land. Throughout we remain practical, since knowing what and how to pack is often the most useful information for a trip. This chapter is divided into two sections: "Mistakes along the Way" (covering the "ugly" collaborator, the noncollaborative collaborator, and getting the "lay of the land") and "Paths to Follow," which suggests directions to pursue.

MISTAKES ALONG THE WAY

The "Ugly" Collaborator

One of the first challenges is deciding whether or not to collaborate at all. Should I even consider such an endeavor? Among mental health care providers this is often a difficult question to answer. Those who want to collaborate with health care professionals are often discouraged from doing so by their colleagues. In Larry Mauksch's experience, "Some therapists thought that I was a traitor for working with physicians. Their view of traditional medicine was pretty negative. 'You're just going to deal with drugs; they don't really care about their patients; you're going to compromise your values.' They seemed one-down to the 'priesthood' of medicine and protective of mental health's turf."

It is virtually impossible to enter a new culture without being influenced by certain cultural stereotypes. With regard to collaboration, many of the stereotypes mental health professionals have about physicians and other health professionals are negative. Physicians are often characterized as hurried professionals who do not care about their patients and are primarily interested in money and power. Interestingly, health care professionals also often have a skewed perspective on mental health care providers. Therapists are seen as secretive, vague, "touchy-feely," and unable (or unwilling) to provide concrete help.

In the 1950s, the "ugly American" emerged as a description of the American tourist who enters other countries with a suitcase full of cultural stereotypes and behaves disrespectfully toward the "natives." To add insult to injury, the ugly American often approached his or her host country as a "missionary" might approach a "heathen" (Doherty, 1986), introducing them to Coca-Cola, Mickey Mouse, and other "benefits" of our more advanced culture. Mental health professionals can make a similar mistake by entering the culture of medicine as an "ugly" collaborator, trying to convert health care professionals to their pet theories or teach them how to be "really" caring. However obvious it may seem that such a mistake should be avoided, it is the one most frequently cited by therapists who collaborate. Recalls Barry Dym, "Sometimes I would push too hard, be too proselytizing. When I think about mistakes I've made, I think of the uneasy relationships I had with some physicians in the beginning. I was arrogant and did not realize that doctors had a lot to teach me." Similarly, John Rolland remembers being "too strident with physicians, maybe writing off a physician when he or she may actually have been afraid of collaboration and what it might mean."

The Noncollaborative Collaborator

Therapists who are new to a medical setting may feel uncertain about whether they have anything to offer. This feeling often underlies their tendency to be too zealous. The medical culture, with its intimidating language, heightened pace, and, at times, intensified focus on life and death, can leave therapists wondering where they fit in. To compensate, they may try to prove themselves by asserting their expertise long before it is invited, or they may withhold expertise as if it were secret knowledge. In either case, the underlying feelings of insecurity may block the therapist from being able to work collaboratively.

Such compensations may also reflect a developmental issue. New professionals in any field may feel they need to prove their competence by showing that they know as much or even more than their senior colleagues . . . even if they don't. This common problem is exacerbated when the mental health professional is not only new to his or her own discipline but new to the medical context. Trying to develop one's identity as a psychologist, social worker, family therapist, or other mental health professional while also trying to enter a non–mental health context is a daunting task. As a result, the therapist may mimic the very behavior of health care professionals that he or she deplores as noncollaborative.

Jeri Hepworth recognizes this experience:

> I think a mistake that all of us have made in the beginning is try-
> ing to prove that we are as good as physicians. To do that, I had
> to prove I was different from them and that I had special skills. So
> I didn't share enough, as if to say, "This is special information that
> you (the physician) wouldn't understand." Much of this was in
> response to the idea that the physician always has the answer and
> so should I.

Without realizing it, the therapist may contribute to a split between the bio- and psychosocial domains by implying that relational, emotional, and psychological issues are off-limits to physicians. Susan McDaniel recalls, "My biggest problem was not being truly collaborative. I thought my job was to be an expert on the family, and the doctor's job was to be an expert on medical issues." Indeed, many beginning therapists in a medical setting, even as they feel that all psychosocial problems are "dumped" on them, may overlook the health care provider's psychosocial expertise.

"Family Therapy 101" teaches therapists that they are never outside the system they are treating. They are always a part of the system and as a consequence influence and are influenced by it. Mental health professionals usually run into problems when they forget this. By trying to force a parent to change, the therapist may replicate with the parent the very behavior that he or she wants the parent to stop doing with a child. A similar problem can occur when a therapist first enters a medical context or begins to collaborate with physicians and health care professionals. The therapist may want to foster collaboration but behave in ways that do not encourage the necessary give-and-take that creates collaborative relationships. Therapists in this position need to slow down, take a giant step back, and get a better lay of the new land they have entered before deciding how to behave (Ross & Doherty, 1988).

The Lay of the Land

The family psychiatrist Donald Bloch reports that a physician colleague responded to his ideas about collaboration by saying, "You're going to put us out of business." The colleague was half-joking. His half-seriousness is worthy of note. Many health care professionals may feel that involving mental health care providers in their practice may be an encroachment upon their areas of expertise and responsibility.

The impact of involving a mental health care provider in a medical practice should not be underestimated. It can be a bit traumatizing to all concerned—physicians, nurses, nurse-practitioners, administrators, support staff. Macaran Baird reports that when he first entered a rural practice and started collaborating with mental health professionals and families, the greatest resistance came from support staff, many of whom did not like having the waiting room cluttered with so many people: "Why do you have to see Mr. and Mrs. Jones and their family when Mrs. Jones has the problem?" Administrators may struggle as well, with issues as diverse as billing, chart structure, and allocation of space. While it is important to be cognizant of how the mental health care provider is affected by the medical culture, it is equally important to recognize the impact that person may have on the culture in turn.

The mental health professional needs to take an ethnographic approach to the medical culture. The ethnographer enters a new culture with a desire to learn from it. The best way to learn from others is to maintain an attitude of respect and curiosity (Cecchin, 1987).

The importance of respectful curiosity cannot be overstated. To be curious is to approach something with an attitude of "not knowing" (Anderson & Goolishian, 1988; Goolishian & Anderson, 1990) rather than an attitude of having something to teach. To be curious is to inquire, to question, and to communicate a desire to understand the culture. This is the first task of any mental health professional entering any medical setting. We noted earlier the differences in language and communication between medical and mental health cultures. There are other differences of equal importance that are valuable for the mental health professional to understand (also see McDaniel, Campbell, & Seaburn, 1990)—particularly time, space, and teamwork.

Time

In primary care medicine, the average patient visit is 12 minutes (American Academy of Family Practice, 1995). Time is driven by the exigencies of practice size (the average physician has several thousand patients in his or her practice) and financial constraints. Because of how they are paid for their use of time, physicians are penalized if they see patients for longer periods of time, even if doing so is the most effective way to provide care. They are reimbursed for expensive tests and procedures but not for talking. Exploring psychosocial issues in any depth with a patient may be costly: the physician falls behind with other patients and is not paid for his or her additional time.

Mental health professionals also feel overwhelmed by the demands of patients and the limits of time. But in a medical setting, seeing a patient for an hour is luxurious. One of the authors recalls incredulous physicians often asking, "What do you do with all that time?" The sense of urgency that often surrounds "doctor time" can be felt in the impatience that therapists experience when frustrated referring physicians do not understand why their patients cannot be seen immediately.

It behooves the collaborative therapist to be respectful of the time crunch in a medical setting and to keep open slots in his or her own schedule for emergency referrals and consults. Being readily available allows collaborative relationships to develop. By the same token, being accessible to health care providers may bring about opportunities to educate them about "therapist time." As one physician said to a therapist after sitting in on a session, "How do you do this all day?"

Space

The therapy room is relatively large, often reflecting the mental health professional's model of working with not only the patient but the family and important others. Furniture in a therapy room is designed to make the patient and family feel comfortable and at home. Many therapy rooms are dominated by the therapist's chair, often a larger desk chair that befits his or her authority in the room.

An exam room, in contrast, is small and sparse. There is a chair for the patient, perhaps a small desk, and a "rolly" chair (a stool on wheels) for the physician, but little room for anyone else. The therapist often has a cushioned chair in which he or she can lean back and present the reassuring illusion that he or she has nowhere else to go. The physician's stool has no back and is built for movement, not rest. He or she is on the move and may glide across the room at any moment to examine the patient or leave to check on a different patient in another room. The physician always has an exam table with disposable paper for the patient to lie on. Fewer and fewer therapists have couches, and those who do have them less for therapeutic reasons than for decor. We know of no therapists who ask their patients to sit or lie on paper.

Therapy space and medical space serve different purposes and, in a sense, speak different languages about the role of the professionals who work in these spaces. Therapists entering medical settings quickly learn that space reflects certain key values: the doctor-patient relationship; the instrumental, action-oriented nature of the medical encounter; and working efficiently. By contrast, therapy space, and therapists, may look inefficient, slow-paced, and without clear purpose to medical professionals.

All of these stereotypes may fade over time. But they do serve to remind therapists that different worlds utilize space in different ways. The structure of space in a medical context reflects how people working in that setting operate. It is important to recognize these differences because they may carry unspoken expectations about how the therapist is supposed to function as well. Typically, physicians and other health care professionals expect the same concrete, direct, practical interventions from therapists that they expect from themselves.

Teamwork

The family physician Austin Bailey (personal communication, 1993) has noted that family-oriented mental health professionals have exceptional skills at working with larger numbers of people, while physicians feel most comfortable working with individual patients; on the other hand, family-oriented therapists typically see families alone, while physicians always work in teams. Mental health professionals may enter medical settings armed with the "good news" of working together only to find that physicians and other health care professionals may have more experience working in teams than they do.

When a patient comes for a visit in a primary care setting, he or she is first met by a nurse who will weigh the patient, take the patient's blood pressure, and prepare the patient to see the nurse-practitioner, physician's assistant, or physician. The medical record serves as a collaborative document that connects the health care team in service of the patient. Consequently, the patient may see the physician for one visit and follow up with the nurse-practitioner at the next. Information about the patient is held in common. The patient is cared for by the team, all of whom are familiar with the patient's health history and needs. Such teamwork also exists in a hospital setting, where it may even be intensified—for instance, in an emergency room.

The health care team is typically organized hierarchically with the physician at the top. This structure may mitigate against the equity of input that is often the goal of collaboration. But the key point is that professional teamwork is normative in medicine. By contrast, therapists commonly work in teams only under more exceptional circumstances, such as the assessment and treatment of serious or chronic mental illnesses and substance abuse.

It is important for mental health professionals working in a medical setting to understand this norm. It provides a more advanced view of what collaboration can be. Exposure to health care teamwork will shape how the therapist works with health care colleagues. Over time it will also alter how the therapist defines his or her role in the health care setting (see chapters 7 and 8).

PATHS TO FOLLOW

Despite mistakes and wrong turns, there are collaborative paths to follow that can make the road less risky and even enjoyable. The most basic advice comes from the family physician Thomas Campbell, who says, "Think about entering the medical system in much the same way that you would think about joining with a family." Many of the same skills that make the initial phase of therapy successful can be used when starting to collaborate.

Face-to-Face Contact

Joining a health care "family" can be facilitated in a variety of ways. William Doherty suggests starting by developing a relationship with one health care professional. For those who do not work in a health care setting, inviting a referring physician to lunch can be an effective way to begin. Better yet, have lunch with a physician at his or her office. One therapist who worked in a rural mental health center started asking patients who their physician was and then getting permission to talk to them as a routine part of beginning therapy. This simple contact often led to more referrals, consultations, and conversations.

For mental health professionals employed in health care settings, it is vitally important to have a health care professional as a guide. The health care professional can orient the newcomer to the language and culture of the setting and help him or her make friends. This simple step is often overlooked. Therapists often feel they must "show their stuff" first. Such an effort is almost as ineffective as a therapist trying to get a new family in treatment to change before learning anything about them.

On entering a teaching setting, such as a residency training program, the first question to ask is, which physicians are interested in psychosocial issues? Collaborative teaching is a must; without it, the mental health professional, usually known as the behavioral scientist, remains isolated and regarded as having important but peripheral expertise. Teaching together is often an effective way to learn about one another and from one another. It greases the wheels for clinical collaboration.

"How Can I Help You?"

This question dominates every medical encounter between a patient and health care provider and defines the health care relationship more than any other question. It is also the most relevant question for a mental health professional to have on his or her mind when starting to collaborate with a health care professional. Anxiety or insecurity may tempt the mental health professional to first ask, in attitude if not in words, "What can I teach you?" A lengthy explanation of the patient's "underlying problem" is sweeter music to the therapist's ear than to the health care professional's.

Typically, health care professionals are more interested in what the therapist can do than in what the therapist thinks or hypothe-sizes. It is important for the therapist to be practical. For example, a physician refers a 14-year-old insulin-dependent diabetic girl to a therapist. The physician explains that the teen is noncompliant with the insulin and thus at constant risk of diabetic coma (ketoaci-dosis). The physician further explains that he has tried everything to get her to comply. The physician has educated the girl about the health risks involved; he has referred her to a nurse-practitioner to learn how to do injections and test her blood sugar levels. The physician wants the girl to take responsibility for her diabetes. She listens and agrees but does not follow through. The physician wants the therapist to work with the girl so that she will become more compliant. A therapist who is new to collaboration may be tempted to respond:

> Maybe compliance is not the key issue here. It sounds like the girl may need to rebel as an adolescent. That is a pretty normal thing to do. Furthermore, in all likelihood the family may function in ways that encourage the girl not to take her insulin. Maybe the girl is caught in some marital conflict between her parents that we are unaware of. By not complying, she can draw her parents' attention to her and away from their marital discord. It could be any number of things.

Remembering the simple injunction to be practical and helpful, the therapist may curb the urge to make such a response and say instead:

> I'd be glad to work with you to help this girl manage her diabetes better. What I would suggest we do is this: I want to meet with your patient and her parents; since she is at such risk, they may need to be more involved until she is able to manage things on her own. If you could come to that visit, it would emphasize the seri-ousness of the problem and let them know that we will be work-ing together.

By responding in this manner, the therapist communicates in a direct and concrete way, respecting the physician's concern about compliance while at the same time expanding the system of care to include the parents.

Being practical and helpful, though, is not just a matter of know-ing what to say in a given situation. It is also important to be famil-iar with the growing body of literature in the field of collaborative health care. A variety of resources are available, including a jour-nal, *Families, Systems, and Health* (formerly *Family Systems Medi-*

cine), that every collaborator should have on his or her bookshelf (Subscription Dept., Box 460, Vernon, N J 07462).

Families as Collaborators

John Rolland has said that the most important—and often over-looked—hierarchical problem in collaboration is not between pro-fessionals but between professionals and families. Inadvertently, mental health and health care professionals can form a parental dyad that replaces the family as a primary support for the patient. One of the authors recalls a case in which the family was defined as too "dysfunctional" to be helpful to the patient. The professional collaborators forged ahead, in many ways effectively treating the patient's problems. Much later in the process, though, the same collaborators lamented that their patient was so "needy and dependent." They had unwittingly "adopted" the patient, remov-ing him from his natural supports and substituting a costly profes-sional support system.

The family, however defined by the patient, needs to be con-tacted early in any collaboration. Their involvement may vary from active attendance to periodic phone contact. One therapist who works in a primary care medical clinic starts every visit with a par-ticular patient by going out into the parking lot to talk to her spouse because he refuses to enter a "doctor's office." Stimulating whatever resources may exist in the natural support system is a vital part of any understanding of collaborative practice. Without it, even the best professional collaboration may in the end only teach the patient and family that they need more professionals in their lives to function effectively.

Therapist, Heal Thyself

The therapist's own self is his or her most important resource. Unfortunately, mental health and health professionals are not trained to care for themselves. Burnout among health care profes-sionals is a common problem. It is a fire fueled by beliefs that mit-igate against self-care among professionals. A study of health care professionals dealing with AIDS patients revealed such beliefs, which included:

- Health care professionals should have no personal needs or feelings.

- Health care professionals should always be immediately available to meet the needs of their patients.
- Health care professionals should be able to produce health, or at least make a difference. (Jaffe, 1986)

Mental health professionals are not immune to similar views about themselves and their work. Add to the stress of such unrealistic self-expectations the typical dilemma of being the only one of your kind in a medical context and it is not surprising that feeling isolated is a common experience. Being the "only one" may heighten the health care providers' expectations about what their one mental health provider can do. And being the "different one" may leave the mental health professional feeling like a foreign exchange student on the first day of school.

Taking care of oneself is a key part of remaining effective as a health care or mental health professional (see chapter 7). Connecting with other mental health professionals working in medical settings is one form of self-care. The Collaborative Family Health Care Coalition has developed a network of local chapters to support mental health and health care professionals who collaborate (see appendix A).

Keep That Passport in Order—The Role of Licensure

With the governmental legitimation provided by a passport, one can travel more easily in a new culture. Indeed, without it, travel may be virtually impossible. In mental health the equivalent of a passport is a license. Although for many traditional mental health disciplines—psychiatry, psychology, social work, psychiatric nursing—licensure does not pose a problem in most states, it may be the most challenging issue other mental health care providers face when entering a medical system. A large percentage of mental health professionals interested in collaborating with health care professionals come from disciplines that are not universally licensed, such as family therapy and counseling. Family therapists, for instance, are not licensed in 13 states.

As health care reform continues, credentialing will become an even more important determinant of which professionals will function inside the health care domain. In many health care systems, all mental health referrals must go through the patient's primary care physician. In addition, insurance providers often approve only referrals to mental health providers who are on their "panel," a list of approved providers who are typically from traditional licensed disciplines. (It should be noted that in many areas even licensed mental health professionals have difficulty getting on panels that have been closed.)

It is important for all mental health care providers to educate themselves about these gatekeeping processes. To collaborate, it is important to develop workable relationships with primary care physicians and others. But it is equally important to recognize that such a relationship can be blocked if the larger system decides that a mental health care provider's "passport" is not in order.

Many states are actively addressing the issue of professional licensure and other forms of credentialing. Mental health professionals should contact their state representatives to learn about pending legislation. Unlicensed mental health professionals should organize in their locales to educate legislators and influence legislation. Two national bodies, the American Association for Marriage and Family Therapy (AAMFT) and the National Board for Counselor Certification (NBCC), have both identified the issue of licensure as a top priority. Most professional organizations are also organized at the state and local level, where initiative is equally important. The future of collaboration may be dramatically shaped by the decisions about licensure and other credentialing issues currently being made around the country.

CONCLUSION

Not all the twists and turns of any new venture can be fully anticipated. It is the unexpected ones that create both the challenge and the richness of collaboration. Certain personal qualities are useful when the checklists and advance advice do not seem to apply. Remaining open to newness and differences, maintaining a sense of humor about oneself and one's expertise, going slowly, and reducing by half one's expectations of oneself and others can make a tremendous difference in both the quality of one's work and the enjoyment derived from collaborating.

CHAPTER 7

The Influence of Collaboration on the Mental Health Professional's Identity and Practice

COLLABORATION BETWEEN mental health professionals, physicians, and other health care professionals is akin to "structural coupling" in biology (Maturana & Varella, 1988). Professionals who collaborate over time are like organisms that join up, form a relationship, and then work continuously to maintain that relationship and help it grow. This is not a purely benign process. It can be both sublime and exasperating. Both partners, or "organisms," exert themselves and perturb the other (in many ways!); consequently, each changes constantly in order to maintain a mutually beneficial fit. Maintaining such a fit is a dynamic process, full of push and pull, give and take.

In this chapter, we focus on the most common ways in which collaboration shapes mental health professionals as they continuously shift and adjust in order to maintain workable relationships with their medical and health care partners. We organize our discussion around four important areas that exemplify how the mental health professional's identity and practice are influenced by working with physicians and other health care providers: the experience of marginality, the impact of biological processes, the expansion of conceptualizations of treatment, and the redefinition of professional role.

Changes in these areas have many implications for how the mental health professional practices in collaboration with physicians and other health care professionals. We provide suggestions for clinical practice that are drawn from our own work and the experiences of those we have interviewed. Let us begin with perhaps the greatest challenge facing mental health professionals working in medical and health care settings—the experience of marginality.

MARGINALITY AND THE ISSUE OF POWER

Mauksch and Heldring (1995) conducted a survey of over 200 behavioral scientists teaching and practicing in departments of family medicine; more than 90% were Ph.D.- or master's-level mental health professionals. The purpose of the survey was to understand how nonmedical professionals experience their work in medical settings. Of note, the survey showed that mental health professionals who had worked in academic family medicine between three and six years were less satisfied than their colleagues who had worked fewer than three or greater than six years in a medical setting. The researchers hypothesized that mental health professionals with three to six years' experience in academic family medicine may

> feel less connected to their family practice surroundings than their less and more experienced colleagues. They feel less cohesive with their physician faculty than either more or less experienced colleagues. . . . This "middle time" (3–6 years) might be construed as a passage or transition when behavioral scientists assess their compatibility with family medicine. (p. 107)

While the mental health professionals surveyed in this study were taken from one particular group and may not represent all mental health professionals who collaborate, they do represent mental health professionals working in a field (family medicine) that has a long history of collaboration. For that reason, the experience of mental health professionals from this survey may be instructive for any mental health professional who collaborates. In particular, the identity crisis implied by the "midlife" experience of behavioral scientists may point to two issues commonly faced by all mental health professionals working in medical settings: marginality and power.

Barry Dym, for one, felt marginalized early on when he first started to collaborate. "I felt right on the margin of the family therapy field and the medical world, not in the center of my profession and not really recognized. At times, I felt I was constantly in a one-down position." As these comments indicate, mental health professionals working in medical settings can feel marginal in several ways. First, they may feel marginal in relationship to their own field. There may be no other psychologists or social workers or family therapists working in a given medical setting, and no opportunity to talk with like-minded professionals who share their language and socialization. One psychologist noted the difficulty even in social situations with friends who were psychologists: they had few things in common professionally, and her friends could not understand why she was working in a medical clinic.

Second, mental health professionals may feel marginal in relationship to the field they are entering, medicine. It can be difficult to enter a medical system; everything from the language to the letters after one's name may demonstrate that the mental health professional is not native-born. At times, mental health professionals can feel very isolated. One of the authors recalls working out of his briefcase for several months because there was no room for him in the clinic. He hoped exam rooms would be available when it came time for him to see patients, and the billing office was unsure of how to handle his patient charges. The staff members most aware of his presence were the transcriptionists, who were upset that his dictation was so long. Entering a medical setting from a position on the margins calls for thick skin, patience, and persistence.

Third, the feeling of being marginalized can reflect the relationship that exists between the professional fields themselves. Collaboration is still in its infancy. It is attractive to professionals from fields that encourage a spirit of adventure and experimentation. Many of the most significant efforts at collaboration have been between family therapists and family physicians. Family therapy has been characterized as a field on the margin of psychiatry (Shields, Wynne, McDaniel, & Gawinski, 1994). Its conceptual base and approach to treatment are often seen as divergent from the more traditional theory and methods at the broad center of psychiatry. Family physicians have faced similar difficulties. Medical students are routinely discouraged from becoming generalists, and family medicine residents often feel lower in the medical hierarchy when they do rotations on other specialties. With health care reform and the emphasis shifting from hospital-based medicine to primary care medicine, this attitude is changing. Nevertheless, it will always be true that both family therapy and family medicine began on the margins of their respective disciplines.

The overall impact of marginalization on the mental health professional can be a feeling of isolation, identity confusion, and limited power (Cole-Kelly & Hepworth, 1991). Mental health professionals may not feel they are full partners in the decision-making process where they work, either owing to the employer-employee relationship they often have with their physician colleagues or, if in medical school, the greater likelihood that they are not in decision-making roles.

Nursing has long struggled with issues of power. Lorraine Wright, a nurse educator and family therapist at the University of Calgary, directs the Family Nursing Unit, which educates nurses to work with whole families who are experiencing difficulties coping with illness. She believes that nursing's relatively low position in the hierarchy of medicine has mitigated against nurses being able to realize their full professional potential. To help establish a stronger sense of nursing identity and independent competence, she has organized her Family Nursing Unit so that it is run entirely by nurses. There are no physicians on staff.

We believe that the reality of structural hierarchy does not mitigate against clinical collaboration. But Wright's experience does remind mental health professionals that a fully collaborative system must account not only for how patients and families are treated but for how the organization or discipline is structured (see chapter 13). There is evidence for hope in this regard. In departments of family medicine, some behavioral scientists are making the gradual ascent to positions of power in their residency programs. For example, Jeri Hepworth is associate director of the family medicine residency program at the University of Connecticut. Richard Holloway, a family psychologist, is a past president of the Society of Teachers of Family Medicine. In the private sector, some clinical practices are being established in which mental health professionals and medical professionals are equal partners. A notable example is the North Coast Faculty Medical Group in Santa Rosa, California, where Donald Ransom is mental health director; this practice supports full financial partnership among mental health and medical professionals.

Because collaboration still exists on the margins of health and mental health care, mental health professionals continue to wrestle with issues of inclusion and influence. Some feel it may be dangerous to persist in a collaborative effort as long as mental health care has a subordinate position to medicine. They worry that mental health professionals may be giving away expertise and thereby reducing their power rather than enhancing it.

We feel that this perspective is shortsighted. It does not recognize that without developing a relationship with emerging health care systems the future of psychotherapy as a field of endeavor may be at risk. This perspective also underestimates the power of collaborative health care to make a difference in patient care and health care costs. What is called for is a "both/and" rather than an "either/or" approach. Mental health professionals must develop collaborative approaches to health and mental health care and also work to have greater access to and influence within the health care systems in which they work.

It is important for mental health professionals to remember that, in the words of Donald Bloch, we are willing to move to the margins because we are trying to create a "new center." That new center brings together not only mind, body, and relationships but also the professionals who have been divided over the treatment of those domains. In the process, we must do everything possible to organize health care delivery so that the practice of collaboration has a collaborative structure to support it (see chapters 13 and 15).

In the meantime, mental health professionals can do several things to combat marginalization:

- Continue training in collaboration (see chapter 14).
- Cultivate relationships with other professionals who collaborate.
- Maintain professional affiliations.
- Educate one's own professional organization regarding the value of collaboration.
- Join existing professional organizations that promote collaboration (see chapter 6).

BIOLOGICAL PROCESSES

Collaboration with medical professionals introduces mental health professionals to a fundamentally different way of thinking: the biomedical model. At the center of the biomedical model is the assumption that disease can be reduced to "measurable biological processes" (Engel, 1977, p. 130). The physician's job is to analyze and isolate various factors until the disease-causing element can be identified and treated. Many mental health professionals exposed to this model for the first time regard it with distaste, even disdain. They are put off by biomedicine's reductionistic tendencies. However, their own focus on psychological and interpersonal processes as the key to human problems and solutions often leaves the human body out of the equation entirely.

However much mental health professionals deny it, working with medical and health care professionals reminds us that patients have bodies; they live inside their skin as much as they live inside relationships, thoughts, and emotions (Seaburn et al., 1993). The corollary of this fact is that therapists have bodies too. William Doherty indicates that his shift to a biopsychosocial paradigm included the realization that he was a "biopsychosocial being." We live in a world of concentric circles that begins with cells and organs and organ systems and extends to self and relationships and social context. To ignore any circle is to ignore a vital system that influences our lives and the lives of the patients and families we care for.

With a growing sensitivity to biological processes in one's patients and oneself, the mental health professional should bear in mind several practice issues:

1: *Ask about the patient's and family's physical health routinely.*
   Patients and families often underestimate the role that illness may play in their individual and family lives. One of the authors recalls an initial visit with an adult woman and her mother in which the focus was on the young woman's recent psychotic symptoms. Neither of the women could identify any recent stressors that might have accounted for the daughter's unusual thinking and behavior. It was not until the end of the hour that the mother announced that she could not attend the following session because she would be out of town being treated for a malignant tumor behind her eye.

   Illness is a powerful theme in many families and should be assessed as a routine part of therapy. A medical genogram (three-generation minimum) is one method for gathering such information (McDaniel et al., 1992; Rolland, 1994a). Common questions to ask include:

- Who in your family has been ill?
- What illnesses have they had? Acute? Chronic? Terminal?
- What has been the outcome of each illness?
- What is your family's style of coping with illness?
- How do you make sense of these experiences?
- Who is most involved when someone is ill? Least involved?
- How are physical symptoms dealt with by your family in general? By the women in the family? By the men?
- Who is your physician?
- What has your relationship with health care professionals been like?
- What other life-cycle or developmental issues are you and your family dealing with at this time?

In our experience, answers to these questions give the therapist not only an understanding of how the family deals with illness but an understanding of how the family may deal with other forms of adversity.

2: *Recognize that mind–body interaction is a two-way street.* Among mental health professionals there is general acceptance that the mind influences the body's functioning. Griffith and Griffith (1994) argue convincingly that the body is an articulate spokesperson for what is happening in the lives of individuals, couples, and families. Medical family therapists have taken increasing interest in somatically fixated patients, patients whose lives are organized around physical symptoms and whose bodies are the channels for expressing their emotions (Griffith & Griffith, 1994; McDaniel et al., 1990; McDaniel et al., 1992; Seaburn, 1995).

Mental health professionals who work in medical settings or who collaborate closely with health care professionals gradually learn that the opposite is true as well. The body influences the mind in ways that are equally powerful. It is important for mental health professionals to help patients and families address interpersonal processes that affect physical health and well-being. But to do this alone is to miss half the story. Biological processes or physical illnesses are often powerful "family members" that shape the life course of families as much or more than other factors (Gonzalez, Steinglass, & Reiss, 1989;

Rolland, 1994a). To overlook how the body impacts individual and interpersonal processes is to run the risk of supporting many patients' worst fear—"Am I to blame for my health problems? Is it all in my mind?"

It is useful for mental health professionals who work in medical settings to be aware of how the body influences emotional, psychological, and interpersonal functioning. Table 7.1 lists common conditions in which the body affects the mind.

TABLE 7.1

COMMON HEALTH PROBLEMS THAT AFFECT PSYCHOSOCIAL FUNCTION

Disorder	*Symptoms*
Central nervous system directly affected:	
Alzheimer's	Forgetfulness. Lack of dependability. Laissez-faire attitude.
Brain tumor	Variable depending on site of tumor. Can be emotionally labile, aggressive, passionate, forgetful, fatigued.
Stroke	Variable depending on site of stroke. Same as for brain tumor. Many strokes affect motor function (increasing dependence) and speech articulation and recognition (aphasia).
Central nervous system indirectly affected:	
Diabetes	Mood fluctuations. Need for increased regimentation of diet, activity, and sleep. Mental slowness with high blood sugar; agitation with low blood sugar.
Hypothyroidism	Mental slowness, fatigue, apathy, hypersomnia, flat affect.
Hyperthyroidism	Hypersexuality, physical weakness, insomnia, mood lability.
Renal failure	Fatigue, forgetfulness, limited diet, may need to be on dialysis (3 times a week, 3 hours at a time). Restricted travel.
Anemia	Fatigue, forgetfulness, physical weakness.
Cardiac	Decreased exercise tolerance. Fear of heart attack. Easily fatigued.
Hormonal—male	Decreased energy.
Hormonal—female	Irritability, mood lability, dietary restrictions, hot flashes.

3: *Utilize the therapeutic value of medications.* Many psychotherapists, especially family systems–oriented therapists, begin their work in medical settings with a bias against the use of medications. This perspective is often derived from professional training that may have fostered animosity toward the medical model of treatment, which is seen as a dismissal of more important problems, or a dismissal of the patient as a person. In our interviews with therapists who work in medical settings, the issue of medication usage came up repeatedly. To a person, their viewpoint had changed with experience. Nevertheless, though few therapists question the need for and value of medications such as antidepressants, many continue to question the use of benzodiazapines (Valium, Librium, Tranxene, Xanax, etc.) because of their potential for addiction. This attitude, however, is shared by most primary care physicians, who also struggle with the value of prescribing such medications for the treatment of anxiety.

It is estimated that 10% of all patients who seek help in primary care settings in this country are suffering from depression (Duer, Schwenk, & Coyne, 1988). Seventeen million people suffer from major depression each year (Preston, O'Neal, & Talaga, 1994). Depression is responsible for more days of work lost per year than physical illness (Ormel, Von Korff, Ustan, Pini, Korten, & Oldehinkel, 1994). While only one-third of these people seek treatment, 80% of those who do seek treatment experience relief (Preston et al., 1994).

Studies have also shown that antidepressant medication is more effective when used in tandem with psychotherapy (Beck, 1976; Klerman et al., 1984). Not only are patients more likely to comply with antidepressant medication if their partner is involved and supportive, but psychosocial factors are the greatest contributors to depression. Studies show that depressed persons whose relatives demonstrate a high degree of critical comments are more likely to relapse than those who experience a low degree of criticism (Hooley, Orley, & Teasdale, 1986; Vaughn & Leff, 1976).

A collaborative approach is critical in treating many depressed patients because of the biopsychosocial nature of the problem. When antidepressant medications are indicated, the mental health care provider must have a working understanding of their value so that he or she can collaborate effectively with the physician. The mental health care provider must also address the psychological and interpersonal factors that are contributing to the depression or mitigating against its effective treatment. Two valuable resources for mental health professionals are *Concise Guide to Somatic Therapies in Psychiatry* by Guttmacher (1988) and *Handbook of Clinical Psychopharmacology for Therapists* by Preston, O'Neal, and Talaga (1994). Tables 7.2 and 7.3 indicate medical conditions that could cause depression and provide a guide to the types of antidepressants and their dosages.

CONCEPTUALIZATION OF TREATMENT

Mental health professionals who work with physicians and health care professionals are often humbled by the impact that illness has on patients, families, health care providers, and themselves. What is readily apparent is that many patients and families must navigate their lives with chronic illnesses, such as hypertension, diabetes, epilepsy, heart disease, cancer, and AIDS, that won't go away. To these must be added those patients who suffer from chronic pain or other persistent physical concerns or disabilities for which there may or may not be a medical diagnosis. Such patients

TABLE 7.2

MEDICAL DISORDERS THAT CAN CAUSE DEPRESSION

Addison's disease	Infectious hepatitis
AIDS	Influenza
Anemia	Malignancies (cancer)
Asthma	Malnutrition
Chronic fatigue syndrome	Multiple sclerosis
Chronic infection	Porphyria
(mononucleosis, TB)	Rheumatoid arthritis
Chronic pain	Syphilis
Congestive heart failure	Systemic lupus erythematosus
Cushing's disease	Ulcerative colitis
Diabetes	Uremia
Hypothyroidism	

Note. From *Handbook of Clinical Psychopharmacology for Therapists* (p. 62) by J. Preston, J. H. O'Neal, and M. C. Talaga, 1994, Oakland, CA: New Harbinger Publications.

TABLE 7.3

TYPES OF ANTIDEPRESSANTS AND THEIR DOSAGES

Drug (brand name)	Dosage (mg per day)
Tricyclic	
Amitriptyline (Elavil)	75–300
Clomipramine (Anafranil)	75–200
Desipramine (Norpramin, Pertofrane)	75–300
Doxepin (Sinequan, Adapin)	75–300
Imipramine (Tofranil)	75–300
Nortriptyline (Pamelor, Aventyl)	50–150
Trazodone (Desyrel)	150–400
Selective serotonin re-uptake inhibitors (SSRI)	
Fluoxetine (Prozac)	20–80
Paroxetine (Paxil)	20–60
Sertraline (Zoloft)	50–200
Effexor	37.5–75
Monoamine oxidase inhibitors (MAOs)	
Isocarboxazid (Marplan)	20–30
Phenelzine (Nardil)	45–90
Tranylcypromine (Parnate)	20–40

Note. Adapted from *Handbook of Clinical Psychopharmacology for Therapists* (p. 70) by J. Preston, J. H. O'Neal, and M. C. Talaga, 1994, Oakland, CA: New Harbinger Publications.

pose challenges to physicians and nursing professionals and are often referred for mental health services.

These patients are also our best teachers. What they teach us about how to do therapy may differ from what we have learned in our training. Typically, a good psychotherapist wants to facilitate change in the problems his or her patients face. What does the therapist do when the problem afflicting the patient and family is a health concern that won't go away? "Working with chronic illness deeply affected my work with all my patients," said Barry Dym. "I became less interested in changing people fundamentally and more aware of what was constant; helping people to live with themselves, whether it was due to an illness or a character trait." Larry Mauksch learned another lesson:

> One of the . . . things that working with doctors and health care professionals has taught me is the difference between care and

cure. I came into mental health and collaborative practice with a desire to cure. That's the way I defined success; if I wanted to be accepted in the medical context, I had to "fix" things. That was a setup for me to fail with many of my patients. With many patients I focus much more on care than cure. This provides a sense of relief and peace of mind for me. I focus on tolerance and coping in life and [spend] less time talking about curing what can't be cured.

For many patients cure is an elusive goal that can never be reached. The most valuable work is providing care. This should not be confused with "support," important though that may be. Active caring is a different approach from that of trying to eradicate a problem that won't go away. At its most fundamental level, caring involves a willingness to stay with people in the uncertainty of their life situations and to struggle with them to make the daily act of living better. Reconceptualizing treatment to accommodate the persistence of health problems and the goals of health care has several practical implications for the mental health professional:

1: *Clarify with the referring physician or health care professional what the current goals are for the patient's health care.* A referral for therapy often implies a mandate to change things, preferably as soon as possible. This may be contraindicated, particularly if the health care goal for the patient is "stabilizing" a current health problem. In such a situation, rapid change may compromise the patient's overall health.

Mr. and Mrs. Gonzales were referred by Dr. Wong for work on their marriage. Dr. Wong told the therapist that the couple was having difficulty communicating. She felt they were holding in a lot of feelings related to Mr. Gonzales's recent heart attack. Dr. Wong said, though, that she felt the couple had been having problems even before the heart attack. The therapist asked how Mr. Gonzales's recovery was going. Dr. Wong indicated that the patient was having unstable angina, which they were trying to manage with medication. Given the unstable nature of Mr. Gonzales's condition, the therapist and Dr. Wong both agreed that pacing would be very important in the therapy. Opening emotional issues prematurely could be detrimental to Mr. Gonzales's health; by the same token, the tension in the couple's relationship due to lack of communication was also unhealthy. The therapist and Dr. Gonzales planned to communicate regularly to monitor the balance between stability and change that was called for in the treatment.

2: *Actively elicit the patient's and family's illness story* (McDaniel et al., 1992; Rolland, 1994a; Seaburn et al., 1992). It is important to take an "ethnographic" approach to a patient's health problem and the personal and family stories that surround it (Stein & Apprey, 1990). By respectfully entering the world of the patient and family, the mental health care provider is best able to learn what will be most helpful, what will be most healing. Often the storytelling process itself is healing. As Stein and Apprey indicate, "to help people to be able to tell their own story and to work with and within these stories is the core therapeutic function" (p. 227). Through the "storying of experience" (White & Epston, 1990), patients and families create a framework for understanding and coping with illness. The capacity of the therapist and health care provider to be witnesses to the suffering of patients and their families is central to providing care; indeed, it is frequently the fountainhead of healing, if not curing (Kleinman, 1988).

For many patients and families consumed by an illness, their illness narrative provides the best access to the rest of their lives as well. In telling the tale, the patient and family reveal much of who they are and how they are, as a whole and as individuals. The medical genogram provides an excellent structure for eliciting the patient's and family's stories. Questions that build on medical genogram information are included in appendix B.

3: *Facilitate agency and communion in the patient's and family's approach to health problems and in the professionals' collaboration.* "Agency" includes the individual's tendency toward self-protection, self-assertion, and mastery; "communion" includes union, cooperation, and being one with other organisms. Bakan (1966) first introduced these concepts in his analysis of human existence in Western culture. Agency and communion are "two fundamental modalities in the existence of living forms, agency for the existence of an organism as an individual, and communion for the participation of the individual in some larger organism of which the individual is a part" (p. 14). In Bakan's view, no living organism can survive without a blend of both agency and communion.

Implied in Bakan's concept is the idea that a balance of agency and communion is necessary to foster any organism's overall health. This perspective is brought into sharper focus by McDaniel, Hepworth, and Doherty (1992) as they apply these concepts to the patient's and family's experience of illness. In their view, agency refers to "a sense of making personal choices in dealing with illness and the health care system, both of which often contribute to a patient's feeling of passivity and lack of control" (p. 9). Of equal importance, communion has to do with "emotional bonds" and a sense of "being supported by a community of family members, friends, and professionals" (pp. 9–10).

By eliciting the patient's and family's illness stories, the health and mental health care providers are given an inside view of how much agency and communion family members feel in the face of their shared problem. Loss of agency often occurs when people try to change the unchangeable.

Mr. and Mrs. Swenson were referred by the psychologist in the Cancer Center to a family therapist because of difficulties the family was having with Mr. Swenson's stomach cancer. The Swensons and their five adult children came to the first interview together. Mr. Swenson's cancer was in an advanced stage; he was not likely to live longer than a few more months. Yet in the first 15 minutes, his children's anger exploded in the room. They were upset that he was not attacking the cancer more aggressively, that he was not "reading more about it," "changing his diet," and generally fighting the disease. After several minutes, Mr. Swenson responded by saying, "I know what you mean; it's like I should be digging a ditch or something."

The Swenson family was struggling for control over something that was beyond their control; in the process, they were left feeling angry and frustrated. The family needed help identifying how they could have agency in a situation that left them feeling helpless. The therapy focused on recognizing what the family could do and what was beyond their control. This helped the family make peace with the terminal course of Mr. Swenson's illness. By doing so, they were able to prepare themselves to care for Mr. Swenson at home in his final days. This included physical care as well as emotional leave-taking.

The Swensons are a good example of the interplay of agency and communion. Agency is fostered as much by coming together as a family as by anything else. Patients and families often feel buoyed simply by being together. A natural strength inherent to the family may emerge in the process of interacting with each other.

Health and mental health professionals can experience the same problems as families dealing with an illness (Rolland, 1994a; Seaburn, 1994); they can also feel a loss of agency and communion. Interestingly, these losses are often due to the same difficulties that cause families to lose agency and communion. Professionals trained to "cure" may not know what to do when curing is impossible. Professionals who feel helpless or burned out are often hesitant to talk about what they are dealing with for fear of how they will be seen. Providers can feel isolated when working with difficult patients and families. The more isolated they feel, the less agency they feel as well.

Fostering agency and communion is a key part of any work with patients and families in a medical setting. It is also a key part of any collaboration between health and mental health professionals, who should continuously assess their own sense of agency and communion during the ebb and flow of caring for challenging patients and their families. Table 7.4 presents suggestions for facilitating agency and communion that recognize the isomorphic relationship between how families cope with illness and how professionals cope with families dealing with illness.

REDEFINITION OF PROFESSIONAL ROLE

Many health and mental health collaborators have tried to define their relationship in ways that adequately describe their functioning. These have included "clinical family" (Stein & Apprey, 1990), the "primary health care team" (Dym & Berman, 1986), the "primary health care network" (Seaburn et al., 1993), and the "generic health care team" (Bloch, 1993a). What each of these labels has in common is the recognition that something new and different is created when mental health and health care providers work together

TABLE 7.4

FACILITATING AGENCY AND COMMUNION

Patients and Families	*Professionals*
Agency	
Help them differentiate between areas over which they can have agency and areas over which they cannot	Regularly assess your expectations of what you can accomplish in patient care
Whenever possible, facilitate family member involvement in treatment planning and patient care	Routinely discuss these expectations with health care collaborators
Enable the family to identify other areas of family life and routine that need to be maintained and supported	Maintain a healthy balance between work, family, and recreation
Help the patient and family access beliefs and values that enable them to find balance between uncertainty and hope	Nurture the values and beliefs that enable you to provide care in an atmosphere that is often demanding and uncertain
Communion	
Include as many family members as possible	Routinely talk to friends and/or colleagues about the rewards and pressures of patient care
Facilitate communication within and across generations about the illness and its impact on everyone	Discuss and respect differences in theoretical perspective
Normalize affect, especially sadness, fear, anger, and guilt	Talk to your health care colleagues about how challenging patients may impact your capacity to collaborate
Encourage acceptance of different styles of coping	

over time. The role of the mental health professional collaborating with physicians and health care professionals is gradually redefined in a way that at first is unsettling. Recalls William Doherty:

> When I first saw patients with residents, I expected that at the end of the visit the patient would contract for therapy and want to come back. Oftentimes this did not happen. I might not see the patient again at all. At first, I didn't know whether or not I had done a good job. When I realized that the resident was very satisfied with what I did, I began to understand that I was serving a different or broader function than just providing therapy to patients, as I might in a private practice.

Most mental health professionals who enter a medical context begin by thinking of themselves as just that—a mental health professional doing therapy in a medical setting. Over time that definition changes. Mental health professionals learn that they are part of a larger team of providers involved in varying degrees with each other and with patients, often over an extended period of time. This team may include primary care physicians, nurse-practitioners, physician's assistants, nurses, dietitians, medical specialists, and others. Providing psychotherapy to patients and families is only one part of the therapist's role on such a team. The needs of the team of professionals help define the mental health professional's role as much as the needs of the patients.

The primary dimensions of the mental health collaborator's role include being a coprovider, a consultant, and a specialist.

Coprovider

The coprovision of patient care is the essence of teamwork—particularly because most patient problems present a blend of biomedical and psychosocial concerns, such as chronic or terminal illness, pain management, depression, drug and alcohol abuse, somatic fixation, and eating disorders, to name a few. The therapist, physician, nurse-practitioner, and others form a communication web in which each professional plays a vital role, realizing that no one of the team members can stand alone. In the words of Larry Mauksch, "There is a reward that comes from systems problem-solving that is at the core of what collaboration is all about. There is something humbling about that. It reveals the limits of my power and the need to work in tandem with others."

The team members can simultaneously feel "small" in their individual capacities to "do it all" and "large" in what they can accomplish by working together. For the beginning therapist in collaboration, coprovision of care means rethinking patient "ownership." Jeri Hepworth suggests that the insecurity of a therapist who is new to collaboration may stimulate the desire to "own" patients, to have a hierarchically elevated position over one's coproviders—to, in a sense, be the "lone ranger" who fixes the patient and the problem all by himself or herself. This temptation is a natural response to being new in a medical setting and wanting to be successful and appreciated by medical colleagues. But this approach is essentially noncollaborative and fosters animosity among one's colleagues (not to mention that it doesn't work!). Coprovision of care calls for mutual support, clarification and reclarification of roles, respect for the expertise of colleagues, and a willingness to constantly shift team leadership roles based on the needs of the patient.

Consultant

Wynne, McDaniel, and Weber (1986) expanded the definition of the systems therapist to include consultation. A systems consultation model in a medical context focuses on the needs of the medical provider in a unique way (McDaniel et al., 1992). The therapist's "customer" is the physician or other health care provider who may consult with him or her about a challenging patient or situation.

Such a consultation may be specifically patient-focused. Common dilemmas that lead to a patient-focused consultation include patient noncompliance, difficulty managing a patient during an interview, patient affect or behavior (angry, demanding, critical, sad), diagnostic questions, family assessment or preparation for a family meeting, and pre–mental health referral planning. In such situations, the physician may feel stuck. The mental health professional's role is to help the physician do his or her own problem-solving. It is useful to facilitate the physician's exploration of various elements of problem-solving that may be relevant to his or her situation, including:

- Relationship-building: Has the physician established an adequate working relationship with the patient and/or family?
- Assessment: Has the physician elicited the patient's and family's story well enough to identify, understand, and address the problem?
- Agenda-setting: Have clear goals for treatment been established?

- Mutual agreement: Do the physician and patient/family share a common treatment plan?
- Management and intervention: Has an action plan been implemented?
- Closure: Has the plan been effective and the problem resolved? (Botelho & Harp, in preparation)

Frequently, the core consultation task is to help the physician or health care provider identify which problem-solving area is most appropriate to the situation. For instance, a physician may seek consultation when he or she is frustrated with a patient who is not complying with a treatment plan, such as maintaining a diet to manage diabetes. Consultation may help the physician recognize that he or she may be trying to intervene before an adequate relationship has been established with the patient. In this way, the mental health collaborator functions as a consultant to the process of the physician's developing relationship with the patient.

At other times the consultation may be focused on the physician or health care provider. Physicians may face difficulties working with patients that are due in part to personal, relational, and family-of-origin issues (Mengel, 1987).

Dr. Melendez approached a therapist colleague about a patient he was having difficulty caring for. The patient was recently diagnosed with stomach cancer. Despite the assurances of medical colleagues with whom he had consulted, Dr. Melendez wondered whether he should have been able to diagnose the cancer sooner. He found himself thinking about the patient often while at the same time having difficulty talking with him during medical visits. Dr. Melendez talked about his own father's death from cancer, which his mother felt should have been diagnosed earlier. This discussion helped Dr. Melendez separate his own family's experience from his patient's experience enough to provide effective care for the patient.

Consultation of this kind should not be confused with psychotherapy. The consultation needs to remain focused on the patient care issues at hand. If it becomes apparent that the primary focus of the consultation is the personal concerns of the physician, then the therapist should discuss the possibility and value of psychotherapy for his or her colleague.

Most consultations are a blend of both patient- and physician-focused concerns. Such consultations may be thought of as relationship-focused since they emphasize the interaction between the professional and the patient and family more than intervention. No matter what the focus, the consultation itself may vary in structure (see chapter 8).

We are focusing on the mental health professional as consultant, but the consultation process is actually more mutual than this orientation implies. The mental health professional is just as likely to be in a consultee role with the health care professional. Patients often present complicated medical issues to mental health professionals in medical settings. Consultation with physicians and other health care providers not only reduces the mental health professional's anxiety but helps the therapist understand the patient better. By the same token, the patient's health care provider is often an excellent consultant to the mental health professional regarding how to engage and work with patients and families. In a sense, the mental health professional can borrow from the trust that has been established between the physician or health care provider and the patient.

Specialist

The idea of being a specialist may seem like the antithesis of being an effective team player. But their specialized knowledge and skill are key reasons mental health professionals are important members of any collaborative health care team. When a primary care physician detects a problem with a patient's heart, the physician will refer the patient to a cardiologist, whose specialty serves as an extension of primary care. In a similar fashion, health care providers will refer to the social worker, family therapist, psychologist, psychiatrist, counselor, or other mental health professional so that they and their patients can benefit from the mental health professional's areas of expertise and skill.

These areas of specialty may include everything from parent-child problems, play therapy, and marriage and family counseling to smoking cessation, relaxation techniques, or assessing for psychosis. Patients are often referred to mental health professionals so that these and other specific issues can be addressed more effectively. When the nature of the patient's problem appears to fall exclusively in the psychosocial domain, it is tempting for the mental health professional to work solo. But like the cardiologist who accepts a referral from a primary care physician, the mental health provider has a responsibility to maintain open communication and contact with the referring health care professional. The service provided by the mental health professional may seem like a separate thread. From a broader vantage point, though, it is but one strand in a larger web of health care.

CONCLUSION

The mental health professional's development gains in both diversity and richness as his or her role is redefined. This process of role redefinition mirrors the broader impact that working collaboratively has on the mental health professional's practice. This broader impact includes a different vision of what health and mental health care can be. This vision is more integrated and complete in its view of patient and family problems; it is also more inclusive of those health and mental health professionals who are needed to implement integrated health care. As Susan H. McDaniel has stated, "In a really good collaborative situation, two plus two equals more than four. The whole is definitely greater than the sum of its parts."

PART III

Implementing Collaboration

In this part, we examine the efforts of mental health and health care professionals to collaborate in a variety of settings. All of these efforts represent creative and effective blendings of the various key ingredients of collaboration. Part III begins with a look at "The Spectrum of Collaboration" (chapter 8). The spectrum provides a flexible range of possible roles that the mental health care provider may play when collaborating in any setting.

Then we examine four different contexts. Chapters 9 and 10 describe the familiar world of primary care and private practice. Most mental health care providers have operated independently or in small groups providing general or specialized mental health services. They do not usually practice in the same space as physicians but do often receive referrals from their medical colleagues. Chapter 9 highlights the increasing importance of collaboration in these settings and provides examples of successful partnerships. Chapter 10 is written by one of the authors (Alan Lorenz) who is a family physician also trained as a family therapist. He walks the reader through a 'primary care medical practice designed specifically to include on-site mental health consultation and collaboration.

In chapter 11, we describe a context that is less familiar to mainstream mental health: residency programs that train family physicians. For over 20 years, a small group of mental health professionals from psychiatry, family therapy, psychology, social work, and nursing have taught and practiced in these training settings. Much groundbreaking work in collaboration has occurred in these programs where mental health professionals are engaged in a variety of collaborative roles.

In chapter 12, we turn away from the primary care medicine world and focus on specialized medical settings. We describe the trends in providing care in hospitals and in acute, intensive environments. One of these trends is that traditional high-technology settings are becoming more patient-centered and collaborative with their "customers." Finally, in chapter 13, we turn to the critical issue of collaboration in managed care, the wave of the present and the future. This chapter provides a comprehensive overview of managed care and discusses the important implications for mental health professionals wishing to collaborate in these settings.

Throughout part III, we provide practical suggestions that highlight the nuances of collaborating in each of these contexts.

CHAPTER 8

Fostering Flexibility: The Spectrum of Collaboration

THE SPECTRUM OF COLLABORATION represents the broad range of collaborative options available to mental health and health care providers when working in partnership with patients and families. The color spectrum as seen in a rainbow comprises color bands that are distinct yet connected. Each color blends gradually into the next color. The spectrum of collaboration is similar in that the various "bands" of collaboration are distinct, reflecting different needs and functions, yet each band is an extension of the others, allowing for flexibility of professional functioning and movement across the spectrum.

Doherty, McDaniel, and Baird have developed the notion of "levels of collaboration" (Doherty, 1995). These levels reflect the influence of location of services and system design on the capacity of the mental health care provider and health care practitioner to work together. The spectrum of collaboration focuses more specifically on the ability of professionals, patients, and families to create collaborative relationships, which may be influenced by factors such as location of service but need not be limited by them. A basic premise of the spectrum is that various forms of collaboration are possible no matter what the circumstances.

The primary bands on the spectrum of collaboration are: parallel delivery, informal consultation, formal consultation, coprovision of care, and collaborative networking (Figure 8.1). These bands represent the *breadth* of collaboration that may be available in any given clinical situation.

Parallel delivery occurs when the division of labor is clear and the problems addressed do not flow into each other in any significant way; mental health and health care professionals are connected typically through a referral and benefit from the knowledge that a partner is available, though each functions independently. Informal consultation focuses primarily on the consultant (mental health or health care) helping the consultee (mental health or health care) address a clinical concern; typically, the consultant has no contact with the patient or family. In formal consultation, the consultant may have direct contact with the patient and family; the relationship with the consultee is more contractual. Coprovision of care involves sharing professional responsibility for patient care; the professionals often see the patient and family together. Coprovision of care is generally not hierarchical, although professional leadership in treatment may vary depending on the problem. Collaborative networking expands the provider team to include

FIGURE 8.1

THE SPECTRUM OF COLLABORATION

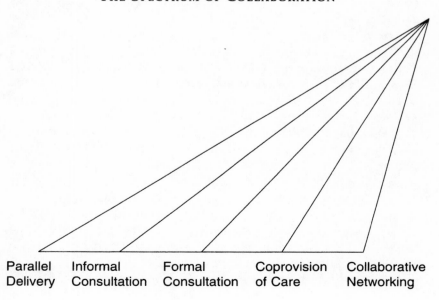

Parallel   Informal   Formal   Coprovision   Collaborative
Delivery   Consultation   Consultation   of Care   Networking

extended family and other medical specialists or educators, as well as community resources.

Collaboration at any point on the spectrum involves varying degrees of *depth*. Just as each color band has a range of hues that reflect varying degrees of richness and vibrancy, collaboration at any band on the spectrum may be more or less intense. Depth of collaboration reflects not only frequency of contact among those who collaborate (mental health professional, physician, other health care professional, patient, and family) but intensity and meaningfulness of contact as well. In that sense, depth of collaboration reflects how much each of the collaborators changes because of their interaction together. Possible changes include healing, growth, insight, and the development of new skills or perspectives.

Many factors contribute to depth of collaboration. How the key ingredients of collaboration are implemented in a particular setting or professional relationship are obviously important determinants of the possible depth of collaboration. If the professionals have no agreed-upon way to communicate with each other, or their financial arrangements mitigate against working together to develop a relationship, then depth of collaboration will be greatly affected, though not eliminated.

We want to emphasize three other critical factors that influence both the depth and breadth of collaboration in any clinical situation: the nature of the problem being addressed, the amount of patient and family involvement and/or distress, and the degree of professional "stuckness."

The nature of the problem being addressed often has a direct impact on the breadth or depth of collaboration. Some problems present very little overlap between the psychosocial and biomedical domains. A patient may see a therapist for career counseling and visit his or her physician or nurse-practitioner infrequently. The patient may have ideas about what he or she wants to do professionally and the support of family regarding career decisions. Such situations call for parallel delivery of care with little or no contact between professionals or involvement of family and others in treatment. The work with the patient may be gratifying, but it may not have either the breadth or depth of working with a patient who has a chronic, terminal disease, such as AIDS.

By contrast, the course of treatment for a patient suffering from a disease like AIDS may be long and complicated. Communication between participants in the collaborative network of primary care providers, medical specialists, mental health professionals, and other community professionals may be complex and frequent. Involving the patient's family and other loved ones may call for careful and sensitive planning between the patient, therapist, and primary care provider. The patient's experience may lead all participants to face their own mortality in a different way. In both of these situations, the nature of the problem being addressed plays a key role in both the breadth and depth of collaboration.

The involvement of the patient and family in care is the second critical factor. Developing a working partnership with a patient and family is the most fundamental form of collaboration. Upon that foundation all other collaboration rises and falls. The patient and family are the people whose lives are most affected by the problems being addressed. They are the ones who understand their experience best and often have the greatest influence on the success or failure of any care plan. For that reason alone, the patient (at a minimum) and the family (whenever possible) should be included in all treatment planning. Their distress may signal not only an increased alarm about the problem but concern that professionals are not involving them adequately in efforts to solve the problem. By expanding the care team to include family, a healthy complexity of viewpoints is added to the process, a complexity that can generate new directions or solutions. Also, family involvement invariably adds a dimension of intimacy and history that both broadens and deepens the work.

Professional "stuckness," the third critical factor, is often the primary reason providers expand the treatment team by referring, consulting, or otherwise involving additional professionals in a patient's care—particularly the care of challenging patients with mental health difficulties. In our experience, physicians and other health care providers are often more motivated to seek a mental health referral than the patient is. They are eager to try something new since nothing else is working. The mental health care provider may not recognize this dynamic until the first patient interview. When asked about his or her reasons for coming to therapy, the patient may answer, "I don't know. My doctor thought it was a good idea." Just as the patient's physical ailment may be a symptom of other nonphysical problems, a patient referral to a mental health care provider may be a "symptom" of professional distress on the part of the health care provider.

Mental health professionals who become psychosocially fixated and overlook biomedical aspects of a problem can also become stuck. By turning to a medical or health care colleague, the mental health professional may broaden his or her perspective and the clinical logjam may be loosened. The degree of professional stuckness or distress often determines how intense or frequent the contact between professionals needs to be.

The struggles of the professionals involved also may bring other dimensions of meaning to the collaboration. These struggles include family-of-origin issues, difficulties with the uncertainty that is always a part of providing care, and exploration of professional identity, to name a few. The influence that collaborative partners have on each other's personal and professional growth is one of the most valuable rewards of collaboration. One of the authors recalls working together for over a year with a physician colleague and her young male patient who was dying of cancer. Both were deeply affected by this patient's struggle with the reality of his eventual death, his efforts to decide whether to continue living, and his painful attempts at resolving unfinished conflicts within his family. The physician and therapist met from time to time to talk about how this patient was affecting their own lives. They became more sensitive to the ever-present uncertainty involved in caring for patients who are ill, as well as the uncertainty that characterizes living itself. In the end, collaborating in the care of this dying patient pushed them to wrestle with many of their own issues regarding life's meaning and purpose. Though neither arrived at any final answers, both appreciated being in a collaborative relationship that helped them at least address important questions.

We want to make an additional point about the breadth and depth of collaboration. Some believe that the breadth and depth of any collaboration are determined primarily by whether the professional collaborators are located in the same setting. Clearly, where the professionals are located is a key ingredient to any collaboration. And we agree that when mental health professionals, physicians, and health care professionals are located in the same setting, collaboration is greatly facilitated. But we do not believe that colocation of professionals is the single determining factor in effective collaboration.

In our view, effective collaboration is determined by how the key ingredients of collaboration (relationship, common purpose, communication, flexible paradigm, location of services, and business arrangement) are implemented, even if the professionals do not work in the same setting. How these ingredients are blended determines the relationship among the collaborating professionals, patients, and families. It also determines whether the mental health care provider functions as a specialist, consultant, coprovider, or some combination of each. With this in mind, we now look in greater detail at the spectrum of collaboration.

PARALLEL DELIVERY

Parallel delivery of care often occurs when the problem the physician or health care professional is addressing and the problem the mental health professional is addressing have minimal overlap and can be managed effectively without intensive contact between them. Other factors leading to parallel delivery include geographical distance between the providers and limitations due to financial arrangements or insurance coverage.

The contact between the professionals may occur only at the beginning and end of therapy. In such situations, the mental health care provider and physician or health care provider have primarily a "referral" relationship (McDaniel et al., 1992). The physician or nurse may refer to a therapist in the same HMO or to a mental health professional working in the community. A referral relationship may not, however, imply a "split biopsychosocial" approach to care (Doherty, Baird, & Becker, 1987). A split model implies that services are delivered separately, largely owing to divergent paradigms (separation of body and mind). Professionals working in a split model are not yet delivering parallel services. In fact, they are often moving in divergent directions.

The most important feature of parallel delivery is the mind-set of the collaborating professionals. An attitude or spirit of collaboration connects them even when direct contact is unnecessary. Mental health and physical health professionals who work in parallel may not be in continuous contact but may nevertheless feel confident they are moving in the same overall direction (common purpose). This confidence is often based on the response of the patient and family. The patient, couple, or family may take responsibility for their care and work effectively as partners with the therapist and physician or health care professional. They may speak highly of the therapist and physician or health care provider. This often contributes to the professionals' confidence in each other's work even if their direct contact is limited.

Following is a common example of parallel delivery of care:

Mr. and Mrs. Feinstein had been Dr. Vasquez's patients for seven years. Dr. Vasquez delivered the Feinsteins' two children,

Aaron, 6, and Ruth, 3. The Feinsteins enjoyed their relationship with Dr. Vasquez and had confidence in her ability and caring. This confidence was buoyed when Dr. Vasquez helped Aaron through a difficult bout of pneumonia at age two.

More recently, Mrs. Feinstein called Dr. Vasquez to discuss some concerns they had about Aaron's behavior. Dr. Vasquez invited the couple in for a conjoint visit. She listened to the Feinsteins' concerns and suggested that a therapist might be a good resource for them. The couple was reluctant at first but felt more comfortable when Dr. Vasquez said she knew a therapist, Mr. Hoffman, who worked with parents dealing with child concerns (therapist as specialist). Dr. Vasquez said she had referred others to him and felt he did a good job. The Feinsteins were agreeable, and Dr. Vasquez gave the couple Mr. Hoffman's phone number.

The Feinsteins contacted Mr. Hoffman, who worked at a separate location. Mr. Hoffman saw the whole family for the first visit. At the end he asked permission to contact Dr. Vasquez to let her know the family had come and to thank her for the referral. The Feinsteins praised Dr. Vasquez and said it would be okay for Mr. Hoffman to speak with her.

Mr. Hoffman had worked with three other families referred by Dr. Vasquez. Although he had never met her, Mr. Hoffman felt she was a caring physician who made appropriate referrals. He dictated a letter to Dr. Vasquez and also called her to thank her for the referral. He told her that the first visit went well and then shared some preliminary plans for working with Aaron and his parents. Upon receiving the letter and phone call from Mr. Hoffman, Dr. Vasquez felt confident that her patients were in the right place.

Mr. Hoffman saw the family four times over the next few months. During that time the Feinsteins did not see Dr. Vasquez. Also, Mr. Hoffman and Dr. Vasquez had no additional contact.

The value of parallel delivery of care as a form of collaboration should not be underestimated. Physicians, health care providers, and mental health professionals who work in parallel report that just knowing a collaborative colleague is involved and available is very beneficial. Physicians and health care professionals feel more confident asking the patient psychosocial questions when they know they can talk with a mental health care provider if necessary. By the same token, mental health care providers feel confident that biologic or physical factors in the patient's situation can be addressed if warranted. And both benefit from knowing the patient has a solid relationship with each professional; both professionals can learn from these relationships.

There are limits to this form of collaboration. Mrs. Feinstein could return to Dr. Vasquez with complaints about the therapist, as well as complaints about her spouse. Dr. Vasquez may not know how to respond. In the meantime, Mr. Feinstein may call Mr. Hoffman complaining about Dr. Vasquez. The couple may feel their son is "hyper" and may urge Dr. Vasquez to prescribe a medication while Mr. Hoffman is working on parental limit-setting skills. Or one of the Feinsteins may confide in Mr. Hoffman that he or she has had severe headaches and nausea for several weeks but does not want to tell the doctor. Each of these scenarios cries out for greater depth of collaboration between the mental health professional, the physician or health care professional, and the patient and family. Greater contact may begin with professional consultation.

INFORMAL CONSULTATION

Informal consultation occurs when one professional contacts another professional to get advice on a particular problem situation, typically patient-related (mental health professional as specialist and consultant). Informal consultation usually involves one or a few contacts; it is not ongoing in nature. Typically, the patient and family are not seen by the consultant. Such consultation occurs in person or by phone, letter, or E-mail (although E-mail may present serious confidentiality issues). Informal consultation is a common practice among medical professionals, who often call specialists to whom they refer patients, asking questions about a symptom presentation, diagnosis, or treatment plan. Mental health professionals often use their psychiatrist colleagues in a similar way.

Most consultations in a primary care setting where mental health professionals, physicians, and nurses are colocated happen as informal "bumps in the hall" (Hepworth & Jackson, 1985) or "spot conferences" (Blount & Bayona, 1994) that last only a few minutes. One study showed that 92% of physician-therapist consultations in a primary care setting occur in this brief format, and that one-half are less than five minutes long (Coleman, Patrick, Eagle, & Hermalin, 1979). These consultations should not be devalued for their brevity. They are an important part of the choreography of primary care. Informal consultation may develop because of how services in a particular setting are structured, for example, the availability of consultation-liaison (C/L) services in a hospital.

For many health and mental health care providers, an informal consultation is the first opportunity to collaborate with another health care professional. It is their entry point on the spectrum of collaboration. Or an informal consultant relationship between professionals providing parallel delivery of care may emerge after several successful referral contacts. Such informal consultation reflects a maturing of the relationship. In the Feinstein case, for example, Mr. Hoffman may get permission to talk to Dr. Vasquez about physical symptoms Mr. Feinstein is having. Or Dr. Vasquez may call Mr. Hoffman to ask how to handle Mrs. Feinstein's efforts to discuss marital problems during medical visits. Such contacts, even if infrequent, enhance the work of the professionals and instill confidence in patients and families, who value coordination of care. Sometimes more formal consultation emerges from hallway conversations and other informal contacts.

FORMAL CONSULTATION

Formal consultation differs from informal consultation in several ways. The relationship between the consultant and consultee is more contractual in nature. Together they establish clear goals for the consultation (Wynne et al., 1986). The consultant and consultee meet more regularly, and the consultant, by invitation from the consultee and agreement by the patient and family, has direct contact with the patient and family. For example, the mental health professional (consultant) may join the physician or health care practitioner during routine patient visits. The consultant adds notes on the consultation to the patient's chart if he or she is working in the same setting.

The consultee retains full responsibility for treatment. The consultant's role may be to differentiate a mental health diagnosis. He or she helps the consultee develop a more effective relationship with the patient and family. The consultation may also facilitate the referral of a patient and family who are reluctant to enter therapy. Typically, the referral is made to the consultant.

One of the authors who works in a primary care medical clinic recalls being asked to consult with a physician colleague about a patient with chronic foot pain. The goals of the consultation were to provide practical input on how the physician could support the patient's emotional needs, how to involve the patient's spouse in treatment, and how to help the patient manage her pain. The therapist and physician met together to discuss a plan, then both met with the patient. Postvisit discussion between the therapist and physician enabled the physician to clarify what steps she wanted to take with the patient. Over the next several months, the therapist joined the physician, patient, and spouse during a few medical visits and met with the physician alone twice. Eventually, it became apparent that psychotherapy with the consultant therapist would benefit the patient and her spouse. The physician then referred the patient to the therapist.

COPROVISION OF CARE

In the preceding example, the therapist's role changed. He became a coprovider of care with the physician. Coprovision of care is much easier to accomplish when the mental health professionals, physicians, and health care professionals are all located in the same setting. But it can also occur whenever the professional collaborators incorporate regular contact to discuss mutual patients into the structure of their relationship.

Coprovision of care often occurs with patients and families whose problems are confusing, complex, demanding, or long-standing. Such patients may be high utilizers of health care whose charts are thick, whose needs are extensive, and whose care is costly. They may have chronic pain, somatization disorder, chronic illness (cancer, diabetes, hypertension), as well as a full complement of psychosocial problems (substance abuse, relational discord, poverty, abuse). The key element is that the biomedical and psychosocial problems are so interconnected that collaboration is the only way to provide effective care. Coproviders share responsibility for the patient's treatment, negotiating with each other and with the patient and family what role each will play in treatment and how communication between them all will take place.

Coproviders also negotiate how fees will be handled. In fee-for-service situations, coproviders may both charge for visits with the patient. When they see the patient together, they may alternate charges, the physician charging one time, the therapist another, depending on the patient's insurance. In capitated systems (see chapter 13), the providers are paid in advance to care for all their patients. As a consequence, any limits on collaboration due to payment arrangements are eliminated.

Returning to the Feinstein case:

> Twice Mr. Feinstein reported to Mr. Hoffman that he had experienced severe headaches and nausea that frightened him. When asked if he had seen Dr. Vasquez, Mr. Feinstein told Mr. Hoffman he was afraid to; he was afraid there was something seriously wrong.
>
> After a lengthy discussion with the couple, Mr. Feinstein agreed to make an appointment with Dr. Vasquez. They also gave Mr. Hoffman permission to contact Dr. Vasquez to inform her about the symptoms. Mr. Hoffman called Dr. Vasquez, who was very concerned. She contacted Mr. Feinstein to schedule an earlier appointment.
>
> Dr. Vasquez, upon examining Mr. Feinstein, ordered a CT scan. The scan revealed a mass in Mr. Feinstein's brain. The Feinsteins called Mr. Hoffman to inform him. In turn, Mr. Hoffman called Dr. Vasquez to suggest that they all meet to discuss the impact of this news on Mr. Feinstein's health, the steps to be taken next, and how this news affected the marriage and family. At a conjoint meeting at Dr. Vasquez's office, the physician, therapist, and couple agreed that they would meet periodically as a group to assess future steps, to clarify what each would be doing, and to be sure they were all working appropriately together. Dr. Vasquez and Mr. Hoffman also talked more frequently by phone to support each other and to confer about the case.

At this point, responsibility for the care of Mr. Feinstein and his family is shared, although areas of focus and even leadership may vary depending on whose expertise is most applicable. For the mental health care provider, particularly one working in the same setting with physicians and nurses, coprovision of care often leads to a fundamental redefinition of his or her role. Rather than retaining a fully separate identity as a mental health professional, the therapist begins to see himself or herself as part of a health care team. The therapist also begins to understand more clearly that mental health is just one aspect of overall health.

There is an ebb and flow to coprovision of care. At times the professionals may talk to each other several times a week, or the patient and family may see either the physician or therapist more often. The professional collaborators may need to see the patient and family together routinely during periods of crisis, such as the diagnosis of a new illness or the exacerbation of parenting problems that affect an adolescent's willingness to administer insulin for diabetes. At other times, many months may go by as the providers only speak briefly with each other in the hall or maintain contact through chart notes, phone calls, or letters. This level of collaboration is common when the patient's problem is stable but still needs attention. When an illness moves from the crisis phase of evaluation, diagnosis, and initial intervention to the chronic phase of adjusting and attempting to resume normal routines of living, the intensity and frequency of contact usually decreases (Rolland, 1994a).

This ebb and flow is determined by the needs of all those involved in the collaboration—the professionals as well as the patient and family. If any of the collaborators feels "stuck" or in need of reassessing treatment goals, contact and communication among them all may need to increase. In this way, the hierarchy of care is flattened and each participant influences the course of collaboration and care.

COLLABORATIVE NETWORKING

Collaborative networking recognizes that a community of professional and natural supports may be needed to effectively care for some patients and families (Combrinck-Graham, 1990; Landau-Stanton & Clements, 1993; Seaburn et al., 1995). It reflects a collaborative effort that is interagency as well as interpersonal (Heubel, 1993). Landau-Stanton, Clements, and their colleagues (1993) describe an elaborate model for collaborative networking in the care of HIV/AIDS patients. In their model, professionals related to every level on the biopsychosocial hierarchy are identified and included, from the cellular and interpersonal to the community and spiritual domains. Blount and Bayona (1994) describe this as "distributed teams" working collaboratively and "cooperating in a task by contributing from different locations or at different times" (p. 175).

In our view, the mental health professional (now blending specialist, coprovider, and consultant roles) and primary health care or medical professionals retain key roles at the center of this network of care (Seaburn et al., 1993). In conjunction with the patient and family, they coordinate overall treatment and function as case managers, information interpreters, advocates, care providers, and more.

For instance, if Mr. Feinstein is diagnosed with a cancer, the physician may need to involve a surgeon, oncologist, and radiologist, who in turn have their own medical and health care teams. Mrs. Feinstein may feel more comfortable with Mrs. Washington, the nurse-practitioner who has taken care of her for years. Mrs. Washington may meet with Mrs. Feinstein regularly to help her adjust to her husband's diagnosis. Dr. Vasquez and Mrs. Washington may work together to refer the couple to a community support and information group.

Mr. Hoffman may help the Feinsteins maintain their relationship and talk to their children about their father's illness. The therapist may also contact Aaron's school to talk with the principal, school psychologist, and teacher about Aaron's needs during this difficult time. Mr. Hoffman may even convene a meeting of family and school professionals to discuss these matters. Information from that meeting may be shared with Dr. Vasquez and Mrs. Washington. The therapist may also be in regular contact with the family's rabbi to coordinate support that addresses the spiritual dimension of illness and trauma.

Dr. Vasquez and Mr. Hoffman may need to work with Mr. Feinstein's employer or the department of social services if he becomes disabled and must go on disability or seek other forms of financial aid. The professionals may convene an extended family meeting that includes the Feinsteins' relatives to explain Mr. Feinstein's condition and treatment. This would provide an opportunity to garner ongoing family support for the Feinsteins and clarify what role the family could play in the course of care.

In many cases such as this, the professional collaborators meet informally to discuss the uncertainty of the situation and the possibility of death. These discussions may help each of them better define what he or she can or cannot do for the patient and family. Meeting together may also enable them to be more open to and supportive of the patient and family as they wrestle with their own anxiety and doubt.

Key members of this larger network may be convened (in person or by conference call) with the Feinsteins to facilitate connectedness, coordinate care, and create a common purpose. This networking process may be greatly affected by the exigencies of reimbursement, that is, the health care program in which the Feinsteins are enrolled. Nevertheless, the collaborative networking approach supports a broad definition of the factors that contribute to patient and family health or illness.

CONCLUSION

Flexibility is central to the spectrum of collaboration. Professionals involved in collaboration must move across a wide range of possible roles in order to interact effectively with other professional collaborators, patients, and families. In the Feinstein case described in this chapter, the mental health care provider functioned as a specialist, consultant, and coprovider of care. Such flexibility enables the mental health professional to adapt to the needs of any given situation.

The spectrum of collaboration encourages the mental health care provider to collaborate regardless of the practice setting in which he or she works. The options for collaboration described in the spectrum are based less on location of services (or providers) than on the relationship between providers, patients, and families, no matter where they are located. The kinds of collaborative relationships that develop are influenced by where the providers work and how motivated they are to collaborate. But some form of collaborative relationship is always possible, no matter what the setting is. It is the collaborative relationship that is central to providing effective care for challenging patients and families, and central to creating a professionally and personally rich experience for the providers involved.

CHAPTER 9

The "Real World":
Collaboration in Primary Care

THIS CHAPTER EXAMINES collaboration in primary care environments where providers in both the health and mental health areas see a wide range of patient problems on a daily basis. We first describe what is meant by primary care health or mental health and the current trends in these settings. Then, using "real-world" examples of collaborative practice, we illustrate the integration of the key ingredients across the spectrum of collaboration. Some reflections on the key ingredients follow. The chapter concludes with recommendations on collaboration in primary care.

PRIMARY CARE—CURRENT REALITY AND FUTURE TRENDS

Primary care practices fall into two broad categories, both of which are undergoing rapid change and redefinition as health care in this country is reformed. The first is the traditional private practice setting. On the health care and medicine side, the vast majority of these are practices specializing in family medicine, general internal medicine, pediatrics, and sometimes obstetrics. Solo practitioners or small groups of two to three physicians establish their

159

own businesses and provide services. Depending on their style of practice, they develop arrangements with mental health providers to be employees of the practice, rent space in the practice, or maintain close referral relationships if they are not in the same space. Decisions about specific services a patient needs are made by the physicians.

On the mental health side, most psychotherapists practice solo; though they may share space with colleagues, the degree of collaboration within such practices varies considerably. Collaboration with primary care medical providers by these mental health practitioners is often limited to receiving referrals. The exception, particularly in recent years with the advances in clinical psychopharmacology, is collaboration with psychiatrists. Most mental health care providers in private practice develop a relationship with a psychiatrist to provide medication consultation and treatment. However, in some settings—particularly in rural areas—where the number of providers of all kinds is limited, psychiatry services may be few or nonexistent. Primary care providers across the board prescribe over one-half of all psychotropic medications administered in this country.

The second category of primary care setting is the public sector. Since the mid–1960s, community health centers have provided services to low-income families, providing acute medical care but also focusing on preventive screenings, immunizations, and disease prevention. Nurse-practitioners, physician's assistants, and other so-called midlevels provide many of the services in these settings. In addition to receiving psychological assessment and treatment, people using these clinics often have limited resources and require help navigating through governmental aid systems. In the 1970s, a number of demonstration projects attempted to place health and mental health services in the same location in a community (Burns et al., 1982). However, these centers were deemed expensive and funding was discontinued.

Community mental health centers were established in the 1960s, largely to support the effort to deinstitutionalize the chronically mentally ill and place them back in their home communities. In the 1960s and 1970s, these centers expanded to treat a broader range of emotional disorders as well as provide preventive mental health care and psychoeducation programs to the communities. Psychiatrists, often working part-time, assessed patients, prescribed medications, and provided brief consultations on medication management. In the last 10 years, with shrinking resources, community mental health programs have returned to their original purpose and now primarily focus on the chronically mentally ill. Although they frequently share clients, these programs have not had a history of formal partnership with community health centers. (Some notable exceptions, particularly in rural areas, are highlighted later in this chapter.)

Until recently, practitioners in both community health and mental health systems have typically begun their careers in these settings. However, owing to low salaries, large caseloads, and often difficult working situations, they have often left to establish private practices.

Regardless of the setting, all of primary care is now being influenced by the shift to managed care and its emphasis on how health care is financed. Health care reform efforts are dramatically reshaping how practitioners in primary care view themselves. The influence of managed care has made employers, third-party payers, and hospitals major decision-makers in an ongoing effort to exert cost and quality controls (see chapter 13). Physicians are forming larger groups and networks to maintain decision-making autonomy. These networks often involve both primary care and specialty groups. Within primary care practices, relationships with midlevel providers as well as office and nursing staff are being strengthened to create economies of scale and maintain competitiveness in the marketplace.

This trend in medicine has been developing nationally over the last four years—with several states, California, Minnesota, and Washington among them, leading the way—and has had a major impact on mental health services. Private providers are being advised to form larger, multispecialty groups, which appeal to employers and managed-care carve-out companies. As individuals, they are advised to assess their particular skills and develop a "market niche" in which they can position themselves to add value to overall health care. Public health and mental health services continue to receive reduced government funding and are likely to come under increased scrutiny in a time of balanced budgets and conservative fiscal policy.

These trends present an alarming picture. It will be challenging to implement the kind of collaboration we are describing in the primary care practices of the future. The move to "carve out" primary mental health care from primary medical care may not provide incentives to collaborate. The incentive on the health side will be to keep psychosocial issues out of the picture as much as possible and, when that is not possible, to make a referral into the mental health "risk pool." This risk pool is comprised of providers working on referrals from a behavioral managed-care carve-out company who will not be reimbursed for communicating with the health care provider, only for direct contact with the patient. The reimbursement for even direct contact is often significantly lower than the fee charged. In addition, providers will keep relationships with managed-care companies, therefore keeping treatment focused and limited to as few sessions as possible. Any somatic symptomatology will be immediately referred back to the primary care provider. The incentive structure will not reinforce collaboration in these arrangements.

We believe the carve-out trend will go only so far before providers and consumers demand more integrated models of care. Already many therapists in private practice are choosing to stay outside the system, often lowering their fees and refusing to sign on with these companies that regulate their behavior. A few efforts are being made to carve in mental health care. It will be a challenge for these highly competitive businesses to look far enough ahead to see the potential gains of integration and collaboration.

Organizations like the Collaborative Family Health Care Coalition have formed to advocate for a completely different way of organizing these services. This organization advocates an integrated model in which mental health and medical professionals share risk and resources to benefit the consumers. The issues involved in collaboration in managed-care settings are described in more detail in chapter 13.

EXEMPLARY PRACTICES

In this section, we use examples of current collaborative practices to illustrate applications of the key ingredients of collaboration discussed in chapter 3, as well as the spectrum of collaboration described in chapter 8. The examples, drawn from a variety of primary care settings, cover many of the issues involved in establishing and maintaining effective collaborative arrangements.

Urban Primary Care Settings
Auburn, Washington

In Auburn, Washington, a suburb of Seattle, a group of seven family physicians, three internists, and one surgeon run a private practice. Kathryn Cruze, a certified mental health counselor, has been a member of the practice since 1987. Her experience highlights the importance of negotiating clear financial arrangements early on and establishing communication norms. Her experience also reflects the variety of activities other than direct patient care in which a mental health professional can be involved, adding value to the practice.

In joining the practice, it was important that Cruze consider the business arrangement and carefully question the medical care providers' needs and style of practice. She met with them and looked at two possibilities: renting space, or being paid a set percentage of collected fees. They decided on the second option. It seemed to be the easiest way to figure shared expenses, and Cruze would not have to pay the practice separately for support services. Secretarial and billing services were shared and considered part of the overhead. It is critical to discuss and clarify such business practice questions—only relevant in a shared-location model—before getting started. It is also important to continually renegotiate the terms of the arrangement as the needs of the parties evolve.

The second important lesson in Cruze's early experience was to do what is known in marketing circles as "pull" instead of "push" marketing. A mental health care provider "pushes" by spending a great deal of time early on educating the providers about what he or she can do for them. In chapter 5, William Doherty describes the missionary zeal with which he approached physicians, assuming that they were uninformed and needed to be shown the significant benefits of psychosocial interventions. By contrast, a therapist who "pulls" considers the physician a primary customer. The therapist spends time establishing rapport, asking detailed questions about the customer's world, and gaining an understanding of what the customer considers to be "challenging clinical interactions," those encounters with patients and families that are frustrating for all concerned. Often a therapist can help providers, patients, and families deal with complex situations involving chronic illness or life-threatening events.

Cruze stresses the importance of communication with physicians and nurses to maintain effective collaborative relationships. Since she is colocated, she can work out of the same medical chart. The notes she dictates for the chart are written up on keyed colored paper and not released unless the patient gives written permission specifically for the disclosure of mental health notes. Charting in the medical record allows the health care providers to keep up with the general goals of treatment, progress toward those goals, and other information such as side effects of medication. Cruze gains understanding of the significant medical problems being addressed by the physicians. She also can generate hypotheses about the level of patient and physician concern by the frequency of visits and by reading "between the lines" in the notes.

Cruze plays a number of other roles by sharing a location with health care and medical providers. Because primary care is provided in teams (physicians, nurses, nurse-practitioners, physician's assistants, secretaries, receptionists, transcriptionist, lab services, X-ray services), a mental health practitioner can provide consultation services to individuals on the team as well as to the practice as a whole. When the mental health care provider is a part of the practice, there is a limit to the mental health services a therapist can provide directly to staff. However, employee assistance–type services (e.g., brief consultation and referral for personal problems) can be very valuable to the practice.

Cruze also provides case management services to the patients and their families. She acknowledges that this role can consume a great deal of time negotiating entitlement programs, working with nursing homes, or making other referrals. If the business arrangement does not allow compensation for such services, the therapist is at risk of feeling used. Yet another role she plays is in crisis intervention and debriefing critical incidents in the practice. In the middle of a busy clinic, a suicidal patient can receive direct intervention and/or referrals by the therapist. If a patient who has become "special" to the practice dies, the therapist can initiate a debriefing with staff to discuss their reactions and feelings. These roles benefit the patients involved as well as the practice as a whole.

Roanoke, Virginia

Brambleton Family Physicians is a group practice in Roanoke, Virginia, that has been in operation for 20 years. Four physicians see a full range of medical problems but do not practice obstetrics. Roanoke, a medium-size city with three hospitals, is a referral center for southwestern Virginia. Most of the physicians were trained in the Roanoke Family Practice Residency, a training program at the local community hospital. In the first two years of establishing their medical practice, the Brambleton physicians asked a family therapist, Susan Molumphy, Ph.D., to join them and set up her practice in their office. She did so and has maintained an independent practice in that setting since 1978. Working together while the fields of family medicine and family therapy were "growing up together" has provided an excellent context for the development of a close collaborative relationship. And working together over 20 years has resulted in a professional "marriage" that is extremely effective in coordinating patient care as well as highly satisfying to the providers.

To communicate the collaborative nature of the practice to the public, Molumphy's name is listed in the group of physicians on the exterior sign. Her office, which is down a separate hallway from the main waiting room, is also listed separately on the sign. Her office location is repeated on the inside sign along with those of the other medical practices in the building. A new patient who goes to the receptionist for the medical practice is told to wait for Molumphy to come out and get them from the waiting room. The perception is of medical and mental services being provided under one roof.

Molumphy and one of the physicians, Wayne Grayson, M.D., have a particularly close collaborative relationship. They share a waiting room, which both describe as a significant advantage for patients following through on a referral to see the other provider in consultation or for assessment. Patients can come to a familiar setting and "blend into the crowd." Grayson and Molumphy describe their personal relationship as equally essential to effective collaboration. According to Grayson:

> We were just close. You need someone to trust that can counsel your patients through a tough time that you just can't do. I think family practitioners who have not cultivated a therapist they can work with are not being all they can be or doing all they can to help their patients get well.

Adds Molumphy:

> You learn to trust the fact that we are in this together. I can't practice medicine, but over the years you share so many patients together, you trust the physician's and your own intuition about who will need medicine. I can even make a recommendation about what medicine will be needed. Wayne trusts me to do that.

Time, working together in a shared location, and addressing complex emotional patient stories certainly contributed significantly to the cultivation of such a highly developed collaborative relationship. The decision to involve Molumphy directly in the evolution of the practice culture also made a contribution. For instance, she has always been involved in celebrating birthdays and other social traditions adopted by the practice.

A theme shared by the Roanoke practitioners is their belief in the competencies and abilities not only of each other but of their patients and clients. They clearly perceive their roles not as "fixing things" but as helping people heal from the bumps and bruises of life. It is likely that this common purpose has contributed to a deepening sense of collaboration over the years.

The following case example illustrates the process of collaboration in this practice.

> A 50-year-old man came to Grayson's office originally interested in smoking cessation. He had also been on a regular dose of Xanax for several years. Grayson did not attempt to change the medication dosage but worked with him through several failed attempts to stop smoking. Grayson consulted with Molumphy informally about the situation but did not feel the patient was ready for a more involved discussion about the factors contributing to his difficulty. After the third attempt to stop smoking, he asked the patient to consult with the "in-house therapist"; the patient reluctantly agreed. Grayson described this consultation to the patient as a possible benefit to both the patient and himself in learning about how to be an effective resource. Subsequently, the patient's wife became involved in the treatment and issues in the marital relationship, which had not been previously addressed, were brought to the table and dealt with effectively. The wife's support in changing the patient's smoking behavior was critical. After a relatively brief time, he was able to stop smoking and develop more satisfaction in his marital relationship.

Grayson strongly believes that the location of Molumphy's office within the practice encouraged the patient to follow through with the referral. More important, Grayson described Molumphy's involvement as an extension of his involvement. Further, because of the relationship with Molumphy, Grayson was able to talk specifically with the patient about how the therapist could be helpful both to the patient and to him.

Grayson and Molumphy exemplify a seasoned collaborative relationship of great depth. Molumphy and the physicians or nurses feel free to call each other day or night to consult about a patient or to gain support for themselves in a difficult situation. Molumphy does not get a signed release to talk to the medical providers if the patient is part of the practice. However, with providers outside the practice she routinely obtains a release. While some may question this practice, it reflects the degree of trust in the Roanoke practice's arrangement.

To illustrate the relationship Molumphy has with the practice, she described a young woman with terminal illness whom she had treated over time. Because of the nature of her illness, this woman was treated medically in a specialty setting and was therefore not a medical patient of the family practice. When the young woman died, Molumphy came into the office and the staff knew her sense of loss without her having to say a word. Even though not directly involved, the staff had followed the course of the illness and provided the collegial support that Molumphy needed at that time. This kind of relationship, developed over time, exemplifies some of the benefits of long-term collaboration with primary care providers.

Rural Primary Care Settings

The integration of medical and mental health services has been most prevalent in rural areas where resources of all kinds, including mental health services, are often limited. Physician shortages are common in many areas, forcing individuals to travel significant distances for services. Many rural areas lack specialty mental health professionals. Physical distance and lack of public transportation present barriers to care even when resources are available. Service integration therefore is an important strategy (Beeson, 1990).

Highlands, North Carolina

In Highlands, North Carolina, a small resort community with a year-round population of 2,000 that expands to much more in the summer, five family physicians maintain a practice. In 1986 Carrie Henderson, a clinical social worker and family therapist, was asked by the local hospital to set up a practice in the community. She opened an office in the same building as the physicians and received 80% of her referrals from them.

The issue of establishing a joint business arrangement was not relevant in this situation. Several different ingredients were important to Henderson in establishing her practice. First was the importance in a small community of establishing clear, direct guidelines about who talks to whom about what. Unlike Molumphy, Henderson emphasizes written releases of information from all patients to discuss their care. She always asks the patient whether she can communicate with the health care provider; only in rare circumstances is her request refused. She then obtains a written release to talk with the physician. When maintaining a collaborative practice in a small community, this issue becomes even more important. It is more difficult to "hide" in a small community, where the rumor and opinion mill is usually strong. Nevertheless, Henderson says that her explanations to patients about why she wants to establish links with their primary care physician are always met with agreement. She states that the collaboration "is not something I have felt an urgency to describe in detail, it is something people expect."

Once communication links are established and agreed upon, the issue of how a therapist talks with a physician becomes important. Henderson uses letters, phone calls, and face-to-face meetings when necessary. Since she and the physicians maintain separate offices, they do not use common charts. She emphasizes that immediate feedback to the referring physician or nurse is important, even if only to share first impressions. The importance of ongoing communication is illustrated in the following case example.

Dr. H referred a woman to Henderson with anxiety and panic symptoms. He had started the patient on a low dose of a benzodiazapine and recommended to the patient that she develop some awareness of the triggers for the panic symptoms and coping strategies for dealing with them. The patient was reluctant to see a therapist, but because Dr. H assured her he was going to stay involved and in close communication with both patient and therapist, she agreed. Henderson saw the patient for several months, with little noticeable improvement. At that point, the patient wanted to drop out of treatment and became angry, even somewhat suicidal. She complained to the physician that the psychotherapy was not being effective. Dr. H was able to support the therapist's efforts and convince the patient to continue looking for solutions. He was in close phone contact with Henderson to relay the patient's concerns. Further psychological testing helped both providers and patient discover significant depressive symptoms that the anxiety and panic disorder had covered. At that point, a combination of antidepressant medication and the involvement of the patient's spouse in treatment resulted in progress and eventual resolution of the original anxiety symptoms.

This case illustrates coprovision of care. Complexity is often directly correlated with progress or lack of progress and the resulting frustration for patients and providers. During the two months prior to Henderson's involvement, and the three months before the change in treatment plan, the patient was very symptomatic and everyone was frustrated. As a result, the providers agreed to stay in regular weekly contact with each other, and more often if necessary. The patient was actively involved in the treatment plan and saw both providers. The possibility of having a joint meeting was discussed, and all agreed that could happen if needed. Open communication between the providers seemed helpful to the patient in reducing some of her frustration. Even though what would help was unclear, how the treatment team would go about addressing the patient's problems was clarified. When the patient became understandably frustrated and angry, this contract proved especially helpful to both the patient and the providers. It served as a reminder that no one was giving up and that the search for solutions would continue. When the patient on two occasions wanted to drop out of therapy, assurance from Dr. H helped gain the patient's agreement to continue the treatment until some progress was made.

Prior to their co-involvement in this case, Henderson and Dr. H had not worked together. During the first three months, there were some confusing moments about their relationship with the patient and with each other. Developing clear communication patterns and having the common purpose of caring for the patient helped develop trust and served to keep the providers from being "split" by the patient's natural frustration. In addition, the effective relationship and communication that Henderson and Dr. H developed in working with this patient made it easier to work together on other cases.

Jackson Hole, Wyoming

Two thousand miles away in another rural setting, Jackson Hole, Wyoming, Michael Enright practices with Buzz Bricca and three other family practitioners. Until recently, Enright rented office space from the physicians. Because Enright and his physician colleagues were able to develop a good working relationship, Enright decided to purchase the space and become part of the practice. He wanted both the patients and the physicians to see him as a colleague. At the same time, he wanted separate, autonomous space that would be quieter and lend itself to more traditional psychotherapeutic interventions such as biofeedback. His solution illustrates an attempt to respect the clinical requirements of different providers while maintaining a connection between them. Although Enright works with other practitioners in town, the geographical distance prevents the development of the same kind of collaborative relationship he has with Bricca and his colleagues.

Enright's advice about collaboration echoes the standard three pieces of advice given by most realtors: location, location, location. In primary care settings, location may be the ingredient that influences the others most. Sharing a location significantly enhances communication about personal beliefs or paradigms, common goals, treatment strategies, dealing with change, and financial issues.

Enright, unlike Cruze, uses a double charting system. He does not write directly in the medical chart, though his verbal feedback on patients is often recorded by the physician in the medical chart. He maintains a psychosocial record that is kept in a locked cabinet in his office.

Enright also emphasizes the importance of developing relationships with physicians and with the staff in the medical office as well as in the local community hospital.

> Any psychologist who is going to collaborate with a physician needs to understand how the physician looks at a problem. It is easy to get all locked up in thinking the "medical model" is bad. If you are judgmental about that, you are not going to do much collaborating. . . . Being able to read a medical chart, understanding what people's expectations are, understanding that they don't have a whole lot of time to spend, knowing what you have to offer, are just a few examples of what it takes for effective collaboration.

Jackson Hole does not have a psychiatrist, so the family physicians with whom Enright works prescribe antidepressant psychotropic medication when it is indicated. Enright realized they did not have the time to keep up with the latest thinking about use of these medications, so he subscribes to journals, such as *Clinical Psychopharmacology*, to help himself, the providers, and ultimately the patients use medications more effectively. He passes journal articles around the office and has found that the physicians who know of his special interests will send articles to him as well. This provides an excellent practical example of how collaborative relationships can increase the learning of all involved.

Enright also describes a rationale for working closely with nurses and other staff. First, taking advantage of the shared location often requires holding brief conversations between patient visits or even interrupting a physician during a patient visit. Since the nurses monitor patient flow, any interruption in efficient patient care might be perceived negatively by them. It was important to Enright to build trust with the nursing staff and develop an understanding of how therapists can add value to the ongoing treatment of patients. Second, in all primary care practices, there is collaboration between the nurses and the physicians. Nurses, nurse-practitioners, and physician's assistants provide direct care in the office or over the phone. As a result, they know the patients and families well. They often are the key providers with whom to collaborate because they are more centrally involved in a patient's care than anyone else.

A third reason to work closely with nurses is their effectiveness as referral sources and partners in care, as illustrated by the following example. Enright was treating a woman using biofeedback and stress management training. She had not seen a physician and did not want to take any medication. Enright was not able to convince her to see a physician but had a nurse from the practice take her blood pressure reading at each visit. This reading was consistently high, and it was clear that no amount of biofeedback or stress management training would decrease the risk of a stroke if the patient continued to avoid medical intervention. After the nurse talked with her about getting an evaluation for hypertension, the patient eventually followed through and did so. Her fears of starting medication were gradually alleviated.

Primary care medicine is delivered by a team that includes nurses, nurse-practitioners, and physician's assistants. Receptionists and administrative personnel also have an impact on patient care. Therapists working in these settings need to view the practice as a whole, treating everyone as a partner in care.

Mental health professionals are not typically involved in hospital care. Enright realized that the physicians in Jackson Hole met with patients they had hospitalized every morning, shared information about cases they had in common, and sought advice from colleagues. He established himself as someone interested in consulting on the mental health aspects of hospitalized patients. Willingness to meet, often early in the morning, with physicians and their patients gained him respect as a coprovider who was willing to come onto the "medical turf" and assist in quality care. He is able to bill for some of these services as consultation or therapy visits. His flexibility also helped him establish relationships with providers, share diagnostic and treatment ideas, and establish communication systems, all of which are helpful in the outpatient setting. In addition, since hospitalization is a crisis point for patients and families, the connection made with them during inpatient treatment greatly facilitates follow-up outpatient therapy.

Carrie Henderson and Michael Enright are two examples of mental health care providers who have established collaborative practices in rural areas. Their experiences reinforce the importance of building relationships, establishing clear communication processes, and keeping role definitions flexible in working with a medical office staff or in an inpatient setting. Therapists who increase their knowledge base in these settings are only broadening their repertoire.

Community Mental Health Settings

Relationship development between community health and mental health centers has similar components to relationship development between individual practitioners. However, two differences are important in getting started. The first is a commitment between the leaders in both settings to model a trusting, collaborative relationship and to set up the meetings necessary to start the ball rolling. Community health and mental health centers are usually separated geographically, and their different cultures may foster negative assumptions about each other. For these reasons, collaboration at the top is critical. Charlie King, director of the health center in Albion, New York, made initial efforts to work with the local mental health center, but only when Mary Richards became director of that center did joint meetings occur. These meetings were held monthly at the mental health center, over lunch. The individuals involved contributed their time; attendance was voluntary. The meetings focused on the common interests of the professionals and on how to collaborate on shared patients.

A similar story was told by Susan Walter and Fred Donovan,

directors of the health and mental health departments in Martinsburg, West Virginia. Donovan said that one of the major barriers was the attitude of his staff toward the health department. However, his work with Walter and their combined efforts to place a mental health case manager on-site at the health department resulted in dramatic changes in the capacity of the two organizations to work together. Understanding the challenges faced by each partner in the collaboration has resulted in some innovative solutions. For example, the mental health department was having difficulty getting critical blood work done on patients taking Clozaril. A support/therapy group, whose members were all using this medication, met weekly at the department, so the health department began sending a laboratory technician to the group to draw blood. This practice had benefits for the patients as well as the providers.

The second key to health and mental health centers working well together in community settings is illustrated in the example of the Martinsburg case manager. Placing liaison individuals on-site provides a conduit for information and ideas to flow back and forth between the two systems. Joint meetings like those held in Albion can greatly aid communication but are no replacement for a person who keeps a foot in both worlds. How a liaison person is chosen is obviously critical. In Pembroke, North Carolina, at the Robeson Health Care Corporation, Jennie Lowery, director of the mental health center, received a federal grant to place a counselor in the health center to work with pregnant women who had substance abuse problems. The program, in its fifth year, is going well now but had a rough beginning because medical providers were not involved in the project development or the hiring of the counselor. This contributed to several turnovers in the counselor position. In retrospect, Lowery says, she would have worked harder to include the medical providers in the planning, building a relationship with them before instituting the program.

Pediatrics and Pediatric Psychology

Many pediatric practices have close relationships with mental health professionals who come to the pediatric setting to provide services. Often referrals are made to mental health professionals to evaluate developmental progress in children, provide screening and testing for common problems like attention deficit disorder, or provide brief parent training around child-focused difficulties. One such setting, in Chapel Hill, North Carolina, has been operational since 1980. Carolyn Schroeder was teaching child psychology at a local university. She was asked by a group of pediatricians to provide consultation on children who they identified as having behavioral or developmental problems. Schroeder provided some of the direct service herself and supervised students who saw children and their parents. She initiated a psychoeducational program involving practical advice for common childhood difficulties, a lending library of reference material for parents, and a call-in hour each day staffed by graduate psychology students. This call-in hour was highly utilized by parents. The success of the collaboration led the pediatricians to want a permanent child psychology on-site service. They convinced Schroeder to leave a tenured position at the university and open a practice in their office.

Schroeder considered an employee arrangement but decided to maintain autonomy and establish a private practice. The pediatricians let her use space in the practice and did not charge any overhead. She shared their offices and used exam room space. After two years, the service expanded to the point that a separate suite, attached to the pediatric office, was built. Then she began to rent the space and added a social worker to the practice.

In the last 15 years, the practice, known as Pediatric Psychology Associates, has grown to include six psychologists, two part-time psychiatrists, and a social worker. They have developed consultation forms with their pediatrician colleagues to communicate about cases. An assessment report is provided immediately to the pediatricians by the psychologists. For ongoing cases that follow a parallel delivery pattern, a quarterly written report gives the physicians updated progress information. Referrals continue to come from the pediatric practice but comprise only about one-third of the children seen. The rest of the clients come from self-referrals and other physician referrals.

Recently, owing to space constraints, the mental health care providers moved across the parking lot from the pediatricians. Even though their new offices are only 30 yards away, the pediatricians report a loss in the capacity for informal consultations and face-to-face communication about coprovider issues. The mental health care providers, although admittedly enjoying the quieter and larger space, also report a loss in the ability to "bump in the hallway" and to feel like they are in a collaborative practice. They plan to create a service that would put one of them on-site for an hour a day to rebuild the bridge that was damaged in the move.

ESTABLISHING COLLABORATIVE RELATIONSHIPS: ONE PHYSICIAN'S STORY

Although this chapter is directed to therapists, this section is the story of a physician who intentionally set out to create relationships with mental health care providers so that she could provide more comprehensive and coordinated care to her patients and families. The process is instructive to therapists who want to create a network of collaborative physicians.

Deborah Davis is a family physician who works with Kathryn Cruze in Seattle. Interested in women's health issues and in pediatrics, Davis asked colleagues to recommend effective mental health practitioners and started making referrals to them. When talking to therapists, Davis looks for "common ground," which helps her determine whether to continue to collaborate with them. She has three criteria for establishing common ground. First, what is the therapist's view of medications, particularly anti-anxiety agents, in the treatment of situational problems? Second, does the therapist have a commonsense orientation to problem-solving that keeps psychological jargon and theory to a minimum? Third, and most important to her, is the mental health professional oriented to patient strengths and competence? She selects potential collaborators who share her paradigm of looking for the "health strivings" and positive efforts people make. With her common-ground criteria in mind, Davis will ask a therapist to have lunch with her to discuss the particular case they share and also to discuss his or her general orientation to patients. These initial meetings provide Davis with an intuitive feel for, and sense of comfort level with, the other provider.

Over the first two years Davis was in practice, she got to know the kinds of patients she was going to have, the kinds of mental health issues she would handle herself or refer to a therapist collaborator, and the therapists with whom she felt she could collaborate. She currently collaborates with five therapists, including Cruze. Because her patients frequently want to see a female therapist, four of her collaborators are female and one is male. Davis considers the personal attributes and professional interests of each of the therapists in making a referral. She understands that the match between therapist and patient is a critical variable in effective care.

The cost-awareness issue is also an important variable in Davis's referral choices. She assesses the patient's insurance plan to see who it will reimburse, at what rate, and for what problems. The economic factor is critical for Davis in her selection of the right collaborator for a particular case.

Davis estimates that about 20% of her visits include a significant psychosocial issue, the treatment of which could add value to the overall care of the patient and family. If she does not have the time or expertise to treat the issue by herself, she feels confident in matching the patient needs with a particular therapist. She attributes this confidence to her early work establishing relationships with them. Doing so took more time initially, but now her referrals involve only a short telephone conversation with the therapist outlining the issues in the case, the degree to which each provider will be involved in treatment, and how they will communicate with each other and with the patient and family about the collaboration. Davis's patients express satisfaction with the team approach and the ease with which information can be shared.

Deborah Davis provides an excellent model for being proactive about collaboration. She took initiative to develop professional partnerships based on a paradigm of care. That paradigm placed the patient at the center of her considerations. Collaborative relationships were then built on the common purpose of effective patient care.

ADVICE FOR THERAPISTS PRACTICING WITH PRIMARY CARE PROVIDERS

1: *Treat medical providers as customers equal to patient/clients.* Learn what they need before you try to help.
2: *Initiate discussions about how communication will occur between providers.* For example, find out what information your collaborator would like to have over time. It has been our experience that such process-oriented conversations often do not happen. In general, we recommend that you use the same practice skills you would employ with patients and families in clarifying goals, purposes, roles, and plans in your work with health care providers. Further, provide specific timely feedback to the medical providers on treatment plans.
3: *Develop working relationships with the staff of the clinic—nurses, receptionists, etc.* Consider yourself a consultant not only to individual providers but to a system of providers with its own culture. Seen as a consultant to the practice, you can serve in

other roles as well. These include providing referral information on support groups in the community, debriefing crisis situations, and providing support to the staff on personal issues.

4: *Get involved in hospital settings.* Hospitalization is often a crisis
time when people are most open to mental health interventions. It is also a place where primary care physicians need
help. Your willingness to come out of an office and into an often
confusing, chaotic environment to help medical providers is
important.

5: *Accept that not everyone wants to collaborate.* Look for who is
interested, who is courteous, who asks questions, and who
doesn't have the "fix this person" attitude. Develop a thick
skin for conflict, and use it as an opportunity for relationship
development.

6: *Ask physician and health care collaborators to consult with you.*
Physicians learn a lot about patients and families over time. If
asked, they will often share their knowledge, even if they don't
have the confidence or the language to express it. Asking them
about their patients brings you useful information, validates
them for knowing, helps form the relationship, and helps both
the health care provider and the patient see themselves as
more competent.

7: *Use words like* consultation, stress, *or* family challenges *and
avoid therapy or even counseling in the early stages of involvement
with patients, families, and medical providers.* Encourage physicians to ask psychosocial questions early and involve you
early in a difficult process with a patient.

8: *Beware of the potential for splitting.* Encourage the medical
providers to let you know if they get complaints or confusing
statements from the patients about your therapeutic interventions or suggestions. Find ways to keep working together with
the patients without being split.

CONCLUSION

Health care reform will increase the importance of the role of primary care physicians. Managed-care plans all utilize these medical
providers as the key to cost-effective, preventive, quality care (see
chapter 13). Primary care physicians, particularly family physicians, have traditionally been trained to recognize and treat psychosocial difficulties themselves. They will continue to be the de

facto mental health system. However, with increased demands on their time, they will need to look to other sources to provide that care. To do this, they will need increased training in collaboration skills. On the mental health side, few therapists have been trained to work effectively as consultants and coproviders with primary care physicians (see chapter 14). If both medical and mental health professionals can develop an attitude conducive to collaboration, the primary care setting is an ideal arena in which to develop the skills and relationships necessary to make that happen.

CHAPTER 10

Views from the Inside: Setting up a Collaborative Primary Care Practice

THIS CHAPTER DESCRIBES one model for collaborative primary care practice. Material for it is taken predominantly from a family practice in rural upstate New York.* Some material in the chapter is borrowed from other similar practices. The health care providers consist of two physicians, a psychologist, and two nurse-practitioners. The physicians work part-time, the psychologist works in the office one day a week, and the nurse-practitioners work nearly full-time. This arrangement is typical for many rural primary care practices. Approximately one-third of family physician offices have an on-site mental health professional (Cassata & Kirkman-Liff, 1981; E. Feldman, personal communication, August 15, 1994, survey of New York State family physicians; T. Campbell and S. McDaniel, personal communication, 1993, survey of family medicine residency graduates in Rochester, NY; D. Kaplan, personal communication, 1984, survey of family physicians in the state of Washing-

*Canal Park Family Medicine in Palmyra, New York, where Alan Lorenz, the author of this chapter, is currently practicing. Nancy Ruddy, a psychologist, practiced with him at this site, and her comments were particularly useful in preparing this chapter.

ton). Our intention is not to present this example as the only way to set up a collaborative primary care practice, but rather to provide an in-depth example of starting such a practice. This model can then serve as a base from which to evaluate potential collaborative partners and practices. A series of questions to aid in this endeavor concludes each section.

The chapter is organized differently from previous chapters. We follow a hypothetical patient through her first contact and then subsequent visits to our office. We view her experience through her eyes. The patient is a composite of three different actual patients; some of the details have been changed to protect their anonymity. At various points we interrupt her story to allow the providers to comment on their experience or their rationale for certain structures or behaviors. The physician is a trained family therapist with substantial collaborative experience. The clinical psychologist is also a family therapist, with prior experience in primary care. The chapter is ordered chronologically: first contact, initial impressions, first visit, referral, coprovision of care, and follow-up.

FIRST CONTACT

PATIENT: My physician retired about one year ago, and no one in my family has needed to see a physician during this time except me. Over the past year, I have seen only specialists, who recommended I establish myself with a primary care physician. After my previous primary care physician retired, I was not sure what to do, until a new office opened up in town. This seemed to be the most convenient, and over the course of the past year I have heard some good things about the practice. I arranged with my HMO to be assigned a new physician in this office. I was intrigued when I called to make my first appointment that they not only asked if I was a new patient but if anyone in my immediate family had been to this practice.

As the term implies, an appreciation for family is one of the cornerstones of family medicine. Family medicine is one of three primary care specialties; the other two are pediatrics and internal medicine. At this time, more graduating residents are selecting family medicine than either of the other two specialties (American Academy of Family Practice, 1995). All three primary care specialties recognize the importance of the patient in his or her context, yet family medicine pays particular attention to the role of the family. With the current trends in health care, virtually everyone who has a physician has a primary care physician. The primary care physicians in managed-care plans serve as the focal point of care delivery and the gatekeeper to other health care services.

The charting by family in our office reflects our high regard for the role of families. Family is broadly defined as any group of people bound by blood, legal, or emotional ties, though for charting purposes we define family by household (anyone living in the same dwelling). All family charts are numbered and kept in numerical order. This large manila folder contains a genogram and the separate family member charts (see McDaniel et al., 1990). These individual charts list pertinent medical information on their cover (past medical and surgical history, active problems, and medications). Inside the individual chart, all the progress notes are on the right-hand side. Progress notes for visits with the nurse-practitioners and physicians are on white paper, and behind these notes, in a separate section labeled "Counseling," are mental health progress notes. These are on pink paper with a "Confidential: Do Not Photocopy" stamp on them. On the left-hand side of the individual chart are laboratory studies, X-rays, consultations, and so on.

Family charting ensures that a single genogram (see McGoldrick & Gerson, 1985) is available for all family members for all visits. This genogram expands over time as different family members make visits. An initial three-generation genogram can be done in minutes; it is updated every one to three years or as necessary. Probably the main objection to doing family-oriented primary care is that obtaining psychosocial information takes too long. We believe these few minutes represent time well spent. The genogram has proven itself to be a practical instrument for succinctly gathering and organizing both pertinent family medical history and pertinent psychosocial information. Furthermore, family members often ask questions about themselves during someone else's visit. Having their chart available makes answering these questions easier. The only significant problem associated with family charting is the occasional difficulty of finding the chart. This may happen when one family member comes in the office right after another and the chart has not been returned from dictation yet because there is a backlog in dictation. There is no problem finding the chart if chart notes were handwritten or the chart was immediately refiled. The numbering system for family charts also solves the problem of keeping track of family members with different last names.

Assessing a Potential Collaborative Practice

- Does the practice have a family orientation?
- How is psychosocial information gathered?
- How are the charts organized?
- Do the charts have genograms?

INITIAL IMPRESSIONS

PATIENT: With a lot of trepidation, I walk in the front door. I notice the names and degrees stenciled on the front glass: two M.D.'s, two N.P.'s, one Ph.D. Given my current situation, I could certainly benefit from speaking to a psychologist—not that I would ever admit that to anyone. I am greeted by someone at the front desk and again am asked not only if I am a new patient but if anyone else in my immediate family comes here. Still intrigued by this question, and after supplying the usual demographic and insurance information, I look around and see two waiting rooms. To my right are several young parents who are talking together while their children play on a small climbing structure in the center of the waiting room. One child is sitting at a small table with crayons, coloring. To my left is what appears to be the adult side of the waiting room. Here there are a number of people from all walks of life, some of whom I recognize. A few are reading magazines, some are talking, and some are just waiting. For the most part, there are very few individuals in the waiting room, and most people are with a family member or friend. I choose a magazine and sit on the adult side.

Our office is a full-service family practice. One of the early definitions of family practice was that family practitioners do not discriminate on the basis of age, sex, race, culture, or health problem. In other words, we see patients from birth to death and for a wide assortment of health-related issues, including mental health problems. Current estimates are that primary care health providers supply mental health care to 50% of the people who receive such care in this country. It is a big part of our day. Given this volume, the most important specialist to have on-site is a mental health professional.

Our waiting room is divided in two, mostly as an accident of how the building was originally designed and then subsequently remodeled. The design has worked out well in many respects. Some adults prefer not to wait in the same waiting space with very active children yet enjoy being able to see the children playing from across the room. It is also nicer for the children to play in a safe area where their parents can gather and talk. This arrangement often makes for the same kind of impromptu parent support groups that occurred in the original Peckham Project (see Johnson, Jeppson, & Redburn, 1992). We think that most people like to see a variety of other people in the waiting room.

> PATIENT: After a short wait, the nurse comes around the corner and calls out my name. I get up, am greeted, and follow her. Together we walk down a wide central hallway where my height and weight are checked, and we enter a room on the right. The room contains two comfortable, yet practical, cloth chairs, a floor lamp, the usual rolling doctor's stool, and an exam table. An Impressionist calendar hangs on one wall, and a print of Van Gogh's *Irises* is on the other wall. I am most struck by how homey the room is with the lamp and the clutter of magazines and children's books stacked on the circular tray around the lamp pole.
>
> My blood pressure is checked, which always makes me apprehensive, and I am relieved to hear that it is very good. The nurse asks me why I have come in today. I tell her, "This is my first visit here, and I wanted to have my blood pressure checked." Then I blurt out, quite to my own surprise, "I have breast cancer, and my oncologist told me I needed to have a primary care doctor too." The nurse responds with an empathetic look and after a pause asks if I am on any medications. "I'm not, but my oncologist wants to put me on Tamoxifen, and I wanted to get a second opinion." The nurse asks if I am allergic to any medicines, and I tell her, "I think I am allergic to penicillin." The nurse closes our conversation with, "The doctor will be with you in a few minutes." She then closes the door and leaves me to recover my wits.

The health care provider section of the office contains nine exam rooms; one of these rooms is a surgical room that can double as an exam room when things are busy. The six smallest exam rooms are 10 feet by 10 feet, and the other three are larger. The exam rooms were specifically made this large so that each room could accommodate two comfortable chairs along with the exam table and the doctor's stool. At about 70% of our office visits, another family member is present. This fact underscores the need for at least two chairs, and sometimes we bring in other chairs or rolling stools for other family members. We find that having this architectural design encourages family members to come in. Their presence

often saves us considerable time since they may be able to contribute significant details and observations. Of course, there are
times when we ask family members to leave the room, such as during an exam, but by and large we find it very helpful to be able to
accommodate additional family members (see Doherty & Baird,
1983).

We find it is helpful to meet patients while they are fully dressed.
We think this promotes a more balanced relationship between
provider and patient. In general, the health care provider has considerably more power in the relationship, a fact made even more
dramatic by having the patient get undressed before the provider
greets him or her. Furthermore, when the patient is female and the
health care provider is male, and even more so when the patient is
a black female and the health care provider is a white male, there
are so many power issues at work that anything possible should be
done to enhance the patient's sense of power. Having an adequate
number of exam rooms facilitates the health care provider's ability
to see patients continuously without being slowed down by the
time it takes for the patient to get into and out of a gown. If the
health care provider can go from room to room or step out and
make phone calls while patients change, he or she is using time
efficiently while also promoting empowerment.

Assessing a Potential Collaborative Practice

- Are family members welcome during patient visits?
- Are exam rooms big enough to accommodate family mem-
  bers?
- Are there family meetings?

FIRST VISIT

PATIENT: After a short wait, there is a knock and the door opens.
The doctor enters, strides over, and introduces himself with his
hand outstretched. I shake his hand, relieved to have the visit
beginning. I notice that he is not wearing a white coat and is
younger than I am. He begins by restating my name and asking
how I am doing. I say, "Fine," though I really don't feel fine. He
then observes that this is my first visit here and wonders how it is
that I have come to this office. I reply that it is convenient, and I
always used to see Dr. Burns until he retired. He listens, nods, and

says that he usually likes to start by getting a little background information. That relieves me even more since I am nervous about discussing my breast cancer.

He begins by asking how old I am, and then whether I am married, single, divorced, or widowed. I tell him my age, and that I am married. He asks my husband's name and age, and I tell him, though I am curious about why he wants to know. Mentioning my husband, for some reason, makes me anxious. He appears to be writing this down on my chart and drawing it in some kind of picture. He moves over and uses the exam table as a desk, and I can see the picture he is drawing. He says it is a kind of family tree or family map that helps him get to know more about who I am.

He asks if my parents are still living and invites me to watch while he draws the map. I tell him that both of my parents are deceased. He asks about how old they were and how they died. My father died of cirrhosis of the liver sometime in his sixties, though I did not have much contact with him after I was a very young child. He left my mother and my brother and sister when I was fairly young. The doctor then shifts to my mother, who died of a stroke about four years after she was diagnosed with breast cancer.

He asks if she had any other medical problems, and I tell him that she had bad circulation and some problems with her heart. He then asks about my brother's and sister's health. I tell him that my sister has had a number of female problems and that my brother seems to also have a problem with drinking. He asks if that seems to run in the family, and I respond, "It seems to . . . with the men anyway." I tell him that my father's father was supposedly also an alcoholic, though I have no memory of him. My brother works but has lost jobs, probably related to his drinking. At this time it is not a health problem, as far as I know. Neither my mother nor my sister, nor myself, drink at all. He then asks if I have any children, and I tell him I have two teenage daughters who are both well.

At the beginning of any encounter, it is imperative to establish rapport with the patient. This is particularly challenging at the first visit since we are new to each other. Obtaining genogram information serves several purposes. It helps to establish rapport between the health care provider and the patient. The patient is given an opportunity to tell bits and pieces of his or her life story, enabling the health care provider to connect with the human side of the patient. A basic, medically focused three-generation genogram often provides a wealth of information. Knowing when to pursue any leads a patient gives you and when to back off is important.

Recognizing the patient's need for privacy promotes mutual respect. Not all of the information needs to be obtained at the first visit, since the genogram will be expanded over the years. Our expectation is that we will see our patients for the rest of their lives (or until we retire).

Our experience has been that at least 10% of the time the real reason for the medical visit is embedded in the genogram. Most patients expect to provide some background information, especially pertinent medical family history. We have yet to have a patient refuse to provide at least a skeleton genogram. In fact, just the opposite is true. A great majority of the patients freely offer this kind of information and welcome an opportunity to relate on a more human basis.

> PATIENT: The family tree part of the visit lasts only two or three minutes, but I feel at the end of this portion of the visit that my doctor already knows more about me than many of my closest friends. At the same time, I feel that none of this information is too private to disclose and that this background information will be very helpful for him to know. Frankly, it makes me feel that the doctor likes me more, even though some parts of my history are embarrassing. I feel like he has known me for a longer time than he really has. The doctor then asks about my own and my husband's occupations, and a short discussion follows.
>
> The focus then turns toward me and my own health. He asks if I have ever broken any bones, and if I have had any surgeries. Now is the time to tell him about the breast cancer. Because of the preceding few minutes, I feel connected to him in a way that helps me relate my story without shaking. It is still hard for me to even say the words "breast cancer," but I retell the story of feeling the lump, thinking it was a cyst, believing it would go away, hoping my husband wouldn't find it, and sneaking away to the free breast cancer screening event at the hospital. I have rehearsed the story a thousand times in my head, and the doctor doesn't interrupt me as I continue the story of my referral from my previous doctor to a surgeon, the biopsy, and telling my husband. I don't tell the doctor about how angry my husband became, and I don't tell him about not telling my children. Next I saw an oncologist, who was very nice but seemed a bit distracted. It was the oncologist who told me I really needed to have a primary care doctor, and that's how I ended up here.

As a health care provider, it is easy to get desensitized to how important a visit to the doctor is. We see a patient every few minutes, but the patient may see a health care provider every few months or every few years. Patients can be quite anxious at the beginning of the visit. They may have rehearsed their story repeatedly and usually tell their story best in the context of their family in an uninterrupted style. If we then go back and fill in the gaps, we get the whole picture more efficiently.

> PHYSICIAN: After just a few minutes with this patient, I have learned a lot about her history and the context of her current illness. She has identified two significant areas. The first is her mother's breast cancer and the course of that illness. Understandably, the patient is concerned about having a stroke, like her mother, and hence is particularly interested in her blood pressure and the potential side effects of the Tamoxifen.
>
> The second significant issue relates to her father's "illness," his alcoholism, abandoning the family, and the patient's current family situation.

Family members are often the most significant resource for any patient, and family members are often the primary caregivers.

> At this point, given the patient's failure to mention her husband and his involvement until late in the conversation, I would assume that the diagnosis of breast cancer has been difficult for him as well. I am thinking that it would be helpful to have him join her for a visit sometime. The patient is here alone, and that says something about the way she is trying to cope with the demands of this illness.

In general, we try to identify both the patient's and family's strengths. We then try to help the patient and family apply these strengths to their current problems. A profound family legacy has been passed on to this patient, and she is in a significant period of transition. It will be important to identify her support system and promote the utilization of her own and her family's strengths.

> PATIENT: The doctor next asks me who knows about my breast cancer. I tell him that my husband and two of my girlfriends know about it. I notice my voice faltering when I mention my husband, and the doctor notices it too. He asks how my husband has taken it, and I say that he hasn't taken it very well. I explain that when things are difficult for him, he often responds by getting angry, and that is what he is doing now. I also feel less appealing to him, like I am some kind of leper. I don't tell the doctor this, but my husband and I haven't had sex since my diagnosis, and I just don't feel like a full human being. The doctor then states that it might be helpful to meet with my husband at some point, since

this seems to be difficult for him as well and he may have some questions. Perhaps he could come in with me for one of my appointments. I say that he works during the day and it is very hard for him to take time off. The doctor responds by letting me know there are some evening office hours.

We have found it very useful to have evening office hours, especially when one or both members of the family work and it is particularly important that as much of the family be present as possible. Family members are strongly encouraged to attend visits for prenatal care, well-child care, and care of major acute or chronic illnesses. Many patients make excuses for a family member not being able to come in with them. They anticipate, often erroneously, the family member's negative response. Having evening office hours eliminates the excuse of not being able to come in because of work.

PATIENT: The doctor next asks me about how my mother's illness went, and I tell him the details of how horribly upset my mother had been about the radical mastectomy they performed. She had many very serious complications, including problems with numbness and tingling in her arm, terrible swelling in her arm, and she really had a difficult time with the disfigurement. I was lucky to have only a lumpectomy, but then the radiation therapy was more difficult for me. The difficult part was the daily reminder that I had breast cancer coupled with the progressive fatigue that went along with the radiation therapy. I became increasingly anxious every day with the radiation therapy, and the radiation oncologist eventually gave me some Valium to calm my nerves. By the end of the radiation therapy, I shook like a leaf when I entered their office. My mother, on the other hand, became progressively more depressed, took a number of different medications, and eventually had a stroke, which they thought one of the medications caused. This left her horribly disabled for the last year of her life in a nursing home. She eventually died of pneumonia. My hope is definitely that I will not end up like her.

This is a fairly common scenario. Many patients come in and want to rewrite their family story to make their life different from their parents'. This is particularly true around issues of major illness like cancer and cardiac disease. Many patients fear they will end up just like their parents. This patient refused to be put on an anti–breast cancer medication, Tamoxifen, because she was afraid it would cause her to have a stroke—like her mother. In fact, Tamoxifen does not cause strokes. But without this family background, it would have been impossible to understand her reluctance to go on the medication. Many people make these kinds of causal links to explain loss and tragedy. Eliciting each patient's understanding of an illness in the context of how they understand others' illnesses is critical to effective treatment.

> PHYSICIAN: I think this patient would benefit from some kind of therapy. However, she seems like the kind of person who may be reluctant to engage in therapy. I start thinking about how to refer her to the psychologist in our practice.

Assessing a Potential Collaborative Practice

• Do providers subscribe to a biopsychosocial model?

REFERRAL

> PATIENT: The doctor then mentions to me that this is a difficult transition for our entire family, and certainly anybody in this situation would be having a hard time. The Valium made sense as a short-term solution to some of these transitional difficulties, but he has some other ideas in mind. One idea is to talk with somebody about the challenges of coping with a major illness and the family resources I could call upon to help me through this. He mentions my husband as a significant resource, and possibly also my friends and children. He also says that my goal seems to be to rewrite my mother's story, and that certainly makes a lot of sense to me. Especially given the ages of my children, I want to be around to see them grow up and have their own children. He says there is someone here in this office I could talk with. He asks if I would like to meet her. I say that I really am not the counseling type, but he says that she is here today and might have a free moment to at least say hello. I agree, and he steps out to find her.

It is often useful to at least introduce patients to the mental health professional in our office. An informal introduction greatly facilitates referrals of patients who think of a mental health professional as someone who deals only with crazy people (and is crazy himself or herself). The simple introduction and hello enhances the referral process and decreases the no-show rate. Indeed, patients rarely fail to show up for the first visit if they have already met the mental health professional face to face.

PATIENT: The doctor then returns with the psychologist, and she says hello and shakes my hand. She seems very pleasant. I have to admit, it is very nice to see this kind of caring where people are willing to help me with all my problems. I really want to get off the Valium, and this seems like a much better option. She seems very nice and says she will be available if needed. The doctor then thanks her, and as she leaves, closes the door. I like her and decide I will come in to see her later.

PSYCHOLOGIST: When I first started working in this office as a psychologist, I had a little trouble adjusting. Providing mental health services in a medical office can be challenging. A medical office is much noisier and more chaotic than the typical mental health services setting. There may be overhead pages and an occasional interruption. The kind of introduction that happened in this case is also not uncommon. Often I actually set up an appointment during the one-minute introduction in the exam room, but sometimes it is just "hello" and "I am available."

The physician availability is very helpful. When I am seeing a patient and I need to talk to his or her health care provider about a medication issue or medical problem, they are easily accessible. Often as not, that is how I need them too, right away. Also, the patients get much better care from all of us when I can speak with their medical providers on a regular basis.

PATIENT: After this point in my appointment, my anxiety goes way down. Since I do not have any pressing health concerns other than the two medications, we spend the rest of the time talking about my use of them. My doctor reassures me about the safety as well as the possible risks associated with the Tamoxifen and gives me some literature to read. We decide that I will think about it and speak further with my oncologist. As for the Valium, we negotiate how to wean me off the medicine at a comfortable pace. He suggests that either he or one of his nurse-practitioner partners call on a weekly basis to see how it is going. I will follow up with him in a month and resolve to make an appointment to see the psychologist next week.

For a primary care practice, we take a relatively luxurious amount of time to get to know patients. We see patients over long periods of their lives, and since we charge considerably less than a specialist per visit, we can see people on a regular basis. Many specialists do not have permission to see patients this regularly and feel they need to take care of the immediate problem entirely in one or two visits. Primary care medicine takes place over a much more extended period of time, as we try to care for the whole person.

In addition to being prevention-oriented, we also try to be problem-focused. This patient's main concerns were anxiety, medications, and family support. At the initial visit, we tried to focus on these issues and hold off on any extraneous concerns.

Assessing a Potential Collaborative Practice

- What kind of prior collaborative experience have providers had?
- How would referrals be made?
- What kind of patients would I see? What kinds of outcomes would I hope for?

If in the same office space:

- Where would I do the therapy?
- Would I have other office space?
- Would I be salaried?
- How much would I pay to rent a therapy room in this office? (In our area, the going rate is $10 per hour.)
- How would I receive phone messages?
- How would billing be managed?
- How would chart notes be transcribed?
- Do I need extra liability insurance?

COPROVISION OF CARE

PATIENT: Coming to what is now a familiar setting makes me considerably less apprehensive about therapy. I check in at the same place, wait in the same waiting room, and am called like any other patient. No one needs to know I am here for counseling.

The counseling room is pretty much as I imagined it would be. A few comfortable chairs, a comfortable couch, some nice prints, a good window, and a small table and phone in the corner. It is nice to see the psychologist again. Even though we just shook hands and said hello, knowing her name and what she looks like makes her seem familiar. We begin with some chitchat about the weather but soon get into a review of what she already knows about me. I feel I am spending my time (and money) more efficiently by her being familiar with my record already. We soon expand my family map with stories as I disclose my husband's history of alcoholism and angry outbursts and my fear of telling him about my breast cancer. It becomes clear how important his reactions are to my own well-being. My husband and I really need to work on all this together. I think he would probably come in with me, as long as the focus is on me. The psychologist offers to make a follow-up phone call to him if needed. I finally feel I am on the road to recovery.

PSYCHOLOGIST: When I joined this practice as the only mental health professional, overall I was very happy, yet there were some disappointments and difficulties. The therapy room was certainly adequate, but I had no other office. There was no place to put my books, no good place to put my purse or laptop computer. I saw a very wide variety of patients, often only for a few sessions. As soon as I had an opening, it was filled. Basically, one health care provider could keep my one-day-a-week schedule full (four or five health care providers could have kept me full all week). In general, the practice was very supportive. I enjoyed lots of contact with other providers and staff, though I also found it necessary to have some contact with and support from other mental health professionals.

In my work here, I find many things about being on-site valuable. As mentioned, the introduction to the patient immensely facilitates making and keeping that all important first visit. In addition, patients really appreciate not having to repeat their entire story. Having the genogram and medical information is enormously helpful and gives me a big head start with every patient I see. The frequent contact with their health care providers allows for constant up-to-the-minute updates. After I review my notes from a visit, the chart goes back to the health care provider, and vice versa. I feel we work well together as a team to care for the whole person, mind and body together.

Assessing a Potential Collaborative Practice

- How would we exchange information—shared charts, regular meetings, phone calls, letters, impromptu meetings?

FOLLOW-UP

The care of this patient and her family proceeded over the next year. She met several times with the psychologist by herself, and many times together with her husband. Her husband was arrested for driving while intoxicated and was referred to an outpatient alcohol treatment program. He began to attend Alcoholics Anonymous on a regular basis and disclosed his fears about losing his wife. The entire family met with the psychologist on two occasions, and the physician joined them all for the second session. The family's concerns for the patient were finally put on the table, and the topic of her breast cancer was no longer taboo. The patient's anxiety slowly abated, but she did experience periodic exacerbations. The pattern of her recovery was two steps forward and one step back. Frequent hallway consultations helped to ensure her steady forward progress. She was weaned off the Valium very slowly.

One of the nurse-practitioners joined the physician and psychologist to provide ongoing education and frequent phone follow-up. The nurse-practitioner, who is female, helped the patient find a breast cancer support group. The patient found it easiest to speak with the nurse-practitioner about the changes in her sexuality and sexual activity. The nurse-practitioner regularly kept the psychologist and the physician up-to-date on these issues.

Initially, the patient met with the psychologist every two weeks, and her physician or nurse-practitioner every two to four weeks. Eventually, we succeeded in addressing all the pertinent issues. After nine months, she completed therapy and now sees her physician or nurse-practitioner every three months.

CONCLUSION

In this chapter, we have taken the reader on a tour through our office from the perspectives of a patient, a physician, and a psychologist. We have elucidated the rationale for the structure and design of our practice and shared some of our own reactions and behaviors. We could not cover all the possibilities and do not mean to suggest that ours is the only way to provide collaborative primary care. Rather, we hope that this story with commentary can serve as a background against which mental health professionals can view potential collaborative partners. It could also serve as a model for physicians and other health care providers setting up or modifying their practices.

CHAPTER 11

Fertile Fields: Collaboration in Family Medicine Residency Programs

WHILE SITTING AT HIS DESK dictating a note about the last patient, he detects a figure in the doorway in his peripheral vision. He turns to see a family medicine resident reticently leaning into his office, waving the palm of her hand, smiling with raised eyebrows as if to say, "I'm in a hurry and need your help." He gestures to her to come in and offers her an empty chair. She leans against a filing cabinet, unwilling to sit down. He pushes the "pause" button, puts the handset down on his desk, and swivels to face the doctor.

> RESIDENT: Hi! Sorry to interrupt. Ya gotta minute? I'm seeing a 38-year-old woman with panic attacks. At first we thought it was her heart. When I was exploring her history, she burst into tears. Her mother died six years ago from breast cancer. Now her husband has bowel cancer and is one month out of surgery. What should I do? Can you see her?

His mind skips. Should he offer to see the patient? Or should he spend a little time turning this interruption into a "teachable moment," leaving the resident to manage the interview herself? He is the medical residency behavioral scientist, the faculty person responsible for teaching physicians in training about the psychosocial aspects of health care.

A scenario similar to this one occurs every day at hundreds of primary care medicine training sites across the country. Since the late 1960s, the American Academy of Family Practice has required that family medicine residencies include behavioral science training. Primary care general internal medicine and pediatrics, the two other allopathic primary care medical disciplines, often include behavioral science education. Residencies in other medical disciplines, such as rehabilitation medicine, oncology, and obstetrics and gynecology, sometimes incorporate behavioral science into the curriculum.

Why are mental health professionals a part of medical training? There is growing awareness in medicine that social and psychological interventions are essential components of patient care. Patients are often critical of physician interpersonal skills. Medical providers are learning that interpersonal, skillful, sensitive physicians are less likely to be sued for malpractice (Beckman, Markakis, Suchman, & Frankel, 1994). Physicians who listen to patients are more able to construct treatment plans compatible with the values and lifestyles of their patients. Effective treatment plans save money and decrease physician frustration. Of course, physicians also know that many of their patients have mental disorders. Moreover, many of these patients have a complicated mix of bio-psychosocial distress and require interdisciplinary care. These same patients often refuse referral to mental health care providers. For all these reasons and more, behavioral science is becoming an essential ingredient in medical training recipes.

In the future, medical training may require more mental health professionals. The greatest demand will come from primary care training sites. In 1995 there were approximately 420 family medicine residencies. To meet the projected demand for generalist physicians, the 1995 American Academy of Family Practice Congress recommends that the annual number of family medicine graduates increase by 900 (AAFP, 1995). To accomplish this goal, the AAFP Congress has called for the creation of an additional 64 residencies by the year 2000. In a similar fashion, educators from internal medicine and pediatrics are gearing up to ensure that roughly half the graduates in these fields go into primary care. In the future, half of the medical generalist workforce will be general internists and pediatricians, and the other half will be family physicians.

Medical training in the future is likely to be integrated into systems devoted primarily to patient care. Historically, medical residencies have been heavily influenced by educational and research designs that hamper the provision of cost-effective, quality care. University medical centers are scrambling to compete for market share. Satellite clinics are being created to feed patients into university hospitals. Across the country, in North Carolina, New York, Michigan, Missouri, Wisconsin, Texas, California, and Washington, medical residents are working in small, rural clinics, being trained by community physicians. This method of training signals a shift to decentralized graduate medical education.

Plans to increase the number of primary care residencies create new pressure to decentralize medical education. "Today virtually every university has a family medicine residency. If the goals of creating so many more training sites are to be met, training will have to occur elsewhere," says Tom Norris, M.D., assistant dean for regional affairs and rural health at the University of Washington School of Medicine. "Community hospitals are downsizing and merging. What we may well see is that training will be incorporated into health care systems," he adds. If these predictions are correct, many mental health professionals working in large health care organizations and rural clinics will have contact with medical trainees. Teaching will become part of their job.

In this chapter, we examine the unique facets of collaboration in primary care medical training programs. The term "behavioral scientist" will be used interchangeably with the term "mental health professional." Although some who work in these multifaceted jobs do conduct research and contribute to the professional literature, most function primarily as educators and clinicians. However, in the culture of primary care medicine, particularly in family medicine, the term "behavioral scientist" has the widest usage.

Our discussion is limited to family medicine residencies. However, much of what we describe is applicable to training in other disciplines, such as general internal medicine and pediatrics. This chapter's ideas represent a synthesis of our combined experiences, existing research, and data from our own national survey. After providing descriptive features of behavioral scientists, we examine dominant roles, relationships, and activities in training settings. We consider how the training environment influences the collaborative experience. The chapter ends with recommendations for those entering into collaborative roles in training settings.

BEHAVIORAL SCIENTISTS IN
FAMILY MEDICINE RESIDENCIES?

The discipline of family medicine has included nonphysicians since it was established in 1967. Recent data show that over 20% of family medicine educators are nonphysicians; half of them are behavioral science faculty (Bogdewic, Garr, Miller, & Myers, 1994). Other nonphysician educators include nurses, pharmacists, social scientists, health educators, nutritionists, and administrators. In 1982, 72% of behavioral science faculty were physicians, mostly family physicians or psychiatrists. In 1990 two studies showed roughly 90% of behavioral scientists to be nonphysicians (Longlett & Kruse, 1992; Mauksch & Heldring, 1995). Table 11.1 shows behavioral scientist demographics from one of these studies (Mauksch & Heldring, 1995).

Most family medicine residencies are associated with community hospitals. Roughly 60% of these community residencies are affiliated with university medical schools. About 20% of residencies are located at universities and another 4% are operated by military hospitals. The size of family medicine residencies varies from four to twelve residents per year.

TABLE 11.1

**DEMOGRAPHICS OF BEHAVIORAL SCIENTISTS IN
FAMILY MEDICINE RESIDENCIES, 1990**

Sex

Male	Female
67% (143)	33% (71)

Age[a]

20–29	30–39	40–49	50–59	60+
2%	32%	51%	12%	3%

Professional Degree

Ph.D.	M.S.W.	Other master's	M.D.	Ed.D.	Other doctorate
63%	14%	8%	7%	4%	4%

Experience in Family Medicine[b]

0–2 yrs.	3–6 yrs.	6 yrs.+
22%	34%	44%

Note. n = 214.
From "Behavioral Scientists' Views on Work Environment, Roles, and Teaching" by L. B. Mauksch and M. Heldring, 1995, *Family Medicine, 27,* pp. 103–108.
[a]Mean age = 42.5.
[b]Mean experience = 6.7 years.

Family medicine residency training takes three years. The core of the training occurs at the family medicine clinic. During their training, residents spend four to eight weeks in block rotations learning the skills of various medical disciplines, such as internal medicine, obstetrics and gynecology, surgery, and pediatrics. Some residencies include behavioral science rotations. Whether training includes behavioral science rotations or not, all residencies integrate behavioral science training into the day-to-day activities of the family medicine clinic. The behavioral scientists working in these clinics function as models of collaborative practice. As training progresses, residents spend larger amounts of time in outpatient family medicine clinics, integrating skills and knowledge from other medical specialties into the practice of family medicine.

To date, no study of family medicine behavioral scientists has focused on collaboration. We created a 14-item pilot survey, partly to provide demographic comparison to 1990 findings and partly to establish some trends to be studied more comprehensively in the future. In contrast to data collected in 1990 by Longlett and Kruse (1992) and by Mauksch and Heldring (1995), most of our questions focus on collaboration in training settings. We randomly sampled 10% of family medicine behavioral scientists listed in a Society of Teachers of Family Medicine database by mailing a survey to every eighth name on the list. Thirty-seven surveys were mailed out, and 19 were returned. Table 11.2 shows some of the results.

Job Satisfaction

A combination of data continues to support the notion that work in family medicine training is attractive and rewarding. Our data suggest that the length of time behavioral scientists stay on the job is increasing. The studies conducted in 1990 (Longlett & Kruse, 1992; Mauksch & Heldring, 1995) found an average of 6.7 years of experience in family medicine training, a two-year increase over the average number of years on the job for 1982 behavioral scientists (Society of Teachers of Family Medicine Behavioral Science Task Force, 1985). (The five authors of this book average 10 years of work in family practice training settings, about the same as the 9.8 years of our sample.)

We asked respondents to describe the "joys and advantages" and "frustrations and disadvantages" of working in a teaching setting compared to working in a purely clinical arena. Every respondent made more than one positive comment, such as "intellectually

TABLE 11.2

COLLABORATION IN FAMILY MEDICINE RESIDENCIES

Nonmedical Trainees

Mental health	Nursing	Pharmacy	Nonmedical trainees
37%	31%	21%	58%

Professional Training of Behavioral Scientist

Family therapy	Psychology	Social work	Education
26%	58%	11%	5%

Generation of Clinical Income Required?

No	Not yet, coming soon	Yes, 30–60% of salary
42%	26%	32%

Other Roles Besides Clinician

Teacher	Consultant	Administrator	Researcher
90%	68%	42%	32%

Method of Communication with Other Health Care Professionals[a]

Charts	Organized meetings	Bump-in-the-hall	Informal notes	Telephone/voice mail	E-mail
3.93	2.21	2.07	3.78	4.36	5.0

Note. n = 19.
Mean years worked in training setting = 9.8.
Mean years worked in collaborative practice setting = 12.5.
[a] 1 = most frequent; 6 = least frequent.

stimulating," "opportunity to witness growth," "more flexibility," "so many opportunities to collaborate," "can share ideas," and "gratifying to know that residents will do better work with the underserved." However, the work is not without its downside. Respondents' common complaints were "not always appreciated by residents," "not enough time," "need more mental health consultants," and "residents' schedules often interfere with teaching." Despite these complaints, behavioral scientists in our study and in the Mauksch and Heldring (1995) study report high levels of satisfaction with their work. The support from other faculty, particularly from residency program directors, is strong. Interestingly, Bogdewic and colleagues (1994) found that nonphysicians had higher levels of satisfaction with their work than their physician colleagues.

Part of what makes work in training settings rewarding is the opportunity to exchange ideas with professionals from other disciplines. The majority of our sample work in settings with trainees from multiple disciplines, expanding the opportunity for cross-fertilization of ideas with others at various levels of professional development. It is common to participate in educational conferences with nurses, pharmacists, and physicians. Each has a unique perspective. Here is a sample summary of one interdisciplinary discussion.

A middle-aged female patient is admitted to the hospital for nausea and vomiting; she has had multiple prior admissions for the same problem, but the causes remain unclear. Physicians wonder if her long-standing diabetes may have interfered with nerve function controlling her stomach and intestines. Pharmacists discuss possible side effects of her medication and list other drugs that may be helpful in controlling her nausea. Mental health professionals ponder the effects of her illness on her husband. Questions about the quality of the marital relationship and potential secondary gain associated with hospital admission are posed. Nurses discuss ways the patient might better manage her nausea at home to avoid hospitalization.

One cannot tell from this summary whether the discussion was competitive or collaborative. Most such discussions are both to some extent. The degree of collaboration in interdisciplinary training settings is largely determined by whether or not the key ingredients are present. As shared experience accumulates, relationships grow in mutual trust and respect. Members of one discipline develop curiosity about the perspectives of others. The inevitable result in training, as in real-life practice, is an expanded perspective that grows into a new model. The biopsychosocial model (Engel, 1977, 1980) embodies multidisciplinary views to help unite professionals in a training setting. George Engel has had a profound effect on collaborative training at his home institution, the University of Rochester School of Medicine and Dentistry. Mental health professionals at the University of Rochester and Highland Hospital Family Medicine Residency Program describe their struggles and growth:

Differences have led to many frustrating conversations with physicians who to us seemed "reductionistic" while to them, we must have seemed "unhelpful" at best. We have benefited from an emphasis in the residency program on the biopsychosocial model. . . . A practical outcome has been the discovery that our patients have bodies. A biopsychosocial approach helped us recognize how often we reify these relational systems and overlook other equally important parts of the patient's experience. (Seaburn et al., 1993, p. 183)

Role Diversity and Collaboration

While the sentiment of those quoted above is echoed elsewhere in this book, the context from which their remarks emerge is unique. In clinics devoted solely to patient care, responsibilities and roles are less diverse. In training settings, clinician faculty have two major purposes: educating trainees and providing patient care. They relate to one another not only as clinicians and consultants but as teachers, students, administrators, curriculum developers, grant writers, and researchers (Mauksch & Heldring, 1995). Our survey results are similar to the findings of Mauksch and Heldring in showing that the roles of clinical consultant, teacher, and clinician are dominant. Indeed, in residency settings, behavioral scientists spend considerably more time consulting and teaching than providing direct service (Mauksch & Heldring, 1995). Moreover, clinician faculty often work with trainees from more than one discipline. We found that 58% of family medicine residencies provide training for trainees in other disciplines in addition to family medicine residents. Surprisingly, mental health was the largest of these other disciplines, with trainees equally distributed between family therapy, social work, and psychology.

We asked survey recipients: "If you have more than one role, how does role diversity affect clinical collaboration? Of particular interest is, how does the combination of teaching and clinical service responsibilities affect collaboration (i.e., complicates things, enhances process, distracts from giving higher quality care, etc.)?"

Eighteen out of 19 respondents indicated that performing multiple roles in an educational setting synergistically enhanced the process of collaboration. Comments included: "Teaching encourages interaction"; "More complexity enhances the process, increases quality of care, especially for difficult, complex patients"; ". . . makes biopsychosocial issues more real"; "Teaching and clinical service means that residents have to refer themselves with their patients." The one person who did not feel that the training setting enhanced collaboration said, "Multiple roles exact greater responsibilities and limit time for collaboration."

Collaboration is also facilitated in training settings because they operate under less constrained financial arrangements than nontraining settings. Faculty are salaried and often do not have to generate clinical income. This arrangement makes it easier to see all patients, irrespective of their insurance benefits. Nine of our respondents indicated that a patient's insurance had no effect on collaboration. Six respondents noted that the time was coming when clinical income would be required. Another 32% reported having to earn 30–60% of their salary. However, even in these latter job designs, a salaried method of payment affords behavioral scientists a level of flexibility hard to equal in fee-for-service settings, where the compensation structure fosters a "time is money" mentality. When training is part of the mental health professional's responsibility, educational time is protected. Our respondents told us that their second-most-frequent method of communication was organized meetings. Such communication would not be as frequent in nontraining settings where patient volume demands and clinical income pressures impede the ability to take the time to talk.

COLLABORATIVE ROLE VARIATIONS ACROSS TWO RELATIONSHIPS

Behavioral scientists have two primary collaborative relationships: with trainees and with faculty. We asked survey recipients: "Is collaboration between you and other faculty different than between you and trainees/students, residents, etc.?" They could answer "less or more frequent," "less or more rewarding," or "longer lasting."

All respondents noted differences in their relationships with residents in comparison to their relationships with faculty. Each relationship had one unique collaborative theme. Collaboration with faculty was slanted toward the provision of medical training. Collaboration with residents focused on patient care. Educational and clinical content was evident in both relationships, but to differing degrees. To dissect these relationships further, we highlight five roles: coprovider, consultant, supervisor, teacher, and coteacher. Other roles, such as administrator, grant writer, and researcher, consume less behavioral scientist time (Mauksch & Heldring, 1995). Next we examine these five roles and contrast them in relation to the two relationships. Although these roles are described as discrete entities, in reality some—such as consultant and supervisor—overlap. Our descriptions represent a synthesis of our experience, our survey results, and the findings of earlier studies (Longlett & Kruse, 1992; Mauksch & Heldring, 1995).

Assessing the Needs of the Referring Physician

The opening scenario to this chapter portrays a constant dilemma for behavioral scientists receiving referrals from residents. Relative to referrals from faculty, the threshold for acceptance of referrals from residents is higher. That is, the longer the resident can retain involvement and responsibility for patient care, the more they will learn. To foster educational experiences, many behavioral scientists refuse to see patients referred by residents without the resident present.

It is important to assess the needs of the physician seeking assistance. This assessment often involves addressing the palpable anxiety commonly exhibited by residents confronted with psychosocial problems in their patients. In the view of medical trainees, most medical problems have discrete diagnostic characteristics and defined treatments. This ostensible clarity in diagnosis and treatment gives the young doctor the "illusion of control." Patients presenting with anxiety, depression, somatization, family problems, or personality disorders create noxious feelings in the young physician. These problems are often hard to diagnose and can seem even harder to treat. Young doctors want to "do it all" and, as a consequence, feel uneasy when confronted with amorphous, complicated issues. Family physicians, who must establish competency across a range of medical disciplines, must learn to tolerate uncertainty, recognize their limits, and provide care in the absence of assured cures.

Residents may also exhibit anxiety owing to their own emotional pain. Sleep deprivation, recurrent feelings of inadequacy, and exposure to trauma and death often combine to create depression and anxiety disorders in medical trainees. Behavioral scientists may provide a resident indirectly expressing his or her own pain with short-term counseling, support, and often a referral. Finally, resident anxiety may be a reflection of time pressure.

Behavioral scientists often greet the referring resident with educational questions: What do you think is going on? If you did not have a mental health resource, how might you work with this patient? How about counseling this patient and videotaping the sessions to go over with me? What is it about this patient that is most difficult for you?

Faculty seek help when they are confused or at the limits of their time or skill. Behavioral scientist responses to a faculty member should reflect respect for the collegial nature of the relationship:

How can I help? What does the patient want from seeing me? What do you think the patient needs? What do you hope will be accomplished? Are you interested in following the patient by yourself with periodic consultation from me? Would you like to cocounsel the patient with me for a few visits?

Behavioral scientists learn to assess the overt and covert concerns of the physician. In short order, a negotiation occurs resulting in the behavioral scientist assuming one of three roles: coprovider, consultant, or supervisor. Discussion of teacher and coteacher activities follow descriptions of the first three roles.

Coprovider

There are four common situations when behavioral scientists accept referrals from residents. First, when the patient's level of distress is severe, requiring expertise beyond the resident's skills, a referral may be accepted. Second, when the referring resident's schedule does not allow for continuity of care, it makes sense to ask for help. This is often the case for first-year residents, whose training rotations prevent them from providing continuity of care for patients in the family medicine clinic. Third, when the resident is graduating, the behavioral scientist often knows the patient better than anyone else and so is best positioned to provide continuity. Fourth, when the resident is overwhelmed by his or her own emotional stress, the behavioral scientist may share care of the patient and provide guidance for the resident.

Behavioral scientists accept referrals from faculty much as they do in nontraining settings. Faculty interests in mental health counseling vary. Some have training and the desire to traverse the psychosocial terrain of their patients' lives. Others are less interested in counseling patients and relieved to have accessible treatment resources. When the degree of patient distress surpasses the faculty member's skill level, referral is a logical choice. As in most medical settings, even family physicians with mental health training can counsel only a small percentage of the patients in need of mental health care.

Consultant

Behavioral scientist consultation with residents has a larger educational component than consultation with faculty. In both cases, informal consultation is more common and often leads to formal consultation. That is, impromptu visits to the behavioral scientist's office or bump-in-the-hall meetings are used to discuss diagnosis, management, or treatment questions. In the medical education world, providing an educationally flavored consultation is called "precepting." The preceptor provides guidance, education, and often clinical assistance to residents as a routine part of day-to-day patient care. Much has been written about the precepting process (Hewson, 1992; Neher, Gordon, Meyer, & Stevens, 1992). In a similar vein, the behavioral scientist may ask questions to assess the resident's level of understanding before providing a few teaching points. However, educational efforts must be tempered by an appreciation for the resident's time constraints.

Frequently the behavioral scientist will recommend a formal consultation, and the patient is scheduled for a meeting with the resident and the behavioral scientist. Included in this appointment is time for the resident to share his or her impressions, ask questions about the interview, and discuss plans for continuing care. The behavioral scientist shares clinical insights, identifies skills demonstrated by the resident in the interview, and asks for the resident's impressions and reactions. This case-based approach helps bring clinical skills and concepts to life.

Consultation in training settings is frequently trilateral. Many patients have a complicated mix of medical, psychological, and social problems. To address all issues, residents may need to consult with a medically trained faculty member and a behavioral science faculty member. Resident discussions with the behavioral scientist may reveal the value of soliciting medical faculty input. Inversely, consultations with medical faculty may result in the medical faculty recommending that the resident see the behavioral scientist. In either sequence, the outcome may be a three-way conversation between the resident, the behavioral scientist, and the medical faculty. During these conversations, the intrinsic rewards of collaboration reach a peak. Three parties are joined in conversation, simultaneously helping a patient and educating one another.

Consultations with faculty are necessarily brief to accommodate their fast-paced schedules. A longer follow-up conversation might be planned. Questions from faculty are typically more focused than questions from residents. Those who have well-developed relationships with the behavioral scientist or who have a particular interest in counseling may use the behavioral scientist as a sounding board. The behavioral scientist may share hypotheses about the cause of a problem, suggest approaches for treatment, and provide information about available resources. A formal consultation is less likely to include the faculty member because of time constraints and financial pressures. Instead, the patient meets with the behavioral scientist, who then communicates impressions and recommendations to the referring faculty physician.

Supervisor

Supervision and consultation are two educational roles that flow into one another. A supervisory relationship is characterized by: (1) ongoing faculty involvement, (2) detailed attention to trainee skill and concept acquisition, and (3) shared responsibility for clinical outcome. Supervisory discussions take more time than consultations. Supervisory relationships are founded on implicit or explicit educational contracts. In graduate medical education, supervisory contracts can be initiated by either a resident or the faculty behavioral scientist. In their excellent text *Collaborative Clinical Education: The Foundation of Effective Health Care* (1993), Westberg and Jason provide a checklist for "systematic practice of a new skill."

- Arrange for a place for learners to practice.
- Arrange for needed equipment or people (e.g., standardized or real patients).
- Make sure that the learners have a clear image of the skills they need to practice (e.g., by doing demonstration).
- Create an environment in which the learners feel comfortable taking risks.
- Begin by simplifying the learners' challenges.
- Sequence the learners' practice.
- Encourage the students and residents to "overlearn" certain skills, as appropriate.
- Be sure that patients are treated with respect and sensitivity.
- Encourage learners to critique their own efforts.
- Provide learners with timely constructive feedback.
- Make sure that the learners are properly prepared before they practice a new skill with real patients.

- Make sure that the learners are appropriately supervised when they first practice a new skill with real patients. (p. 206)

Most family medicine residencies have behavioral science rotations or longitudinal practicum requirements. During rotations, residents assume mental health care provider roles for predetermined blocks of time, usually from two to eight weeks. The University of Rochester and Highland Hospital Family Medicine Residency Program has a behavioral science rotation lasting 16 weeks. Longitudinal practicum arrangements are supervisory contracts stretching over the natural course of a treatment effort. Residents provide counseling during their routine clinics and arrange additional educational time for supervision. In either arrangement, supervision may include one-way-mirror observation and/or videotape review.

In rare situations, physician faculty will ask behavioral scientists to supervise medical psychotherapy. These exceptions include family physicians doing fellowships on behavioral medicine and faculty interested in learning advanced counseling skills.

Teacher

Behavioral scientists spend considerably more time teaching residents than teaching faculty. Longlett and Kruse (1992) determined that, with the exception of consultation and supervision, the two educational methods used most often were behavioral science rotations and formal didactic seminars. The most common group-teaching method in the Mauksch and Heldring survey (1995) was the large-group (more than six people) educational seminar. However, the most common seminar format changes, according to the Mauksch and Heldring respondents, as a function of years of experience teaching. Novice teachers (less than two years' experience) design concept-focused seminars. Behavioral scientists with more than six years' experience mix equal amounts of case material and conceptual content.

Collaborative teaching is appropriate for adult learners. It establishes teacher-learner relationship norms that influence doctor-patient relationship dynamics. That is, the educational process used to teach the resident informs the relational orientation that the resident employs with patients. Respecting this parallel process is an important quality of the collaborative teacher (Shapiro, 1990). Westberg and Jason's (1993) table "contrasting characteristics of collaborative and authoritarian teacher-learner relationships" is provided in Table 11.3. If the word *provider* is substituted for *teacher,* and the word *patient* substituted for *learner,* one sees parallel distinctions between collaborative patient care and authoritarian patient care.

Coteacher

The majority of family medicine behavioral scientists use the Society of Teachers of Family Medicine Behavioral Science Task Force Core Competency Objectives (1986) to guide curriculum development (Longlett & Kruse, 1992). The seven objectives are: (1) biopsychosocial assessment, (2) family awareness and family-oriented

TABLE 11.3

CONTRASTING CHARACTERISTICS OF COLLABORATIVE AND AUTHORITARIAN TEACHER-LEARNER RELATIONSHIPS

Collaborative	Authoritarian
Learners are treated as valuable contributors to their own and to each other's learning	Learners are treated primarily as recipients of teaching
The teacher and learners jointly set the agenda	The teacher sets the agenda
Learners participate in assessing their learning needs	The teacher presumes to know the learners' learning needs
The teacher and learners establish individual and shared goals for learning	The teacher determines the goals for learning
The teacher and learners develop individual and group learning plans	The teacher may develop a learning plan
Learners monitor their own progress and provide feedback to each other	The teacher monitors the learners' progress
Independence and collaboration are fostered	Dependence and competition are fostered
Instruction is learner-centered	Instruction is teacher-centered

Note. From *Collaborative Clinical Education: The Foundation of Effective Health Care* (p. 18) by J. Westberg and H. Jason, 1993, New York: Springer.

care, (3) biopsychosocial management, (4) physician-patient relationships, (5) personal-professional relationships, (6) human development, and (7) sociocultural factors. Ingredients for a successful
educational forum include case material, interaction with residents, and most important, coteaching.

Arguably the most potent behavioral science teaching tool is the
collaborative educational team. Physicians who demonstrate and
teach behavioral science skills are models who sanction the inclusion of behavioral science in medical practice. Physician–behavioral scientist teams impress upon trainees the importance of collaboration. Collaborative teaching often grows out of clinical
collaboration. It is no wonder that some of the most influential
behavioral science educators since the early 1980s are family physician–mental health professional teams like William J. Doherty and
Macaran Baird (1983, 1986) and Susan McDaniel, Thomas Campbell, and David Seaburn (1990).

While most team teaching is done by two faculty, on rare, but
fruitful, occasions behavioral scientists teach with residents. One of
the authors worked with a resident to provide cocounseling for a
patient suffering from agoraphobia. During the 10-month course of
treatment, the resident–behavioral scientist team escorted the
patient through family meetings, counseling sessions, and a series
of desensitization exercises. When the patient began treatment, it
had been 30 years since she had ridden in an elevator or driven
over a bridge. The patient yearned to fly but had never been in a
plane. Step by step, the patient practiced, progressed, and finally
graduated. Fortuitously, the resident was a licensed pilot. Gradua-
tion was a 60-minute flight during which the patient briefly took
control of the plane. At a subsequent seminar, the resident, the
patient, and the behavioral scientist presented their work.

Family physicians coteach a wide range of behavioral science
topics, from family assessment to managing chronic pain to clinical
hypnosis. One ongoing example of collaborative teaching began in
1977. The Clinical Social Science Conference (Smilkstein, Kleinman, Chrisman, Rosen, & Katon, 1981) combines interdisciplinary
teaching with case consultation. Four to six times a year, a patient
is asked to participate in this educational forum. Selected patients
have a wide range of biopsychosocial problems. The patient is
informed that the purpose of the conference is to teach family
physicians about caring for other patients with similar problems. A
secondary benefit is an interdisciplinary consultation. Patients
selected for the conference usually have complex problems that

have vexed the faculty physician, resident, and/or behavioral scientist who provide care. The patient arrives a few hours before the conference for a preconference interview. The interview panel includes a family physician, a psychiatrist, a family therapist or psychologist, and a medical anthropologist. The pre-interview allows the panel to learn about the salient aspects of the patient's health care and personal, family, and cultural history. Pre-interview preparation helps create an efficient, respectful interview in front of the entire residency community. After the interview, the panel engages the audience in dialogue, interspersed with teaching points and clinical recommendations. The patient is not present for this discussion but is scheduled for a follow-up appointment with his or her primary care provider.

Collaboration between faculty members is not limited to teaching activities. Successful teaching may lead to residency program development by the collaborative team. Success in program development is often translated into a research or training grant proposal or a publication describing the evolution of the team's work. The reference section of this book includes several articles and books spawned from collaborative efforts in clinical experiences, team teaching, or program development.

A GUIDE FOR THE BEGINNING PRIMARY CARE BEHAVIORAL SCIENTIST

Evaluate the Setting

The following is adapted from Medalie and Cole-Kelly (1993), who describe four categories of family medicine residency receptivity to behavioral science and collaboration. These probably apply to any medical setting.

1. The director and faculty do not subscribe to the biopsychosocial model.
2. The director and some faculty have a spoken commitment to behavioral science, but in practice little application exists.
3. The faculty embrace behavioral science in theory and practice, but the director is not an active promoter.
4. The director and faculty practice biopsychosocial medicine and demonstrate commitment to integrate behavioral science into training using a nonphysician behavioral scientist. (p. 36)

With these four categories in mind, we recommend that anyone considering work in a primary care residency ask the following questions:

- Does the director and a majority of the faculty apply a bio-psychosocial perspective to patient care?
- Are suitable spacial, financial, and educational resources available? Is office space available? Is there space for counseling? Can videotaping be arranged? Is there money for behavioral scientist continuing education and the purchase of educational materials?
- Will there be protected time for supervision, teaching, and focused practice of counseling skills?

Hints for Peaceful Integration

Ross and Doherty (1988) make six suggestions:

1. Relax and get to know the system and the individuals within it.
2. Remember, "Leadership is non-anxious presence."
3. Never initiate a program without a physician faculty cosponsor.
4. Avoid being set up as a scapegoat. Don't take charge of a project that everyone knows will fail.
5. Maintain your own professional identity and continue to associate with professional colleagues.
6. Make program interventions that are ecologically sensitive. (The proposed change must demonstrate recognition of the system as it is.) (p. 47)

Other Ideas

In addition to the above ideas, we suggest the following:

- Remember that patients have bodies and that the care of these bodies is predictably preoccupying for newly graduated physicians.
- In teaching and in consultation, be practical first. Teach inductively, using case experience to teach general concepts.

- Do not take it personally when residents are absent, appear disinterested, or fall asleep.
- Seek out others doing a similar job and, as the late Dr. Carl Whitaker suggested, form a "cuddle group."
- Find ways to broaden your base as a faculty member beyond fulfilling behavioral science responsibilities. For example, help with grant writing, selecting applicants, resident advising, and developing evaluational protocols.
- Maintain sharp clinical skills. Residents respect those faculty who know what they are doing. Income generation will become more the rule than the exception as grant funding diminishes.
- Remain accessible. Develop referral mechanisms that allow residents and their patients to schedule appointments with you through the appointment secretary. Remain flexible so as to accommodate ever-changing resident schedules.
- Look for opportunities to teach, write, or pursue other projects with physician faculty.
- In time, consider establishing a mental health internship.

CONCLUSION

Collaboration in training settings is a multidimensional enterprise. Compared to other settings, work in training settings is often luxurious. Educational impetus, time availability, and opportunities to work together in both educational and clinical ways combine to make training settings fertile collaborative fields.

Mental health professionals entering the training world must assume more roles than are commonly found in full-time clinical practice. These roles vary in intensity as a function of the relationship purpose and the developmental level of the physician with whom the mental health professional is collaborating. Initially overwhelming and often exhausting, the job of the family medicine behavioral scientist has proven to be a job with lasting appeal.

CHAPTER 12

Partners in the "House": Collaboration in Hospital Settings

THIS CHAPTER FOCUSES on collaboration in settings in which the acuity or intensity of the medical condition cannot be adequately handled in a primary care context. Secondary care is provided in the general community hospitals where primary care physicians care for their patients, with as-needed consultation from specialists. Tertiary care is provided in regional centers where rare symptoms or disease processes can be diagnosed and treated. Some tertiary care hospitals, such as the National Jewish Hospital for Respiratory Illness in Denver, Colorado, provide care to those suffering from certain diseases. A second type of tertiary care is organized around age, such as the various children's hospitals across the country and centers that treat only the elderly. The trend in health care delivery is toward prevention of illness and cost-conscious management in the primary care arena. However, there is still a clear need for hospitals and specialty units to care for patients who need closer observation, multiple specialist input, or assessments and interventions that require technological assistance.

Historically, mental health care providers have worked in these settings. For example, health psychologists provide neuropsychological or personality testing. They also plan systematic research or clinical interventions in areas like smoking cessation, cardiac care, or pediatric illnesses. Psychiatrists provide consultation-liaison services in most general hospitals, offering recommendations about comorbid medical/psychiatric conditions. They also help other medical providers assess complicated diagnoses such as the organic components of dementia. Social workers play a major role in these settings as well; they assess the psychosocial needs of patients and families and coordinate transitional care back to the primary care setting. Finally, clergy provide pastoral care to help with the spiritual dimension of the illness process.

We begin this chapter with a discussion of the current trends in providing health and mental health care in secondary and tertiary settings. We then describe organizational efforts to increase the amount and effectiveness of collaboration in these settings. These organizational efforts have focused on two areas. The first is patient- and family-centered care: How do large, previously impersonal, and technology-focused systems develop processes to treat the patient and family as customers? The second area involves creating equal partnership systems between health and mental health care providers. Since care in hospital systems has emphasized biomedical care, psychosocial issues have traditionally played a secondary role.

We then move from the organizational efforts to improve collaboration to the individual providers who work together in those systems. What attitudes, knowledge, and skills are necessary to practice collaboratively in these arenas today? We close the chapter with practical advice for mental health professionals who want to be more effective collaborating in secondary or tertiary care settings.

TRENDS

Four trends, all interrelated, affect secondary and tertiary institutions, primarily hospitals. The first is the loss of independence as more "vertically integrated" health systems are designed and developed. Hospitals traditionally have functioned as autonomous institutions with stable and predictable business. Rapid changes in the external environment have forced them to look outside the institution to create integrated networks that include primary care groups, employers, and other institutions. A second trend is the move away from care in the expensive inpatient environment. In the past, hospitals have been the center of the health care system, the place where a patient is evaluated and treated with state-of-the-art technology. Now hospitals are viewed as the most expensive part of the system. Currently, the focus is on developing outpatient services along a continuum of care that avoids completely or at least minimizes time spent in the hospital. Third, clinical and operational processes within hospitals are being reengineered, reinvented, and redefined. This process requires close collaboration between internal departments that have previously competed for budgetary resources. Using empowerment models such as total quality management (TQM) and continuous quality improvement (CQI), clinicians and administrators recommend and implement effective changes at the level where care actually takes place. The fourth trend is the focus on consumer satisfaction with care. Many hospitals are developing programs in the area of patient- or family-centered care. The institution and its processes of care are being redesigned to include the patient and family as active rather than passive recipients of care.

Toward Integrated Networks

The renaming of the journal *Hospitals* to *Hospitals and Health Networks* four years ago symbolizes the movement toward integrated systems of care. One of the driving forces behind this movement is the change to capitated payment systems (see chapter 13). Under these prepaid systems, hospital goals change in the following ways:

- From treating illness to maintaining health and promoting wellness
- From caring for individual patients to caring for specific populations
- From filling beds to providing care at the appropriate level
- From managing an organization to managing a network of services

These new goals provide more opportunity for organizational collaboration than before.

The key ingredients described throughout this book will become even more critical as network health systems are formed. Developing a common purpose and maintaining a flexible hierarchy will help individuals focus on the new vision of promoting health rather than providing services solely for illness. Clear roles and communication processes are equally important for practitioners who are not used to making decisions jointly.

Decreasing Inpatient Utilization

Despite the movement away from secondary and tertiary medical care, there will always be advantages to hospital settings. The technology and the number of available specialists at one site have made them excellent resources for handling acute, life-threatening illness or diagnosing and treating unusual medical problems. However, in addition to the high cost disadvantage, they do not treat chronic illnesses as effectively, particularly ones that involve multiple systems. The core business of hospitals has been to provide acute inpatient care. As the core business in integrated health systems changes to primary care, disease prevention, and health promotion, hospitals will become only one resource to achieve new goals. They will become "servants" of health care delivery networks rather than the reverse. Hospitals that clearly recognize this trend are currently creating linkages across the delivery continuum, for example, with home care agencies and nursing homes.

Inpatient mental health services have also been reduced dramatically. Corporate employee assistance programs and behavioral managed-care companies have achieved the greatest cost saving in mental health expenses by reducing inpatient days. Although most of these programs attempt to cut costs in any way possible, some are willing to pay for the development of intensive outpatient services to meet more severe patient needs. To survive, these programs will need to demonstrate significant cost and quality improvements over care in the inpatient setting.

For example, in 1993 Duke University Medical Center had three adult inpatient psychiatric units, one adolescent unit, one dual-diagnosis (substance abuse and psychiatric) unit, and an intensive outpatient program for adults and adolescents with substance abuse problems. In 1995 there is only one inpatient unit, housing both adults and adolescents. However, Duke also has a large intensive outpatient program for adult substance abuse. In addition, the medical center is forming a network of affiliated mental health care providers throughout the region. This kind of rapid downsizing and refocusing of resources is happening throughout the country.

Internal Reorganization

To make the adjustments necessary to create vertically integrated systems and to integrate with other groups or agencies, hospitals are initiating dramatic internal reorganization. These efforts involve "clinical reengineering," defined as planned activities to reorganize patient care to enhance cost-effectiveness and quality of care (Shortell, Gillies, & Devers, 1995). For mental health care providers in hospitals, internal reorganization is creating the same profound changes that their outpatient, private practice colleagues are experiencing. The pressure to do more with fewer resources is only increasing.

One core goal of reengineering is to reduce the organization's focus on providers and to increase organizational focus on positive outcomes for the patients, including reduced cost. In pursuit of this goal, hospitals have created "service lines": care of patients with a specific disease, such as congestive heart failure or stroke, is broken down into the specific activities needed to provide quality care across the continuum, from prevention to recovery. This concept is also being applied to the care of patients who tend to be high utilizers of inpatient resources, such as those with chronic pain syndromes or sickle cell anemia.

This kind of restructuring has created new opportunities for mental health care providers. MaryAnne Zabrycki is a clinical social worker at Duke Medical Center. She approached the Eye Center, a tertiary care treatment facility, with a request to create a collaborative arrangement. Over the last seven years, her collaboration with the physicians at the center has clearly added value to their delivery of care. Her experience is described in more detail later in this chapter.

Toward Patient- and Family-Centered Care

One of our central tenets is the importance of collaboration with patients and families. Effective collaboration between providers is not enough if the needs of patients and families are not a primary focus in developing care systems.

There are good reasons for hospitals to think about more patient involvement. In a survey of over 6,000 adult patients recently discharged from the medical and surgical services of 62 hospitals, the most common complaint was that hospital staff did not tell patients about the daily routine in the hospital (Cleary, 1991). More than one-fifth of patients reported that no doctor was in charge of their care and that they did not receive accurate information about what to expect before and during hospitalization. Forty percent did not have a relationship of trust with any hospital staff other than the doctor in charge of their care. Finally, about one-third of patients reported that very little time was spent in discussing discharge plans. As expected, patients who reported spending little time with their physicians were more likely to report problems related to discharge. Overall, high percentages of patients were significantly disgruntled with their care in the hospital. Clearly, there is much room for increasing the satisfaction level of the consumer of hospital services.

As a result of this kind of data and the desire to increase consumer satisfaction, hospitals are making efforts to directly involve and collaborate with the patient and family. Decentralization of services, cross-training of employees, work redesign, and physical and geographical reorganization of delivery systems to bring care providers closer to the bedside are typical strategies. However, efforts to create efficient systems, such as those we have described, can take priority over efforts to become more patient-centered. Patients can be seen as obstacles to be worked around rather than customers with whom to collaborate.

In the next section, we describe efforts to implement patient-centered models and to design collaborative care hospitals. Two trends are apparent: adding a psychosocial/psychiatric perspective to the team of medical professionals caring for the patient and family, and encouraging the inclusion of the patient's perspective in treatment.

COLLABORATIVE CARE IN ACTION

Medical-Psychiatric Units

Mental health services have not typically been integrated into tertiary care settings. Many community hospitals have separate psychiatric units designed to handle high-psychiatric but low-medical acuity. Others have the capacity to provide psychiatric or psychosocial consultation to medical units designed to handle high-medical but low-psychiatric acuity. These are referred to as Level I and II units, respectively, in a recent review of medical-psychiatric units. (Kathol, Harsch, Hall, Shakespeare, & Cowart, 1992). In this same organization of delivery systems, Levels III and IV depart from the current ward settings and are designed for patients with concurrent and more severe medical and psychiatric problems. Characterized by high acuity in both medical and psychiatric patients, these facilities are staffed by nurses and mental health professionals trained to deal with both dimensions. In Levels III and IV, patients are cared for by co-attendees in both medicine and psychiatry.

This method of dividing the structure of psychiatric units is helpful to the mental health professional interested in collaboration. It corresponds to the spectrum described in chapter 8. Levels I and II require skills in the first three bands—providing consultation to the providers and direct clinical services to patients. Levels III and IV require skills in the coprovider and collaborative networking bands. The opportunity exists for health and mental health systems to draw from the full spectrum of collaboration in creating and experimenting with new models of collaborative care. Medical social workers, family therapists, clinical nurse specialists, health psychologists, and consultation-liaison psychiatrists can help these systems create services that match the continuum of needs in any setting.

Wamboldt (1994) conducted a survey that identified Level III and IV hospitals that provide services to medically and psychiatrically diagnosed children. Twenty-one were classified as Level I or II and eleven were identified as Level III or IV. Most of the hospitals in the latter group were not free-standing psychiatric hospitals but rather were located in general medical settings in major population centers. The advantages cited by the medical directors of medical facilities included accessibility to medical attending physicians; access to ancillary services (X-ray, laboratory); and greater acceptability by patients and families of a primary medical facility over a psychiatric setting. Another key advantage of these units was the ability of all staff to create and maintain an effective treatment environment. Close cooperation and daily contact between psychiatrists, pediatricians, and nursing staff ensured consistency of patient care.

Children and their families were referred to these units for several reasons. Newly diagnosed severe chronic illness, such as asthma or neurologic disease, could receive an initial multidisciplinary workup that integrated thinking from developmental, psychological, and medical perspectives. Children with a medical illness that had been difficult to control on an outpatient basis made up a second group. Examples included children who refused to take medication and engaged in extreme oppositional behavior, or adolescents with diabetes who frequently went into ketoacidosis. A third category of referrals comprised those children in situations that presented a high risk for further problems. A child who has undergone traumatic medical interventions or numerous hospitalizations may benefit from a combined medical-psychiatric approach.

The key feature of the dual-diagnosis units is the inherently collaborative nature of the delivery system. Providers are colocated and share the common goal of providing integrated care to children and their families affected by severe chronic medical illness. The goal, however stated, is to "put the illness in its place." There is frequent communication between providers and patients about treatment plans, which incorporate elements of biological, psychological, social, and behavioral systems. All of the key ingredients discussed in chapter 3 are present in this model. Mental health care providers working in hospital settings can learn about collaboration and how to integrate services to patients with comorbid conditions.

General Hospital Settings
Bryan Memorial Hospital

Bryan Memorial Hospital in Lincoln, Nebraska, is primarily a cardiac care referral center for a population of about 200,000. In its efforts to redesign the work process, it has created a new care delivery model that is patient-focused. One of the major strategies of this model is to break down the departmental barriers between medicine, nursing, social work, and pastoral care, as well as services such as physical therapy and recreational therapy. Instead of referring a patient to any of these services, teams of providers design individualized programs for patients. At Bryan these teams are led by a nurse specialist, who is the case coordinator. But the leadership for the treatment plan and discharge planning is shared by the team.

It was discovered at Bryan that a patient visited an average of seven units during a hospital stay. This diffusion of services with multiple "primary providers" did not help the patient develop a relationship with any one staff member or team of providers. Patients frequently complained about misunderstanding information and feeling distanced from clinicians and staff. The average number of units visited has been reduced to two, with a resulting cost savings. More important, patients now have increased opportunities to develop a relationship with a particular team of providers. Michael Bleich, vice president for patient services at Bryan, said it is the quality of these relationships that truly allows providers to uncover human need and develop trust (Bleich, 1995).

Changing the focus of hospital teams from professionals and staff to patients facilitates the development of shared goals for individual patients and their families. At Bryan social workers, whose role was previously limited to discharge planning, are now integral members of the team. They are able to gain a better understanding of how an illness affects the patient as well as the providers, and they contribute to case planning. They help decide when joint meetings between patients and providers are indicated and who should be at such meetings. They also help structure the discussion, ensure that everyone involved understands the plan, and provide follow-up to make sure it is implemented. They make other resources available to the patient that will help in the transition from the hospital.

One interesting part of the Bryan model is the addition of spiritual concerns to the treatment plan. Traditionally, if ethical or spiritual issues are raised, a referral to a pastoral care provider is initiated. With a team approach, spirituality is everyone's business. Workshops on bioethics for all staff and ongoing discussion groups focused on issues such as death and dying are held to sensitize all clinicians and staff to the broader questions. Communication difficulties between providers and between providers and patients can result from not talking about the intensely emotional issues of loss, disability, and death. Engaging in conversations about these subjects can increase a sense of common purpose between providers from different specialties and build respect and trust. It can also make it easier to talk with patients and their families about these issues.

New York University Medical Center Cooperative Care Unit

Bryan Memorial is in the early stages of transition to patient-centered care. A more established model exists in New York University Medical Center's Cooperative Care Unit. In 1979 this unit was opened to hospitalize patients who did not require the level of acute care needed in a traditional hospital setting. Two collaborative systems were set in place. In the first, a "care partner" stays in the room with a patient and is actively involved throughout the period of hospitalization. Patients and their care partners are housed in a homelike setting with no physicians, nurses, or nurse's aides. Patients are brought to centralized hospital services by the care partner for all nursing and physician assessments and treatments as well as for individualized and group educational sessions. The second collaborative system is the multidisciplinary professional staff, consisting of a nurse-educator, nutritionist, social worker, and pharmacist. This team is responsible for orienting the patients and care partner to the unit at the time of admission, performing an assessment of the appropriateness of a patient for admission, working with the care partner, and developing educational programs for inpatient needs.

This education-intensive program has been carefully studied in the last 15 years. It has proven to be a cost-effective alternative to traditional inpatient programs. There is no evidence that patients hospitalized on the Cooperative Care Unit were rehospitalized more often or needed more emergency services. There is, on the other hand, evidence of greater patient understanding of treatment, adherence to treatment, satisfaction, and self-management (Grieco, Garnett, Glassman, Valoon, & McClure, 1990).

In a paper describing the Cooperative Care Unit as an innovative alternative for patients with chronic illness, Grieco et al. conclude:

> Cooperative Care stands as a strong support for the philosophy that: (a) patients have the right and responsibility to participate in their own health care as full partners, so that they will be more capable of health self-management following discharge; (b) inclusion of the patient's family and support system into the period of hospitalization leads to more humanistic hospital care and enhances the potential for improved post-discharge self management and medical compliance; (c) an integrated, multidisciplinary health-care team providing patient care and education allows optimal utilization of hospital staff responding appropriately to patient needs.
>   Its time has come. (p. 10)

Planetree Alliance

Bryan Memorial and the New York University Medical Center Cooperative Care Unit are examples of single hospitals that have focused on creating a patient-centered environment. The Planetree Alliance creates a network of hospitals with a patient-centered vision. The mission of this consumer health care organization is to "create healthcare environments that support and nurture healing on all levels—physical, mental, emotional, and spiritual." Planetree has formed partnerships with more than 20 hospitals across the country and in Europe. The sites range from small rural hospitals to large urban medical centers and include acute and critical care, emergency departments, long-term care, and outpatient services. Regardless of site, the programs are specifically designed to encourage and support the patient as well as the patient's family, both in the hospital and at home. Specific programs include the care partner program, self-medication protocols, open chart policies, architecture designed for optimal healing, arts programs, massage, and healing gardens.

Membership in the Planetree Alliance allows a hospital to receive consulting and educational services in setting up a patient-centered model, opportunities for networking with other programs attempting to do the same, and access to the Planetree Institute, which offers education and training to health care professionals.

Hospitals that affiliate with Planetree report increased patient, nurse, and physician satisfaction, decreased nurse turnover rates, decreased postoperative infections, and an increase in the number of patients making lifestyle changes conducive to health and wellness. However, not all of the picture is rosy: these results do not often translate into cost savings in the short run. While the vision focuses on collaboration and its strategies are humane, in the cost-conscious health care environment of today Planetree affiliates are challenged by the same financial realities that confront more traditional health care models.

Duke University Medical Center's Eye Center

MaryAnne Zabrycki provides an excellent example of an individual who has developed a collaborative practice in a tertiary care facility. In 1988 Zabrycki was asked by the chairman of the Ophthalmology Department at Duke University to provide social work services to patients and families receiving clinical services in the department. He particularly wanted her to work with the families of children with retinopathy of prematurity. These children, at risk of limited vision from birth, needed to be linked to additional services, including family counseling. They needed to know what to expect from the medical profession and to understand the critical importance of keeping regular eye care visits.

Zabrycki agreed to start working at the Duke Eye Center, a regional specialty clinic caring for the full spectrum of ophthalmology disorders. She immediately began building relationships with the 18 physicians on staff by scheduling 15-minute interviews with each of them. She recalls that some were not only reluctant to give her even that amount of time but generally lukewarm to the idea of social work services. Their reasons varied, but several themes emerged. First, mental health services were perceived as too "touchy-feely" and as capable of harming patients by providing too much "hand-holding." Second, many thought that the only goal of these services was getting people money through disability or workmen's compensation. Many physicians felt that this form of compensation was inappropriate; that it made people dependent on the system; and that it kept them from recovering as much as possible. A third, more subtle reason that emerged over time was that the culture in which these physicians trained and worked emphasized cure and complete recovery. They were uncomfortable discussing cases in which this was not the outcome—that is, cases in which their expectations exceeded their ability to cure. In new resident orientation, Zabrycki asks which of the physicians became an ophthalmologist to tell people they were losing their sight. When there is no response to the question, she explains that her role is to help them enable the patient and family to understand the diagnosis and its impact on daily life.

In her brief initial interviews with the physicians, Zabrycki had a clear vision of how she wanted to present herself and what information she wanted from them. She described herself as a member of the overall treatment team, supporting both patients and providers. She emphasized maintaining an open referral system so that anyone on the team, including the patient and family, could refer to her. She listened carefully to the concerns of the physicians who expressed reservations and was respectful of their position. She informed physicians that when their patients were referred to her by other members of the treatment team, she would seek their input immediately, and that she would work to support their recommendations and care of the patient.

Another method Zabrycki used to understand and develop rapport with the providers and staff was to enter their world to see what it was like. She scrubbed for surgery and observed several operations. She sat with patients in outpatient follow-up visits to understand the flow of the office and what language was used in explaining the diagnosis and prognosis of various ophthalmological disorders. She talks about the staff making fun of her squea-mishness in the operating room but also appreciating her willing-ness to see what their world was like.

A few of the physicians were willing to refer to her right away. Most remained somewhat skeptical. One of her first referrals came from a staff nurse. The patient's physician, though, was skeptical. Zabrycki approached the physician to gather more information about the case and assure him that she would represent him well in front of the patient. She said that if the patient expressed concern about the treatment, or if the patient or family was confused about a medical aspect of care, she would relay that to the physician. This assurance and the successful coprovision of care in this case helped develop the relationship between Zabrycki and this physician. The physician has since referred other patients to her.

Zabrycki met regularly with the chair of the department and the administrator of the practice to review her progress in working with both the families and the providers. She solicited general feedback from them about how she was perceived by the physi-cians, nurses, and staff. These meetings were frequent in the begin-ning and became less frequent as time went on.

Another method she used to develop rapport was to become involved in the residency teaching program. She developed a cur-riculum using experiential methodology to allow resident physi-cians to learn what an ophthalmological diagnosis is like for the patient and family. Most of this curriculum was offered during res-ident orientation. At least once a year she takes residents to the School for the Blind and has the residents simulate having a sight disability. They are better able to empathize with their patients after experiencing the orientation and mobility problems of limited vision.

MaryAnne Zabrycki developed a well-utilized and respected hospital practice in collaboration with the ophthalmologists, nurses, and staff of the Duke Eye Center. Her assertiveness in setting up this program and flexibility in responding to the center's needs, as well as those of the individual practitioners, provide an excellent model for others in medical specialty settings.

COLLABORATION WITH PATIENTS

The Picker/Commonwealth Program for Patient-Centered Care is an excellent resource for understanding the needs of patients and families in hospital settings. The Picker Program began in 1987 in Boston and was incorporated as the Picker Institute in 1994. Affiliated with Beth Israel Hospital, the program's mission was to discover what the hospital experience is like for patients and families and to make recommendations for improving patient-centered care. Hospitals frequently conduct patient satisfaction surveys using checklists, but Picker's intent was to go behind the checklist to expand on the patient's perception. Since 1987 the program has conducted focus groups and designed surveys for over 200 health care institutions and elicited information from more than 45,000 patients. In *Through the Patient's Eyes* (Gerteis, Edgman-Levitan, Daley, & Delbanco, 1993), the authors organized the feedback from patients into six dimensions of patient-centered care, each of which has implications for mental health practitioners wanting to collaborate with medical providers in a hospital setting.

1: *Respect for patients' values, preferences, and expressed needs.* This dimension incorporates two ideas critical to negotiating and collaborating with patients. The first is understanding the patient's beliefs or "explanatory model of illness." Kleinman, Eisenberg, and Good (1978) describe a university professor who insisted that the diagnosis of his condition was pulmonary embolus rather than angina because he associated angina with becoming incapacitated. He was angry with the providers who insisted his diagnosis was angina. Underlying disagreements about the source of ill health or the appropriate treatment can lead to miscommunication and conflict between patients and providers. Asking questions about individual or family beliefs and listening carefully to the answers can lead to a shared meaning of the illness. Thinking of diagnosis not as an objective statement but as a social construct (Glenn, 1987a) is a better way to create a collaborative relationship.

The second critical idea is to prevent unnecessary dependency. Patient reports are mixed on this issue. Some report that they want the clinicians to make all the decisions and do not want to be involved in care. Others want to know the details of every procedure, to be able to read their chart carefully, and to be included in all discussions about their care. Most patients fall between these two extremes in their desired level of involvement. Of the patients interviewed on a Picker survey, 98% agreed that when there is more than one way to treat a medical problem, the choices should be discussed with the patient. Waitzkin (1985) found that patients are more dissatisfied about the information they receive from their physicians than about any other aspect of medical care except high costs and waiting times. This same report found that clinicians tend to underestimate the desire of patients to be involved and overestimate the time they spend informing them of available treatment options.

Mental health care providers can assist patients, families, and health care practitioners in this area. They can help establish protocols that elicit patients' perceptions about their illness and expectations about treatment. They can ask patients what they want to know, who in the family they want to involve in decision-making with them, and what questions they might want to ask in the future. Mental health care providers can educate clinical staff to be curious about patients' cultural beliefs and the impact these beliefs may have on care. They can help staff develop a technique for inquiring about such beliefs that will aid treatment and increase compliance and satisfaction with overall care. They can provide specific skills in negotiating therapeutic strategies with patients and their families.

2: *Coordinating care and integrating services.* Patients in a hospital setting are often confused about who is in charge of their care, what kinds of technical procedures will be done, when procedures will be done, and who to ask for what service. Patient confusion is greater in academic centers but also is reported in nonteaching hospitals. The complexity of care, the sheer number of providers, traditional departmental boundaries, and the lack of time or desire to talk about the process of care delivery contribute to the problem. Coordination remains one of the patient's chief frustrations. Units like those at Bryan and New York University are addressing problems of coordination by creating new structures to keep the team and the patient informed.

One of the authors, a psychologist and family therapist, has consulted to a team on a family medicine inpatient service for the past six years. Once a week he attends rounds to discuss challenging clinical interactions the team has with patients, try to clarify complicated psychosocial or ethical dilemmas, and facilitate family conferences. The inpatient team is composed of a faculty supervisor, three resident physicians in various stages of training, a resident from the psychiatry program, a physician's assistant in training, and a pharmacy student. Members of the team rotate, resulting in a different "culture" almost every week. Many of the patients on this service require consultative services from other medical services while they are hospitalized. These consultants talk to the patients and write notes in the chart with their recommendations. The consultants may not talk directly to the team or the patients about these recommendations, leaving someone on the team responsible for interpretation and decision-making. The family of the patient is also involved, creating more potential for confusion.

We have found that many of the conflictual situations described by the team result from miscommunication within the team or between members of the team and outside consultants or family members. We have created a norm of giving more time to new members of the team to orient them to the expectations of care, to help them understand how the process works, and to clarify what to do if the process is breaking down. In addition, any conflict is viewed as an opportunity to reflect on the actual sequence of events rather than solely as an occasion for assigning blame.

Mental health care providers can play a valuable role in coordinating care. They can ask questions of team members that focus attention on the *process* of care delivery. For example, looking at the team members' relationships with the patient and deciding on that basis who should take a lead role in a family conference is often critical to a successful conference. If team members hold different opinions about treatment options, these differences can be presented to the patient in a way that provides the information needed to make an informed decision. Mental health professionls can assist the team in clarifying for the patient who is delivering care and what the care plan is.

3: *Information, education, and communication.* Patient-centered education is an increasingly important part of hospital care. It has always been a part of inpatient care but often has been designed and delivered based on provider needs rather than individual patient needs. It has been delivered by professionals designated as educators rather than by clinicians. As hospitals move toward integration, educational programs will be folded into ongoing clinical care so that all members of the team will be responsible for providing education to patients and families. Team members must have the interview skills necessary to assess the patient's needs. They also must subscribe to the idea that an educated patient facilitates a good treatment plan. The Cooperative Care Unit at New York University is a good example of this kind of program.

Mental health professionals who have interest and experience in psychoeducational and preventive approaches can help develop programs to educate patients about their conditions, as well as develop strategies to prevent unnecessary hospitalizations. One example of such an approach is the development and implementation of a program of multiple family groups. The member of a family with a significant chronic illness or disease process attends the sessions with his or her family. The purpose of the group is twofold: (1) to provide education about problem-solving and communication processes that may be helpful in coping with the chronic illness, and (2) to allow the group members to learn from each other. There is considerable flexibility in the structure of these groups. Typically, between two and six family groups meet together from four to ten weeks. Some groups have been illness-specific: all patients, for example, have severe asthma or AIDS. In those groups in which different chronic illnesses are represented, the idea is to allow families to focus on the similarities in coping with chronic illness rather than on the technical medical aspects of a specific disease (Gonzalez, Steinglass, & Reiss, 1989).

Mental health care providers can also help medical providers and teams learn how to provide information and education more effectively. Devine and Cook (1986) report that when surgical staff nurses were given training workshops in teaching educational and psychosocial support skills, their patients admitted for elective surgical procedures had shorter stays and required less medication. The program involved a three-hour, two-stage training workshop, plus one hour of additional nurse staff time per hospital stay and was evaluated to be cost-effective.

4: *Emotional support and alleviation of fear and anxiety.* Patients say they want more emotional and logistical support from their providers in the hospital. This kind of support is defined as offering positive affective statements to the patient, helping to normalize the strong emotions generated by a serious illness, offering advice or logistical help, and connecting the patient to a larger network. In focus groups and surveys, patients talk about the coldness of the hospital environment and the difficulty of getting emotional support from staff.

This is an area where mental health care providers have an excellent opportunity to collaborate across the spectrum. They are skilled in recognizing those patients or family members who are having difficulty adjusting to an illness. If they are part of an initial assessment team, they have the chance to meet patients on a routine basis before there are defined problems. This often happens on specialized services such as dialysis, oncology, or cardiac rehabilitation. They can play an integral role in developing educational groups or other preventive measures for those patients identified as high-risk for psychological complications. If there is an open referral system and a problem has been identified, the mental health practitioner is involved. With this arrangement, mental health care is more likely to involve formal consultation or coprovider services to assist the patient and family in dealing with the conflictual issues.

It is not the mental health professional's role in these situations to be a therapist helping people work through long-standing difficulties. The contact in the inpatient environment is usually short, only one to five meetings. The goals are to facilitate expression of affect, to create a plan to deal with what looks like a mountain of problems, and to initiate the plan in the hospital stay.

Mental health professionals can provide emotional support in other ways. They can teach simple progressive muscle relaxation techniques to help patients cope with medication side effects or difficult procedures; offer patients audiotape players with music, comedy, or relaxation tapes; or facilitate meetings that involve medical providers and the patient and family. These meetings often involve discussions of end-of-life issues, creating living wills, and establishing powers of attorney. Mental health collaborators should be able to address these issues as a normal part of their work in a hospital setting.

5: *Involving and supporting family and friends.* There are a number of reasons to involve family members and close friends in the care of patients in the hospital. The definition of family is who-ever patients perceive to be in their closest circle. This could be somebody to whom they are related biologically, legally, or emotionally. Patients depend on their families to look out for their interests. Often this puts family members at odds with the health care provider because they demand more informa-tion or services than are being offered. But family members can also be the best resource to the patient and the provider. If they feel acknowledged positively by the health care team, family members can interpret information and encourage the patient to comply with the treatment plan. They can make sure dietary and activity prescriptions are carried out, and often they have a more objective view of physical or psychological symptoms than does the patient.

The illness does not affect the patient alone. It can also have a dramatic effect on the family. The demands of chronic illnesses like Alzheimer's disease or cancer can create an all-consuming caretaker role for some family members. Particularly in terminal illness or severe chronic illness, the patient often naturally receives most of the attention. Family caretakers, particularly in the hospital, can be overlooked.

There are several ways in which a mental health care provider can collaborate in this area of patient-centered care. First, they can ensure that the ideas and concerns of caretakers and others surrounding the patient are solicited and valued. While the professional brings a wide range of expertise to patient care, the family knows the patient better than anyone. They often know what kinds of information to present and in what way. Involving them as care partners, as the New York University Collaborative Care Unit does, enhances treatment compliance and patient satisfaction.

Second, mental health professionals can provide support to family members themselves. Family members can articulate their own goals and expectations, which can be included in the patient's chart. In addition, mental health care providers can encourage family members to post questions at the bedside for medical providers to address. They can help families connect with other families with similar burdens and challenges. There are a great number of support networks for family members as well as patients. Most of these networks are disease-specific. Two relatively new organizations that are role-specific instead are the National Family Caregivers Association (NFCA) and the Well Spouse Foundation. The NFCA is a not-for-profit organization dedicated to improving the quality of life of America's 18 million family caregivers. For a low fee, a family member can join this organization and receive informational and emotional support. The Well Spouse Foundation, based in New York, is dedicated to providing support to those who provide care to a severely health-impaired spouse. A third new organization, the Institute for Family-Centered Care, is focused on supporting collaboration in pediatric settings. This organization, founded in 1992 and based in Washington, D.C., provides consultation services around program development and policy planning for hospitals and networks wishing to create better linkages between families with a severely ill child and the providers who serve them.

For family involvement to be effective, the mental health professional and the medical providers must communicate about the value of including the family. Medical providers may sometimes feel that family involvement makes care inefficient. If a clear case is made for the positive impact of family involvement on the recovery of the patient, medical providers are more likely to support the plan.

6: *Facilitating the transition out of the hospital.* A panel of experts in 1987 rated topics for advancing routine quality assurance work for older patients. None of the 27 topics received higher scores than discharge planning (Fink, Siu, Brook, Park, & Soloman, 1987). Studies have shown that both hospitals and patients benefit from facilitating the transition out of the hospital, in the following ways: improved patient outcomes (Rubenstein, 1984), increased patient satisfaction (Berkman, Bedell, Parker, McCarthy, & Rosebaum, 1988), fewer hospital readmissions (Naylor, 1990), and enhanced cost-effectiveness (Safran & Phillips, 1989).

In the Picker National Survey, patients reported that they did not receive enough clinical information to prepare them for the transition to home; they were not as involved as they would have liked in making choices about the treatment plan; and their psychological and social needs were not adequately addressed. Many patients and family members cannot predict what problems or questions they will have once the patient is home. Further, if they have remained in a passive role throughout the hospital stay, they may not feel they can be involved in a more active way preparing for discharge. One of the authors who consults with the inpatient team routinely asks patients whether they understand and can carry out the discharge plan that medical providers have outlined. Patients frequently say they do not understand some or all of the recommendations. Cost, transportation problems, misunderstanding the recommendations, and fear are some of the most common reasons. After giving this feedback to the team leader, patients are routinely asked, "Will you be able to do this?" at the discharge meeting. This follow-up question results in more negotiation between the team and the patient and family, and the whole process greatly improves patient satisfaction and compliance.

One example of a multidisciplinary program instituted by many hospitals is the geriatric program at Scott and White Memorial Hospital in Texas. A nurse specialist with expertise in the care of the elderly meets with the patient, family, and health care providers to assess resources and support networks. This nurse then assists in coordination of services and communication with the patient and family. A follow-up visit is made to the home to assess the appropriateness of the discharge plan and make any necessary changes. Using a randomized trial, data from this particular program were gathered. The intervention group's average length of stay in the hospital was two days shorter than that of the controls, a significant difference.

Planning for posthospital care is a complex, time-consuming process that involves the entire team of providers. It requires creativity, a knowledge of available resources, assertiveness in connecting with those resources, and close follow-up. Some specific ideas that involve collaboration with medical providers include beginning to assess discharge needs at the time of admission, encouraging patients to write down questions they might have before leaving, and tape-recording the discharge interview. Skills in the collaborative networking band of the spectrum (see chapter 8) are critical for a mental health care provider in this role.

BARRIERS TO COLLABORATION IN
HOSPITAL SETTINGS

There are at least five barriers to effective collaboration with patients or between providers that are unique to the hospital setting. The first is the attitude of providers toward the involvement of patients and families in their own care. Often they do not share information directly with patients. Providers may talk with each other but present only a summary to the patient and family. When freedom of expression among providers is necessary, private conversations are warranted. But consistent exclusion of the patient and family can also be detrimental to care.

Bill Schwab is a family physician in Minnesota, the father of a child with special needs, and an advisory board member for the Institute for Family-Centered Care. He talks about what he learned from experiencing the medical system as a patient's family member:

> There were multiple providers doing individual interviews and testing with our child, but since many of them asked the same questions, you had the feeling they were not talking with each other. It would have seemed they could have shared some of the basic information so it would not have felt so fragmented and separate for us. In addition, when they got together to discuss the individual reports and look for common themes and direction, we would have liked to hear that discussion so we could have made our own conclusions based on the data presented. When we only got the group summary, we didn't get to hear any minority opinions or disagreements. Ultimately, whose information is this? I think patients and family members should be in the room much more often than they are when their case is discussed.

John Rolland sees providers' general ambivalence about confronting their own and the patient's limitations and vulnerability as one explanation for the difficulty they can have dealing directly with the patient. Hospitals are often the setting for cases that involve life-threatening consequences, severe loss, disability, or change of ongoing health status. "We don't like confronting our own mortality," says Rolland. A second reason may be a fear of losing a "professional edge." If providers allow themselves to become personally touched by patients and families, they may lose the objectivity necessary to treat them effectively. However, Rolland does not find these reasons compelling enough to justify professional distance. Speaking as a psychiatrist and a family member of an ill patient, Rolland agrees strongly with Suzanne Mintz, executive director of the NCFA, who said, "Only if you understand our feelings can you help us learn to cope."

A second barrier is the stereotypical role definition of mental health professionals in a hospital setting. Medical social work is a good example. Many physicians, health care providers, and social workers themselves retain a stereotyped picture of the social worker as a welfare worker, only capable of discharge planning and helping people get into governmental aid programs. Broadening the role possibilities to include consultant, educator, and coprovider is important.

A third barrier to effective collaboration is the current knowledge and skills of mental health care providers working in hospital settings. According to Patricia Meadows, director of social work at Duke University, the role of a medical social worker is radically different from what it was a few years ago. Historically, the primary role has been to take referrals from physicians and assist in planning for the patient's discharge, often without significant input from the rest of the team. According to Meadows, the skills of medical social workers must expand if they are to be successful. Now social workers need to be flexible enough to create different roles and move across departmental lines easily. As described by MaryAnne Zabrycki, they need to be assertive and confident in the value of their input. They need to recognize the many different customers they serve—patients, families, providers, third-party payers. It is important for a social worker to be assertive in carving out a job role that matches the needs of the situation and in providing direction as an equal team member, rather than only taking directions. The capacity to think about and facilitate the effective functioning of the health care team in relationship to the patient is just as important as the traditional role of discharge planner.

A fourth barrier to collaboration is the division between structures and services in hospitals that make it difficult to obtain needed consultation in a timely fashion. Wayne Katon, a leader in the consultation-liaison (C-L) field of psychiatry, feels that mental health consultation is typically requested too late in a patient's hospitalization to be effective. Katon feels that treatment would be more integrated and satisfying to both providers and patients if mental health care providers were involved in potentially difficult situations early in the process. C-L services are most effective when the psychiatrist and the team have developed a relationship over time. It is easier under this arrangement for the mental health professional to be involved early. If that person is present at all staff meetings, the relationship between providers develops.

A fifth barrier is the place of hospital care in the overall health care delivery system. The emphasis is quickly shifting to outpatient care; more and more often, a hospital admission is seen as a failure of the system. When patients are admitted, the goal is to discharge them as soon as possible. One administrator predicts that the hospitals of the future will be large intensive-care units. In this time-pressured context with multiple providers who each have a different view of the problem, finding the time for meaningful dialogue and effective collaboration is a challenge.

RECOMMENDATIONS FOR COLLABORATION IN HOSPITAL SETTINGS

The current trend in health care is away from high-technology, hospital-based medicine. Nevertheless, patients continue to need hospital care. Such care must be provided in a different way in order to meet the current expectations about cost- and care-effective services. Collaborative care is a creative means of pursuing this goal. We offer the following suggestions for collaborating in hospital settings:

1. *Keep abreast of the current trends in hospital care.* Read journals such as *Hospitals and Health Networks, Health Affairs,* and the *Millbank Quarterly.* Understand particularly the projects that promote patient-centered care. Be an advocate for paying more attention to processes that add patient and family input and coordinate provider services.
2. *Approach areas within the hospital setting that naturally include biomedical and psychosocial concerns.* These include cardiac rehabilitation, dialysis, and infectious diseases. Learn as much about the disease processes in these settings as possible.
3. *Maintain an open referral system so that any staff member can ask you for help.* If you keep referrals limited to physicians, you may be missing cases that need attention. If you get a referral from any team member, consider how the rest of the team can be involved.
4. *Be aware of the potential for splitting when multiple providers are involved in patient care.* Try not to take sides with patients and families against medical providers, or with medical providers against patients and families. Advocate for the whole team. Keep communication open between you, the medical team, and the patient and family.

5. *Cultivate collaborative networking skills.* Coordinating services and getting the right people to talk to each other at the right time may be the most therapeutic strategies.
6. *See physicians and other health care practitioners as customers for your services.* Be practical in responding to their needs, but do not take on tasks that are inappropriate or should be shared.
7. *Participate in hospital ethics committees and keep abreast of the ethical issues involved in hospital care.* One role you can fill on the team is asking questions in difficult situations to help clarify the ethical issues involved.
8. *Maintain a dual identity with the team of health/mental health care providers and with your professional discipline.* APA Division 16— Health Psychology, Medical Social Workers, or Consultation-Liaison Psychiatry—is an example.

CONCLUSION

This chapter has provided an overview of collaboration in the secondary or tertiary care environment. Hospitals have been the setting for significant efforts to be more collaborative with patients and families as well as with providers from different specialties. Organizations such as Planetree, Picker, the Institute for Family-Centered Care, the Well Spouse Foundation, and the National Family Caregivers Association are supporting such efforts. However, it would be misleading to say that these efforts are the majority voice in the reform of our traditionally inpatient-focused health care system. Turning health care into more of a business has had both positive and negative effects. It would also be misleading to say that the pendulum swing toward managed care is only shifting costs from inpatient to more creative outpatient or intensive outpatient programs. In truth, it is currently difficult to talk about cost savings, quality service, and humane, collaborative treatment at the same time.

Even though the overall costs for health care in this country have been exceedingly high, we are hopeful that, as actual excesses are recognized and better managed, hospitals and networks that are stable enough to look at longer-term savings and quality provision of care will increasingly adopt collaborative models as a way of accomplishing both goals.

CHAPTER 13

Up-Front Money: Collaboration and Managed Care

In 1933, in the southern California desert, construction companies paid Sidney Garfield 5¢ a day to provide medical care (Belar, 1995). This arrangement marked the beginning of the Kaiser Permanente Health Plan, the oldest health maintenance organization in the country and today's largest HMO. Between 1933 and 1970, managed care grew slowly in the United States, reaching only 3 million enrollees by 1970 (Miller & Luft, 1994a). In the last decade, managed care has grown exponentially. HMO enrollment in 1988 was 32.6 million. Over the next six years, enrollment grew 56%, reaching 51.1 million in 1994, surpassing 20% of insured Americans (Bernstein, Bergsten, Whitmore, Dial, & Gabel, 1994). HMO enrollment is only part of the managed-care picture. Other forms of managed care, such as preferred provider organizations (PPOs) and managed fee-for-service (FFS) programs, are equally as prevalent in America. In 1984 the total percentage of insured Americans who relied on one of these three managed-care forms for their health care was just over 10%. Ten years later, close to 80% of insured Americans were in some form of managed care. Projections place 90% of the insured in some form of managed care by the year 2000, the majority in HMO or PPO plans (Pyle & Brunk, 1995).

This dynamic, multidimensional health care revolution means different things to different people. To many practitioners and health care administrators, the influx of managed care means earning less money, doing more work, and feeling less secure about the future. Others view managed care as a way to save money, increase health care access for consumers, and provide a fair way to distribute limited resources. Some clinicians enjoy increased control of health care decisions and the spending of health care dollars. Other clinicians feel more constricted in their clinical activities. Some consumers resent restrictions on their choice of provider. Others praise lower out-of-pocket costs and preventive measures.

Today, in the midst of a health care revolution, little is certain, save the assurance that more change is on the way. New companies are forming while many are folding. Mergers and acquisitions are reported daily. Competition for market share is intense. While some people hope and pray for a return to the old way of doing things, most agree that managed care, in some form, is here to stay for the foreseeable fortune.

In this chapter, we examine collaboration in the context of managed care. The first section begins by describing managed-care procedures and organizational forms and concludes with a summary of research on managed care and managed mental health care. The second section examines factors affecting collaboration in managed care: organizational purpose, financial arrangements, and operational features. In the last section, we offer strategies for enhancing collaborative designs in managed care.

MANAGED CARE—IN SEARCH OF DEFINITIONS AND PURPOSE

Describing managed care as a single entity is like suggesting that all the world's people speak the same language. Designs and purposes vary enormously and change rapidly. In a parallel fashion, highly varied collaborative designs are evolving quickly. In researching this chapter, we read dozens of articles and interviewed over 20 providers, administrators, and researchers in the managed-care field. We were struck by the range of perspectives and beliefs these authors and interviewees expressed in defining organizational types, describing the value of various managed-care procedures, and discussing collaborative designs. We find that as managed care has matured, collaborative practice is emphasized more and more. What follows is our synthesis, augmented with our own opinions and beliefs.

Why Managed Care?

Attempts to answer this question focus on two closely linked issues: cost and quality. Today the cost of medical care is approaching 15% of the federal budget. Yet for several populations, including the mentally ill, pregnant teens, and the poor, access to and quality of care is worse than in many other Western nations. Controlling overall costs enables the redistribution of resources to those who are underserved. Some managed-care companies are accused of emphasizing cost control over quality. Managed-care profit ventures can produce large dividends for shareholders and hefty salaries for executives. However, most managed-care systems monitor their quality through internal and external assessments. According to the Group Health Association of America (GHAA), HMOs are rapidly increasing service to the poor and elderly. Soon 70% of HMOs will offer Medicare plans, and roughly 50% will offer Medicaid plans (Bernstein et al., 1994).

What Is Managed Care?

The answer to this question follows directly from the question above, "Why managed care?" If care should be managed to control cost and quality, then describing "what" is to be managed should address the same two issues. However, definitions of managed care vary greatly. Many combine "what" is managed care with "how" to manage care. That is, describing the overall purpose of managed care is confused with describing the methods used to manage care. To eliminate confusion, it is important to examine these two issues separately.

In simple terms, managing care involves a contract to assume responsibility for all or some portion of the care needed by a person or a population. *This contract is made before the patient seeks care.* The arrangement departs from fee-for-service designs, under which providers respond to patient needs on a case-by-case basis.

While contract terms may vary from company to company, three criteria must be met to qualify as a managed-care company. Such a company must demonstrate efforts to: (1) control the quality of care being provided to the patients within its contract; (2) regulate the use of financial resources in the provision of that care; and (3) provide comprehensive care for all patients within the company's enrollment.

Next we turn to the ways managed-care companies accomplish these goals.

How Is Care Managed?

One method for managing care is virtually universal and so deserves special mention: defining a network of providers. The definition of this network implies a contract between the managed-care organization (MCO) and specified providers covering issues of cost and quality. Table 13.1 lists common managed-care roles and procedures for cost and quality control.

Managed-care plans vary in their structure. Table 13.2 provides a list of common managed-care plans and organizations.

Various mixes of managed-care procedures are used in MCOs. The type of MCO determines, in part, the complexity and sophistication of this procedural mix (Wagner, 1993). Managed-care procedural recipes run the gamut in their effects on cost control and quality of care (Miller & Luft, 1994a). In a similar fashion, these recipes influence provider behavior, especially provider incentive to collaborate.

Approaches such as utilization management (UM), used in isolation, represent a simple managed-care procedural design. These less sophisticated arrangements are likely to make providers defensive and thus less disposed to the collaborative mind-set. Conversely, complex organizational structures incorporate a variety of procedures, such as flexible benefits, capitated arrangements, incentive plans, continuing education, profiling, UM, gatekeeping, and case management. These organizational designs have more influence over provider behavior. Under this organizational type, providers are more likely to share accountability and ownership for organizational success or failure (Cave, 1995; Devers, Shortell, Gillies, Anderson, Mitchell, & Erickson, 1994). The resulting sense of shared responsibility enhances the need and desire for collaborative activity. Overhead increases along with complexity, but so also does the potential for controlling cost and quality. Again, what we describe applies to both comprehensive managed-care organizations and to specialty plans such as managed mental health care companies.

TABLE 13.1

MANAGED-CARE TERMS: ROLES AND PROCEDURES
FOR COST AND QUALITY CONTROL

At risk: Assuming full or partial financial responsibility for the health care of a population, and assuming a capitated contract.

Benefit flexing: Allocating funds from one budgetary division to another. For example, using inpatient dollars to pay for outpatient care. Case management personnel have the authority to make these decisions.

Capitation: Prepaid health care. Money paid or received, usually in per member per month (PMPM) units.

Case management: The utilization management (UM) and coordination of care for patients with complex needs. The purpose is to provide quality and continuous care at low cost.

Clinical guidelines: Systematically developed protocols to assist providers and patients in clinical decisions. Protocols attempt to incorporate research outcome data, provider preferences, and patient behavior into clinical recommendations.

Concurrent review: Ongoing evaluation and approval of procedures or services, particularly expensive ones.

Copayment: Fee paid by enrollee at the time of the visit. The fee amount influences the willingness of the enrollee to use health care services. Fee structures can be graduated to deter overuse without preventing initial access.

Education: Education may be provided by external consultants or internal continuing education departments.

FFS (fee-for-service): Payment for health care after delivery of service. In managed care, providers often agree to receive discounted fees.

Gatekeeping: A type of case management wherein a primary care physician regulates and authorizes specialty services.

Incentive systems: The reinforcement of behavior, usually with monetary reward. Money comes from company profits or unused capitation. Other forms of incentive include educational opportunities and time off.

Precertification: Required authorization prior to provision of services.

Primary care: Responsibility to provide health maintenance, preventive care, and comprehensive health care over time. Coordination of care by specialists is an essential part of this role.

Profiling: Data used to describe an MCO provider behavior: expenses, referrals, number of visits, consumer survey results. Profiles may compare organization and peer group trends with individual statistics.

Utilization management (UM): Combination of precertification and concurrent review. Sometimes called utilization review (UR).

TABLE 13.2

MANAGED-CARE TERMS:
PLAN AND ORGANIZATION TYPES

Group model: An HMO with an exclusive contract with a group of providers. Sometimes the provider group sees only patients from one plan.

HMO (health maintenance organization): A health care organization that assumes financial responsibility for its enrollees. Payment is made before delivery of services. Health care is usually coordinated by primary care physician.

IPA (independent practice association): An intermediary organization that assumes capitated contracts with an HMO to provide services. Providers are independent or in small groups and paid either FFS or in capitation.

Managed FFS: Indemnity plans using UM. No provider networks.

MCO (managed-care organization): A managed care organization contracts to assume responsibility for all or some portion of the care needed by a person or a population.

Mixed model: An MCO combining a variety of organization types, e.g., staff, network, PPO.

Network: An HMO contracting with large groups and multispecialty groups without an intermediary.

POS (point of service): An HMO feature by which services by non-plan providers are paid, usually at lower reimbursement rates.

PPO (preferred provider organization): A network of providers who negotiate discounted fees prior to delivery of services. UM and profiling are often used.

Staff model: An HMO that employs providers who see enrollees in facilities owned by the HMO.

Research

Published research examining cost savings and quality in full-service managed care is limited. In general, results suggest that managed care lowers cost without compromising quality of care. In their review in the *Journal of the American Medical Association,* Robert Miller and Harold Luft examined "Managed Care Plan Performance since 1980" (1994b). Most savings come from inpatient changes. While some studies showed that HMOs have reduced rates of hospital admission, most studies showed shorter lengths of stay for inpatients in HMO plans. There was no clear trend showing more or less use of outpatient services in the general medical arena. However, "HMOs use an average of 22% fewer procedures, tests or treatments that were expensive or had less costly alternative interventions. Moreover, HMO enrollees consistently received more preventive tests, procedures and examinations or health promotion activities than did indemnity plan enrollees" (p. 1515).

Sixteen studies showed that HMO plan members had either equal or better quality-of-care results compared to fee-for-service enrollees on a "wide range of conditions, diseases and interventions" (Miller & Luft, 1994a, p. 439). The one notable exception, according to the Miller and Luft analysis, was in mental health, where two studies showed HMO enrollees received poorer care. Both of these studies came from the Medical Outcomes Study. In one of them, depression was detected at a lower rate in HMO medical settings compared to detection of depression in indemnity plan medical settings (Wells, Hays, Burnam, Rogers, Greenfield, & Ware, 1989). In the second study, patients in prepaid settings who were receiving care from psychiatrists had more functional impairment after two years than patients seeing psychiatrists in FFS systems. This effect was particularly evident in independent provider associations (IPAs) (Rogers, Wells, Meredith, Sturm, & Burnam, 1993). We discuss the implication of these and related findings later in the chapter.

Enrollee satisfaction surveys showed mixed evaluations. Most HMO enrollees reported lower levels of satisfaction with quality of care and physician-patient interactions than did FFS enrollees. However, HMO enrollees were equally or more satisfied than FFS enrollees with the financial aspects of their care.

The finding that HMO enrollees are equally or more satisfied with the costs of care as FFS participants is supported by data from GHAA. Note the following trends in HMO member premiums. In 1992, HMOs reported a 10.6% increase in premiums; in 1993 an 8.1% increase; and in 1994 a 5.6% increase. Projections for 1995 are a 1.2% decrease in premiums (Bernstein et al., 1994). A limited number of studies and surveys also suggest that HMO premiums are lower than FFS premiums (Miller & Luft, 1994a). In the general medical care arena, it appears that cost-containment goals have been largely achieved. Now more effort is being directed toward improving quality of care and enrollee satisfaction. HMOs know that quality of care and consumer satisfaction are important. The GHAA 1994 performance report showed 97% of HMOs conduct consumer satisfaction surveys. Data from these surveys are used for quality improvement, provider feedback, and, of course, marketing.

MENTAL HEALTH AND MANAGED CARE

The inclusion of mental health benefits and services in managed care recapitulates our country's history of integrating mental health care. Interested readers are referred to several authors who review mental health's history in the context of managed care (Belar, 1995; Bennett, 1993; Mauksch & Leahy, 1993; Mechanic, 1994). Opposition to the inclusion of mental health in insurance benefits has taken many forms. In addition to barriers created by providers and health care administrators, HMO consumers have been unwilling to pay for these benefits when plans proposed their inclusion (Mauksch & Leahy, 1993). Apprehension about affordability is a consistent barrier. There continues to be no consensus on what HMOs should treat and what constitutes appropriate treatment.

The HMO Act of 1973 included requirements for minimum mental health benefits, not to exceed 20 outpatient visits to cover evaluation, crisis intervention, and short-term treatment (Congressional Committee Report, 1975). By the end of the 1980s, many corporations found themselves in a dilemma: Health care costs represented the fastest-growing portion of their budgets (Mauksch & Leahy, 1993). Employees complained of inadequate mental health care. Waiting times were too long, access was too limited, contact was too brief.

In response to corporate pressure for cost control and for improved quality of mental health care, we are seeing the growth and consolidation of the managed mental health industry. Sometimes mental health care is "carved out" of the health care contract with a comprehensive health care company; mental health care is covered under a separate, usually capitated arrangement. The carve-out company is "at risk" for the mental health care of its enrollees. The remainder of the health care is the responsibility of a different health care organization. Linkages between the carve-out managed mental health company (MMHC) and the general health care corporation vary in complexity but in general appear to be limited because most of the key ingredients for collaboration are missing (communication, relationship, location of service, etc.).

These companies are attractive to employers for several reasons. MMHC contracts can be evaluated separately from general medical costs. Employers purchase professional expertise promising reduction in costs. When carving out, companies protect themselves from the financial risks of providing mental health care but are assured that a predetermined amount of money will be spent on mental health instead of being lost in a general medical budget. MMHCs develop networks covering larger geographic areas than those covered by PPOs or group and staff model HMOs (Starr & Findlay, 1994). MMHCs boast cost savings, particularly through savings from reduced inpatient admissions and reduced lengths of stay in the hospital.

Quality of Care—Managed Mental Health Research

Mechanic, Schlesinger, and McAlpine (1995) offer a comprehensive review of the literature on managed mental health care and substance abuse services. Their warning: "Reducing the use of mental health services is no difficult accomplishment; doing so in a way that maintains or enhances quality without shifting costs is far more difficult and problematic" (pp. 47–48). It seems clear that managed care is reducing costs. As mentioned earlier, savings come primarily through reductions in inpatient expenses and the substitution of a variety of outpatient services. However, most of the evidence for cost reduction comes from companies that previously had higher costs. That is, after implementing managed-care approaches, higher-cost MMHCs show greater savings but their expenses continue to be higher than those of previously lower-cost companies. Thus, it remains unclear which techniques to use, with which problems, and in what settings. Some evidence exists, largely from the Medical Outcomes Study (Hays, Wells, Sherbourne, Rogers, & Spritzer, 1995; Rogers et al., 1993; Wells, Hays, et al., 1989) that enrollees in prepaid plans are less likely to have their mental health problems diagnosed, and that the most severely ill are more likely to be inadequately treated. In prepaid plans, a larger proportion of patients were treated by their general medical providers and undertreated by psychiatrists.

Well-designed studies on the quality of care in managed care are almost nonexistent. Mechanic, Schlesinger, and McAlpine (1995) note that short-term success does not necessarily mean long-term savings. They suggest that the nature of prepaid systems, at their best, allows for the flexible use of services. But when standard cost-reduction techniques are applied across the board with little sensitivity to patient needs, quality may suffer.

One finding is repeated in many studies over the last 30 years. The majority of people who seek care for mental illness are seen first, and often only, in the general medical sector. For example, three large, prospective studies examined population behavior in FFS and prepaid plans. The Rand Health Insurance Experiment (5,800 enrollees) (Wells, Manning, Duan, Newhouse, & Ware, 1987), the Medical Outcomes Study (11,200 enrollees) (Wells, Stewart, et al., 1989), and the Epidemiological Catchment Area Study (22.8 million people) (Regier, Narrow, Rae, Manderscheid, Locke, & Goodwin, 1993) all showed that at least half of the population sought mental health care from their general medical providers. These patients feel ill. Their illnesses are not confined to symptom presentations that neatly fall into categories owned by one discipline or another.

Long-term users of psychotherapy seeing mental health specialists (MHS) report poorer general health and mental health than those who seek short-term psychotherapy from either MHSs or general medical providers (Olfson & Pincus, 1994). Similarly, the highest users of general medical care have four to five times the incidence of mental illness as the average user of general medical services (Katon et al., 1992). Mental illness has a greater and independent association with disability than medical illness does (Hays et al., 1995); this is not only a cultural feature but a cross-cultural phenomenon (Ormel et al., 1994).

This research, combined with accumulated clinical experience and patient feedback, is changing service design and delivery in managed care. In late 1994 the Commission on Health Care Services of the American Academy of Family Physicians produced a "White Paper on the Provision of Mental Health Care Services by Family Physicians" (AAFP, 1994). The commission concludes: "A collaborative model, which integrates both primary care and specialty mental health services, can best meet the needs of our patients and introduce substantial cost savings into a benefits package" (p. 4). Historically, treatment of mental health in HMOs has been underfunded. But now full-service HMOs are expanding benefits and offering comprehensive programs that target specific populations (Budd & Gruman, 1995; Hoyt, 1994; Nelson, Mensing, Baines, & Smith, 1995; Strosahl, 1994). In the managed mental health sector, clinicians and administrators are working to build bridges to the medical sector. Even advocates of carve-out models recognize the importance of collaboration (Shusterman, 1995). Finally, accumulated experience, data, and actuarial expertise make it possible to accurately predict the cost of mental health services (McGuire, 1994). This capacity, which takes into account population characteristics and managed-care designs, can help dispel the myths of "out of control" costs surrounding mental health designs.

Managed care is entering a new era of maturity. One hears a common theme in health care jargon—"integrated care," "seamless delivery systems," "one-stop shopping," "continuous and comprehensive care." These phrases are not just marketing slogans. The duplication of services, information loss between providers, and unnecessary administrative expense of discontinuous and disconnected care make it a lower-quality and costly form of care. Health problems rarely exist as discrete, unidimensional entities. An appreciation of the interwoven complexities of human function is influencing the designs of service delivery. Managed care is embracing integration of services as a central organizing principle. In the next section, we examine the characteristics and activities of organizations and individuals who promote collaborative care designs.

CREATING FERTILE GROUND: COLLABORATION IN MANAGED CARE

Establishing collaborative designs in environments that are unfavorable is "like trying to grow palm trees in northern Minnesota," says Michael J. Bennett. Dr. Bennett, a psychiatrist, draws his perspective from more than 30 years in mental health, mostly in managed-care settings. He is corporate vice president for medical services for Merit Behavioral Care Corporation, one of the largest MMHCs. Earlier, he worked as a consultation-liaison psychiatrist teaching general medical providers. Michael Bennett's ideas are recorded in several articles he has written over the years (Bennett, 1983, 1993, 1994). He is a member of the clinical faculty of the Harvard Medical School. Here is a summary of his recent thinking (Bennett, 1994; personal communication, August 5, 1995):

> Carve-outs must build bridges back to primary care and specialized medical care if the needs of patients who seek their mental health care from their medical physicians are to be adequately met. Medical caregivers require support, education, and consultation; classsical carve-outs have little incentive to meet such needs. Reimbursement mechanisms can create competition and undermine collaboration when there is too much emphasis on dividing the pie. Caregivers must learn to work together. Financial models alone will not promote collaborative patterns of care; however,

attitudes and beliefs must also change. Shifts in attitudes and in the paradigms of treatment require training that is sensitively attuned to the variables associated with healing and promoting health in our patients.

Collaborative systems in the managed-care environment will grow and flourish in the proper environment, just as palm trees grow tall with enough heat and sunlight and the correct soil composition. Embedded in Bennett's comments are a few of the components necessary to sprout and sustain collaborative care. In our reading and our interviews, there seemed to be a consensus about the importance of these components. One of the most articulate on the subject comes, in fact, from a palm grove in Minnesota.

Health Partners, a Twin Cities HMO with over 600,000 enrollees, has used collaborative designs for 10 years. C. J. Peek, former director of integrated care and now consulting psychologist for medical management development, offers a formula that summarizes much of what we have learned. He describes a "three world view" (Peek & Heinrich, 1995). The three worlds are: financial, operational, and clinical. Addressing all three of these areas and aligning them to complement one another creates a cultural change within the organization. A new organizational mission or purpose emerges.

At Health Partners, "health psychologists" are located in 19 clinics, including many primary care settings and specialty clinics such as oncology, endocrinology, and temporomandibular disorder clinics. Patients who need specialty or long-term mental health care are referred to a mental health specialty setting. Peek describes the operation:

> The financial and operational systems of the organization have to mirror the clinical approach for things to work well as a whole. That is, benefits and clinic structure must follow the clinical paradigms. For example, the organization is paid in advance as a team for the care of a population of patients. Therefore, when a patient walks into a medical clinic seeking care for a problem that turns out to have significant psychosocial contributing factors, the patient's physician needs to be able to involve the health psychologist as a normal part of the medical team, "just one of our docs," for the medical care of the patient and family. The health psychology visit is therefore considered a medical visit, not a mental health visit, for purposes of cost-tracking and copayments.
>
> Moreover, the health psychologist is right there on-site, with his or her name on the wall just like the physicians and other

providers, and works off the same scheduling system with the same receptionists and waiting areas. The clinic's health psychologists write in the medical chart on the same forms as the physicians and other providers. The health psychologist works out of ordinary medical exam rooms in the medical hallways so that the medical frame of reference for the visit remains in place clinically, operationally, and financially. This is very important to the large majority of patients, who see their health problems as medical rather than "psychiatric" or "all in my head."

As patients learn more about their symptoms, sufferings, and illnesses through treatment in the medical clinic, many come to recognize that they have an important mental health agenda to pursue as part of their overall care. When this happens, they are then usually happy to accept referral to specialty mental health care or ordinary counseling or therapy.

The health psychologists work within the medical culture, making themselves flexibly available for "spot consults," but do see scheduled patients for an hour at first, often with shorter follow-ups once a care plan is negotiated and in place.

No one of the components—financial, operational, and clinical—is more important than the others in creating a collaborative environment. Each of the components has potent influence on the others. Conceived incongruently, any of them could impede or prevent collaboration in the health care organization.

Organizational Purpose

One example of organizational purpose promoting collaboration began in 1974. Five independent southern California medical groups, each carrying prepaid contracts, formed the Unified Medical Group Association (UMGA). According to its fact sheet, UMGA is "dedicated to excellence in the delivery of prepaid healthcare services. The Association provides extensive educational, informational and support services to help its members maintain high quality standards in health care." Its 90 medical groups employ more than 10,000 physicians, providing care to more than 4 million enrollees in prepaid plans. UMGA helped create The Medical Quality Commission (TMQC), a separate nonprofit organization dedicated to research and quality in health care. TMQC accreditation involves meeting behavioral health standards and is required for full membership in UMGA. Among the standards is the development of multidisciplinary teams that include primary care physicians.

UMGA has a behavioral health subcommittee, formed in response to carve-out designs, which UMGA felt were detrimental to quality patient care. The work of this subcommittee spawned another company, closely allied with UMGA and TMQC, the Behavioral Health Medical Corporation (BHMC). BHMC now works with 10 medical groups, caring for 800,000 capitated lives.

One of the original UMGA medical groups was Bristol Park Medical Group. Bristol Park's director of behavioral health care was John Sherman, now the CEO of BHMC. "Behavioral health is primary care," says Dr. Sherman. BHMC therapists work "hand in hand" with physicians. BHMC's consultation to medical groups to develop integrated systems includes therapist training, financial planning, and a medical information system that provides record-keeping, research capability, and communication linkages. Therapists are employees of the groups. Groups contribute portions of capitated funds from various HMO contracts to hire therapists. Groups can also "flex benefits," if medically indicated; approval of service is done on a case-by-case basis, with the treating therapist determining indication. Financial incentives for the therapists are aligned with incentives for the medical groups.

Organizational purpose that encourages collaborative designs is most obvious in HMOs in which financial systems are self-contained, such as staff and group models. The Kaiser Foundation Health Plan (Belar, 1995), the Group Health Cooperative of Puget Sound (Mauksch & Leahy, 1993; Quirk et al., in press), and the Harvard Community Health Plan include programmatic components that promote collaboration. All these plans have internal research divisions and internal training departments augmented by elaborate relationships with universities. Collaborative efforts in these and other HMOs started 30 years ago. Some of these efforts sputtered, and some failed. Failure happened when one or more of the three macro components—financial, operational, clinical—were not aligned to sustain collaboration.

Financial Designs

Financial structures, the heart of managed care, influence provider behaviors and patient behaviors in a variety of ways. In organizational and economic terms, this influence is called *incentive*. Managed mental health systems (MMHS) are often criticized for emphasizing cost control and compromising quality of care. Supporting collaboration while also meeting cost and quality goals is a difficult task. Combining capitated designs with other incentives can promote collaboration while maintaining quality at reasonable cost. When all providers share responsibility for controlling costs and maintaining quality care, then they have the incentive to work together. To better understand this, it is helpful to consider capitation from a few perspectives: (1) methods of provider reimbursement, (2) horizontal alignment, and (3) budgetary boundary permeability.

Methods of Provider Reimbursement

Various provider payment schemes exist: payment for billed charges (FFS), payment of a negotiated fee (PPO arrangement), case fee (managing an episode of care), capitation, and salary are all health care payment schemes (Grimaldi, 1995). When an MCO pays providers on a fee-for-service basis, providers do not share the financial risk of the company. In FFS designs, provider behaviors are controlled through UM and fee negotiation techniques that do not provide incentive to collaborate. Paying providers a salary instills a moderate sense of cohesiveness and integration. When providers share the risk with an MCO or assume full risk for patient care, they feel responsible to one another, particularly if salary levels are contingent on group success. Distributing unused capitation funds or bonus money in an incentive plan is another way to influence provider behavior. Providing incentives to achieve positive clinical outcomes (Burlingame, Lambert, Reisinger, Neff, & Mosier, 1995), positive patient feedback (through surveys), or positive peer evaluations are also ways to motivate providers toward collaborative activities (Grimaldi, 1995). Today equity companies provide stock options for providers, creating even more incentive to work together. Equity companies are predicted to hold the most promise for sustainability and integration (Cave, 1995).

Horizontal Alignment

Horizontal alignment means that financial designs are uniform across provider divisions (e.g., primary care, specialty care, and mental health care). In many settings, primary care physicians are capitated while the specialists are paid on a fee-for-service basis. This is misalignment. The FFS-paid specialists have less incentive to share responsibility for patient care. Increasingly, specialists are assuming capitated contracts. The parallel nature of the contract design between specialists and primary care providers instills a similar sense of connection to the company. Adding an incentive system increases the potential for enhancing collaboration (Devers et al., 1994).

Budgetary Boundary Permeability

As one might imagine, when MCO administrators representing various health care departments attempt to divide up health care dollars, competition is more evident than cooperation. Each person has stories of distress. Their provider salary levels are not competitive. Quality of care is compromised owing to inadequate funding. Providers are overworked. Each complaint is a justification for getting a bigger piece of the budgetary pie. The rivalry between members of the same organization dilutes the feelings of shared ownership necessary to produce collaboration.

MCOs distribute percentages of the budget to company departments. Mental health divisions receive between 1% and 12% of patient care dollars. When MCOs hold funding levels below what is needed to meet the needs of patients, purchasers become disgruntled. They demand more mental health spending from the MCO and, to protect their interests, may decide to contract with a managed mental health company, carving out the mental health component of the budget. When this happens, a "perverse" incentive to inadequately treat patients is created. MMHS providers are motivated to send patients to their medical providers as soon as possible. Medical providers are motivated to refer to mental health specialists. For medical providers, this is a prescription for frustration. Many patients do not accept the referrals, and many others return with intertwined presentations of biomedical and psychosocial distress. It is like saying to the primary care physician, "Attend to the left side of the body, but not the right side."

An example of an organization seeking to provide integrated, collaborative, and truly comprehensive care through a hybrid group/network model is the North Coast Faculty Medical Group (NCFMG), based in Santa Rosa, California. By assuming full risk and controlling all primary and secondary care professional fees, and by sharing full risk on the facilities side of the ledger with a hospital partner, a core group of family physicians, nurse-practitioners, and psychologists have retained the flexibility to structure the delivery of care from the primary care provider's perspective with their fully capitated contracts. NCFMG, a member of the Sutter Medical Foundation, is composed of clinicians who are also on the faculty of the Family Practice Residency Program of Community Hospital, an affiliate of the University of California in San Francisco. The group provides care to a five-county area north and east of San Francisco.

This hybrid model includes about 30 salaried clinicians, including two psychologists, and about 220 contracted specialists, including 41 behavioral health care providers, of all types. We spoke with Don Ransom, NCFMG's behavioral health care director and professor of family and community medicine at UCSF. Dr. Ransom manages the mental health and substance abuse portion of the group's capitation and tracks provider and patient behaviors.

> We try very hard to keep the mental health money included in the general health plan capitation by demonstrating that we can provide comprehensive and high-quality care that is well coordinated with our primary care providers. I manage a mental health budget, a kind of "pseudo-cap," but did not want to take a subcapitation and be at risk. I think that is the wrong model for behavioral health care anyhow and creates perverse (dis)incentives. Keeping the money pooled and under group control means the family physicians and the behavioral health care director can decide together what mental health and substance abuse providers, services, and facilities are best. Being at full risk as a group, we can decide together how to allocate resources for preventive care and specialty care when patients need it. We can also share in the successful management of the plan at the end of the year. Because our mental health providers and primary care physicians have a history of working together and can respond quickly as a team, we have few hospitalizations. In fact, our hospitalizations for drug and alcohol problems significantly exceed our mental hospitalizations, even though the initial budget estimates were substantially the other way around.

Dr. Ransom describes a design that includes "flexibility of benefits," crossing specialty boundaries. This term, increasingly common in mental health contracts, means that case managers (Blase & Kaufman, 1994; German, 1994) within the system are empowered to make financial decisions based on patient needs. When money cannot flow between mental health and biomedical subdivisions, the system is not aligned with the complexities of human function. The financial structure maintains the mind-body barrier.

Operational Features

Imagine for a moment that your city needs a new public transportation system. Four city council members divide up the task, each one taking one quadrant of the city. One council member purchases a contract with the CARE Company—Comfort Area Railways Enterprise—for the northwest quadrant. A second council member purchases a contract with the SMART Company—Speedo Monorail Area Rapid Transit—for the northeast quadrant. A third council member finds the BEST Company—Bus Express Safe Transport—to serve the southwest quadrant. A fourth council member locates the TOTE Company—Taxis Offer Transportation Excellence—for the southeast quadrant. When all the systems are built, the four council members meet to test out the new "citywide transportation system." To their horror, they discover that there is no coordination between the four systems. They have to pay four different fees, schedules do not match, and operators in one system know very little about how to use the other three systems.

This story provides an extreme example of how a lack of coordination creates inefficient and ineffective systems. In health care organizations, operational features need to be aligned between themselves and in conjunction with financial and clinical designs to promote collaborative efforts. In studying MCO collaborative designs between mental health professionals and health care practitioners, we limit our discussion to three variables: leadership, architecture, and culture. Interested readers are referred to Devers et al. (1994); they have developed an "integration scorecard" listing 49 operational features such as human resource designs, financial management procedures, communication and information systems, support services, and strategic planning efforts.

Leadership

"The provider gets the money at the front end in capitated managed care," says Bruce Amundson, former vice president of Ethix Care Northwest, a managed Medicaid company in Washington State with 25,000 enrollees. While Dr. Amundson appreciates the "risk" of assuming a capitation contract, he focuses on the opportunities. Front-end money fosters a proactive stance to patient care. Dr. Amundson convinced the primary care providers to allot $2 per member per month (total capitation was $125 per member per month) to fund a "family health team." The team comprises a psychologist, nurse-practitioner, social worker, nurse-care manager, nurse-midwife, and health educator. Each new enrollee in the Ethix system receives a welcome call during which he or she is asked eight screening questions related to general health, sleep problems, emergency room and inpatient use, and issues associated with high medical utilization. Patients viewed as potentially high utilizers on the screening tool receive a 45-item questionnaire assessing medical, psychological, and social issues associated with high medical use: depression, high-risk pregnancy, general poor health, history of family mental illness, substance abuse, and other difficulties likely to remain undetected or untreated. "We know that 10% of the people will spend 70% of the dollars. So identify the 10%! We see primary care providers as family advocates rather than gatekeepers. They get patients into the best care," says Amundson. Screening information is given to the primary care physician, who decides what should be done. A member of the family team offers consultation or provides patients with education, makes a home visit, and supplies social work or mental health services or referrals.

While the program described above may seem like an innovative idea, its significance is not apparent. The health plan that Ethix contracted to administer *did not include benefits for the services provided by the family health team.* Dr. Amundson approved the use of capitated up-front funds to create collaborative health care designs. Without his vision and approval, such a program would never have been created.

Dr. Amundson possesses many characteristics commonly associated with effective leaders: strong communication and organizational skills, ability to work with groups, desire to empower others, and so forth. Like other leaders we interviewed, Dr. Amundson possesses one characteristic that is particularly useful in creating collaborative designs: He thinks systemically. Dr. Amundson's training and career experiences have required and honed his systemic problem-solving skills. Trained as a family physician, he has received additional training in mental health, including family counseling. His experiences include 15 years practicing family medicine in rural, urban, and training settings, teaching family medicine residents behavioral science skills, and consulting with rural communities to develop health care.

It is not necessary to be trained in family medicine or family therapy to think systemically. Many business and health care visionaries use systemic problem-solving skills. The willingness to do so is evident in anyone who expresses curiosity about different cultures, whether the culture of patients, of providers from other disciplines, or of other organizations.

Architecture

"Health care is fundamentally a relational experience—between patients and providers and between one provider and another. So in a human service system, smaller is better. Larger systems are more complex and more distant," notes Dr. Amundson. The principle that smaller is better is evident in the design of other managed-care systems, such as Health Partners (Nelson et al., 1995), the Group Health Cooperative of Puget Sound (Mauksch & Leahy, 1993), and Group Health Northwest. Service delivery units such as primary care clinics or specialty clinics need to incorporate and align all the factors described in these pages—financial risk, methods of reimbursement, interdisciplinary staffing, combined charts, benefit parity, and so forth. Such alignments create systems in which providers are accountable to one another. This accountability fosters "professional intimacy" (Rogers & Holloway, 1993). Clinics are compact and self-contained yet strongly connected to the surrounding health care system.

Linkages between clinical service units need to be multidimensional, bidirectional, and fast (Devers et al., 1994). For example, clinicians in primary care clinics should have relationships, communication systems, and referral structures with specialty mental health clinics, interdisciplinary settings like adolescent clinics or pain clinics, and inpatient units. Patients moving from one setting to another should feel known to new providers because financial information, clinical findings, and provider questions arrive in the new clinic before the patients do. Health care is continuous, elaborated, and deepened rather than fractionated or started over.

Culture

"The right kind of time at the beginning of a case saves time over the life of the case. . . . Watch the team score, not just your own score. . . . Health care relationship problems exacerbate health problems." Health Partners in Minnneapolis–St. Paul uses these and other case management mottoes to build much-needed common ground between diverse "professional ethnicities" that often do not understand each other and have a history of competition rather than cooperation (Peek & Heinrich, 1995). Health Partners, like other MCOs, works on a variety of levels to create a cultural transformation. In a circular fashion, changes evolve from operational changes and from a variety of training efforts. Training prepares clinicians for new interdisciplinary working relationships. In turn, new relationships introduce new skills, reinforce other skills, and foster a new outlook on health care. The result is the disappearance of "professional chauvinism" (Belar, 1995) and the emergence of an interdependent milieu.

"In developing interdisciplinary teams as our basic 'service delivery unit' (psychiatrists, nurses, adult, child, and chemical health therapists), we evolved from a professional, guild-oriented culture to functional units that are patient-centered," said Richard Heinrich, head of the Mental Health Department at Health Partners. "As mental health professionals contemplate collaborating with medical professionals, they often fear that they will not be valued and respected as colleagues. At Health Partners we have begun a training program that prepares mental health professionals to understand the 'medical culture' and to work in primary care clinics," says Heinrich. The training program comes from a 10-year health psychology pilot program. Health psychologists were recruited and trained to work in medical clinics as part of primary and specialty care teams. The success of this program sold collaborative care to other clinics and paved the way for mental health professionals to work in the medical clinics.

One of the first documented efforts to introduce collaboration into an HMO occurred in the mid–1970s at the Community Health Center Plan (CHCP) in New Haven, Connecticut (Coleman et al., 1979). At the time, CHCP was a small staff model HMO with 14,000 members. In 1974, six nonmedical mental health care providers were placed in several clinics to work with 14 primary care providers. Collaborative contacts were recorded during 16 separate, randomly selected weeks between October 1974 and November 1975. During the first week, the average number of collaborations was 32, compared to 75 during the 16th week. Overall, mental health professionals initiated 52% of the collaborative contacts, and primary care physicians initiated 48%. However, initiation by primary care providers increased over the course of the study. The authors speculate that this increase was due to "greater familiarity and trust between PCPs and MHCs arising out of continued collaboration" (p. 90). Interested readers will enjoy the entire article, which includes data about location and theme of collaboration, distribution of diagnosis, and an interesting discussion. Descriptions of other efforts to train collaborative teams in practice settings have been published (Bhatara, Fuller, & Unruh, 1994; Bray & Rogers, 1995; Katon et al., 1995; Mauksch & Leahy, 1993).

Pilot projects are best staffed with people who want to make them successful. Within primary care medicine, family physicians are the clinicians most likely to have been exposed to collaboration during training. A growing number of primary care internal medicine and pediatric programs are incorporating behavioral science curricula. Compared to primary care physicians, mental health professionals are less likely to have been exposed to collaborative designs in training or in practice. Certification as a family medicine residency requires the inclusion of behavioral science faculty and curricula. No such widespread curricular element exists in the mental health training world, even for the training of psychiatrists. Therefore, mental health care providers, more so than medical providers, must negotiate a major cultural transformation. This shift, despite its potential rewards, is predictably uncomfortable. Care must be taken to help providers adjust to new roles, alternative practice styles, and colleagues from other cultures. Mental health care providers able to come out of their "50 minutes corners" (Mauksch & Leahy, 1993, p. 126) are best suited to become HMO collaborative practitioners (Hoyt, 1994; Quirk et al., in press).

A GUIDE FOR PROMOTING COLLABORATION IN MANAGED CARE

1: *Show that effective, focused care of high utilizers saves money.*
  (a) Get the studies from the library, read them carefully, and have copies to share with administrators.
  (b) Show MCO administrators that half of the highest utilizers have psychiatric diagnoses such as depression and somatization disorder. This 10% consume 40–60% of health care dollars. Mental health care keeps people out of the hospital, shortens length of stay, and decreases unnecessary outpatient testing.
  (c) Educate the purchasers. Employers may know that psychiatric disability means more time away from work than most medical illnesses. However, they may not know that
    . these same patients see themselves as less well and so use more medical services. Seeking medical care often means

costly duplication of service when there is no integration and coordination of care.

(d) Describe how mental health problems go undetected in prepaid medical settings. They are more likely to cost the MCO more money down the road. Having mental health professionals available lessens the barriers to referral and enhances the willingness and ability of primary care providers to detect and refer mental health problems.

(e) Create a financial scenario to make your point. Use common psychosomatic presentations (know the literature first): chest pain, back pain, pelvic pain, headaches, childhood asthma, irritable bowel syndrome. Outline two cost scenarios, one with psychosocial evaluation and one without. The lab tests, studies, and imaging tests included in evaluations without psychosocial components cost much more than one hour of time with a mental health professional.

2: *Use language that has meaning to the listener.*

(a) When talking to an MCO administrator, use phrases like "bottom line," "product line," or "service line."

(b) When talking to physicians, suggest that you can save them some "headaches" or "backaches." Let them know you can help with the "thick chart" patients. Providers will experience less "burnout" and greater job satisfaction.

(c) Collaborative care increases consumer satisfaction. Patients feel cared for. They appreciate "one-stop shopping" and feel less stigma receiving care in collaborative care settings.

3: *Develop financial scenarios to fund mental health service.* In network and IPA HMOs, providers may be contracting with as many as 20 or 30 companies. A simple suggestion is to use between 1% and 10% of the combined capitation to hire mental health providers. The amount of money allotted depends on the needs of the population and the extent of services to be provided. One full-time counselor will be kept busy by three to four full-time equivalent (FTE) primary care physicians. A $50,000 salary should be no more than 1% of combined capitation pools if the practice population is at least 40% prepaid enrollees. A salaried mental health professional can see more people for less money than contracted FFS providers. Incoming mental health professionals should be viewed as part of the team, and their salary arrangements should have similar incentive structures once they are accepted into the practice. They should have access to practice population descriptions to develop programs to best meet population needs (see chapter 15). Profiles of their practice patterns should be provided to help all concerned feel that the mental health professional is aware of cost and service design effects.

4: *Keep up on the behavioral health literature.* Managed-care journals (e.g., *HMO Practice, Managed Care Quarterly*), mental health administration journals (e.g., *Journal of Mental Health Administration*), and health care management journals (e.g., *Health Care Management Review*) regularly include articles on behavioral health care innovations. These are useful in educating yourself, MCO administrators, and physicians.

5: *Use the suggestions listed elsewhere in this book.* As each day passes, a larger proportion of patients in your geographic area will be covered by managed-care plans. Developing good relationships and establishing regular, reciprocal communication structures are only enhanced in value within managed care.

CONCLUSION

In the beginning of this chapter, we suggested that the wide variety of today's managed-care approaches was analogous to the diversity of languages in the world. Despite these many differences, the people cared for across the myriad of managed-care cultures are more alike than different. We are all complex organisms who function in ways that contradict the precepts of mind-body dualism. Primitive attempts at managed care reveal the residue of a Cartesian split. More mature designs, though, promote integration in deference to the intricate nature of the human being.

This chapter describes some features of managed care that are oriented toward collaboration. As managed-care designs evolve, the capacity of providers to collaborate will be held at a premium. Many mental health professionals have felt shackled and disillusioned by isolated, shortsighted efforts to manage care. We believe these ineffective models will become a part of the past and be replaced by the designs described in this chapter. We hope that our readers now have an enhanced appreciation of the central role collaboration must play in managed care.

PART IV

Training and the Future of Collaboration

The future is here. Building on the concepts and experiences described thus far, part IV of this book gives the reader a glimpse of tomorrow and how to prepare for it. The description we provide is not ethereal; nor is it a prediction of activities 20 years from now. We describe initiatives that are emerging today, initiatives that are logical extensions of collaborative practice.

Chapter 14 describes collaborative training for mental health professionals. In chapter 11, we noted that a significant number of family medicine residency programs provide training for students in other disciplines, including mental health. Mental health professionals also learn collaborative skills in other settings. In the near future, we believe that collaborative practice will be a major emphasis in graduate school curricula, internships, fellowships, and postgraduate programs.

Chapter 14 focuses on three levels of training and profiles many existing training opportunities. It also provides a guide for those in search of training and for those who are thinking about developing new training initiatives. This is a rapidly evolving aspect of collaboration. In fact, during the writing of this book we observed significant growth and refinement in training for collaboration on all the levels we are proposing. Not surprisingly, the most exciting training models are in settings where progressive designs permeate the whole organization.

In our final chapter, the reader learns how collaborative models contribute to and are influenced by the surrounding health care environment. Nothing we describe is fantasy. In fact, all of what we describe has existed for several years, but in muted forms.

Economic pressures and managed-care designs are making many professionals, patients, and families anxious about the quality and cost of the care they are giving and receiving. These same pressures and designs also provide both the rationale and the financial means to support the emerging trends in collaboration that will enhance quality of care in a cost-effective manner. Chapter 15 outlines those broad trends and their implications for the future of collaborative practice.

We hope that the last two chapters give the reader solid ideas about how to train for the future and a way to conceptualize the next steps in the evolution of collaboration.

CHAPTER 14

Training for Collaboration

TRAINING IN COLLABORATION has a checkered history. Various programs have tried to develop integrated cross-disciplinary training, but few have passed the test of time, for financial and other reasons (Baldwin, 1994; Baldwin & Baldwin, 1979). Most mental health pioneers in collaboration acquired their knowledge and skills through on-the-job training. Some had previous personal experience with physicians and health care professionals. Others taught themselves, without the mentoring or support of mental health colleagues in the same setting. Only a few received formal training in collaboration. The pioneer collaborators have written enthusiastically about the effectiveness, pleasures, and difficulties of working with their health care colleagues and with patients and families (Cole-Kelly & Hepworth, 1991; Doherty, 1986; Glenn, 1985a, 1985b; McDaniel & Campbell, 1986).

Their work has roused the curiosity of other mental health professionals. However, traditional mental health training programs have been slow to offer courses in collaborative health care. A few programs have summarized their initial work (Hepworth, Gavazzi, Adlin, & Miller, 1985; Muchnick et al., 1993; Patterson & Magulac, 1994; Talen, Graham, & Walbroehl, 1994). Until recently, no training opportunities existed to prepare mental health professionals for this work. Today students and new professionals can build a foundation of knowledge and develop collaborative skills in a variety of ways.

In the United States, the delivery of health care continues to evolve. Some practicing physicians and other health care providers and mental health professionals have developed new relationships to deliver more effective care (Blount & Bayona, 1994; Dashiff, Greiner, & Cannon, 1990; Molinari, Taverna, Gasca, & Constantino, 1994). Now is the time for traditional health and mental health training programs to expand their curricula and clinical training opportunities in this area.

This chapter covers some of the current training opportunities in collaboration for mental health professionals in the United States. We explore the various levels of training available to health and mental health professionals, ranging from self-directed learning to intensive workshops, clinical placements, and entire curricula devoted to training the collaborative mental health professional.

The first level includes workshops, institutes, and course work that introduce the foundations of collaborative practice. These opportunities can be found in mental health graduate degree–granting institutions with a special interest in collaboration, postgraduate training programs, and seminars or workshops at state or national conferences. The second level provides clinical training, typically as practicums, internships, or fellowships. Susan McDaniel (1992), in the special 10th anniversary issue of *Family Systems Medicine*, said, "The most pressing concern of the 1990's is to train psychosocial specialists properly so as to enable them to participate in a biopsychosocial approach to medical care" (p. 280). She suggests that mental health internships and fellowships colocated with primary care providers are the best avenues for such training. These opportunities last one or more years and include supplemental didactic experiences. The third level of training integrates academic course work and clinical experiences and provides the training parallel to physicians and other health care professionals in training. This level involves the greatest time commitment and financial output. We believe it may be the most effective training model for mental health professionals interested in obtaining counseling skills with a collaborative perspective. Only a few of these programs are currently established in the United States; excellent training in collaboration is also being designed and implemented internationally (Graham, Senior, Dukes, Lazarus, & Mayer, 1993; Martinez, 1990).

More often than not, mental health professionals design their own training program using various settings to incorporate theoretical input with practical experience. They attend conferences and institutes and seek the clinical training that best meets their needs. Several faculty and students from across the country described their training to us. We believe their experiences may stimulate potential trainees and trainers to develop similar training opportunities without as much struggle. We conclude the chapter with our suggestions for obtaining and developing effective training in collaboration. Finally, the appendices include conference suggestions, a directory of training opportunities, a glossary of common medical terminology, and a format for chart documentation.

TRAINING OPPORTUNITIES

A variety of training opportunities are available for the new mental health professional interested in collaboration. Creative students can design an excellent experience that may include attending specialized training settings focused on collaborative care. A few such innovative training opportunities are flourishing across the country. For simplicity's sake, we review them in three broad areas: course work, clinical experience, and fully integrated cotraining programs.

Course Work

The health and mental health collaboration literature continues to grow. Becoming familiar with current trends is the most effective and least expensive way to learn the basics. Since collaborative family health care is a new approach for mental health professionals, most traditional mental health training programs do not yet offer organized courses on collaboration. One difficulty faculty face when approached by an interested student is that many teachers have no training in this area themselves. Consequently, they find it challenging to guide the eager student or develop the needed courses. Therefore, interested students may need to design an independent study with faculty support and guidance.

Degree-Granting Institutions

Jenny Speice, a graduate of the doctoral program in Marriage and Family Therapy at Virginia Polytechnic Institute and State University, developed her own independent study: "This area is so new to faculty; I selected what I wanted to read. I decided to write a paper at the end to show that I completed my study. To continue with this interest, I requested that I incorporate special medical family therapy topics into the more traditional marriage and family therapy courses."

Through her study, other students and faculty learned more about medical family therapy and collaboration with health care professionals: "I gave stacks of literature and reading lists to other students. I said, 'Here are some really important things that I think you should know.' Since I left Virginia, people have called and said, 'What was the list of materials you were reading?' I think students are now more interested."

Although Jenny felt more informed through the literature, she lacked the opportunity to discuss this new material and integrate it into her clinical training. She asked her clinic director to assign her medically related cases. Since the clinic had no active health care referral sources, only a few families presented to the clinic with health-related issues. Jenny wanted more training, so she continued her self-directed learning journey. She secured a clinical internship in a medical setting.

Another student designed a different training experience with his fellow students. Gary Bischof, a doctoral student in Purdue University's Marriage and Family Therapy Program, and several of his colleagues proposed a special elective course to supplement the required graduate curriculum. They designed the reading list, generated specific assignments, and asked Douglas Sprenkle, the department chairperson, to sponsor their course.

Bischof said, "We devoted the first four weeks to theory and conceptual materials. The second part was more application. Each student selected a topic to research and to present to the class. Topics covered were AIDS, chronic illness, aging, and enuresis." Since the study of collaboration was a new area for faculty as well, the faculty sponsor and students organized conference calls with experts in the field. These calls brought experienced collaborators into the class to discuss their work. The class read articles written by the experts before the phone conversation. Some invited speakers were Susan McDaniel, Don Bloch, William Doherty, and John Rolland. In addition, the class invited a behavioral scientist, Stephen Bogdewic, from a local Department of Family Medicine and a clinical psychologist from an HMO. "We were unsuccessful getting psychiatrists, nurses, or other physicians. If we had to do it again, we would try harder to arrange for their participation." This group also generated an annotated bibliography for their department's library. "We left it in the student lounge on a family systems medicine shelf."

The format used at Purdue gave students the opportunity to discuss the literature. However, they noted the lack of opportunities for collaborative clinical experiences around health issues. Both Speice and Bischof later attended conferences to meet other mental health clinicians who practiced in medical settings. The Society of Teachers of Family Medicine's Family in Family Medicine Conference finally provided the opportunity to talk with health care professionals. The American Association for Marriage and Family Therapy annual conferences presented them with opportunities to hear mental health professionals discuss case-based materials. They tried to see medically related cases referred to their own clinical setting during their clinical training; however, because this clinical area is still new, experienced supervisors were not readily available. Both obtained a medical family therapy internship to advance their clinical skills.

Some faculty in established training programs are integrating new material on collaboration into their curriculum. Jerry Gale, an associate professor in the University of Georgia's Marriage and Family Therapy Program, designed an open elective in medical family therapy for graduate students.

> I began this course, as many people may say, because of personal experience. My father had several heart attacks and several major heart surgeries three or four years ago. I spent much time with him in the hospital and with my mother and other family members. . . . So it made me interested in what goes on in that setting between patients and their physicians and other practitioners. . . . As a doctoral student, I worked on a project at Texas Tech University at the Health Sciences Center. We interviewed children whom the pediatricians referred for some type of heart problem. So two years ago, I decided I wanted to learn more about this. The good way to learn is to teach a course on it. I started contacting various people. Sherri Muchnick was putting the Medical Family Therapy Program together at Nova University. I joined an electronic-mail academic family medicine list. Through that I developed a new collegial relationship with a faculty member at the University of Arizona–Tucson. I went and visited her program last year.

Gale's story shows the evolving training process for collaborative health professionals and teachers. His journey began with an academic experience in his own training program. The personal experience with his father's hospitalization generated more curiosity. Finally, he decided to teach an elective course. The summer of 1995 was his second year of teaching the course; he plans to include more health care professionals as consultants to the class.

Conferences and Institutes

Those professionals who have completed their advanced degree may want to supplement their traditional training with brief educational experiences. Various annual conferences now include collaborative health care presentations. These annual events provide helpful content material that is not only fundamental but new and creative.

Another benefit of attending annual conferences is networking. With the collaborative approach still in its infancy, many mental health professionals work alone and have no mental health colleagues with whom to share stories. This isolation can make collaborative work in a medical setting even more challenging, not to mention stressful. For professionals new to collaborative health care, as well as those well established in practice, an annual meeting provides the forum to develop and maintain supportive relationships. They often maintain these relationships between conferences through phone conversations and E-mail. Such support or encouragement during difficult periods in one's home institution is invaluable.

We have found several national organizations, some training programs, and other institutions that include short programs on collaborative health care. We suggest attending the following conferences and developing a professional network while there (see appendix C for addresses).

- American Association for Marriage and Family Therapy (AAMFT): The annual conference offers daylong institutes, workshops, seminars, and master's case presentations. The program brochure identifies medically related workshops and seminars.
- American Psychological Association, Health Psychology Division: This division of APA offers special topics on health psychology at the annual conference. In addition, the Association of Psychology Internship Centers publishes a directory of relevant professional psychology internship programs and many postdoctoral programs.

- Collaborative Family Health Care Coalition: This coalition, founded in 1994, held its first annual conference in July 1995. Mental health professionals, health care providers, and health administrators from across the country met to present their current collaboration activities. The program's design encouraged professionals to build networks with colleagues locally and across the country. The number of local chapters continues to increase (see chapter 6 for current information).
- University of Rochester, Postgraduate Family Therapy Training Program: This program offers the one-week, intensive Medical Family Therapy Institute, codirected by David Seaburn and Susan McDaniel. The course provides both didactic presentations and a small-group, learner-centered format. The Departments of Internal Medicine and Family Medicine and the Family Therapy Training Program also offer a three-day, biannual, intensive course for educators entitled "Working with Families in Medical Settings." The workshop is codirected by Susan H. McDaniel and Thomas Campbell.
- Society of Teachers of Family Medicine: The society holds the annual Family in Family Medicine Conference. Most presenters model their clinical and academic work on a family systems approach to health care. The four-day conference, attended by academic health care professionals, is notable for the supportive environment it creates. Small discussion groups follow the formal plenaries. These groups, facilitated by a joint team of a physician or nurse and a mental health care provider, stimulate discussion by the attendees. These discussions not only encourage the assimilation of the materials but foster the development of relationships with new colleagues.

Clinical Placements

Some new professionals attempt to collaborate after reviewing the literature, attending a workshop, or taking a course. Often they find themselves stuck or having difficulties at the interface with their health care colleagues (Shapiro, 1980). Our suggestion is to move to the next step. We encourage them to secure clinical placements where the focus is on collaborative care (see appendix D).

This section highlights the key components of effective clinical training sites. Besides our own experiences in clinical teaching, ideas were provided by several clinicians from collaborative clinical training placements for mental health professionals across the country. We interviewed both trainers and trainees from master's, doctoral, and postdoctoral clinical training sites. All these are colo- cated within family medicine residency training programs.

These programs have several elements in common. Whether the placement is full-time or part-time, trainees report having ample time to work with patients, families, and medical and health care providers. The trainees maintain an average case load of 8 to 20 sessions per week. Each clinical placement gives the trainee the opportunity to conduct mental health counseling and to discuss his or her cases with a mental health supervisor and a health care pro- fessional. Each location offers support from other mental health professionals in the same setting. In addition, these settings offer advanced training for other medical and health care professionals (physicians, nurses, social workers, psychologists, family thera- pists). This cotraining environment produces an atmosphere open to new ideas about providing care. Trainers experienced in collab- oration supervise trainees.

Whether the trainee is beginning mental health training or pur- suing postgraduate training, there are several key components of a good clinical placement: immersion, modeling, mentoring, on-site supervision, and cohort effect. We will review the importance of each component.

Immersion

The key to developing a collaborative relationship with a health care colleague is to understand his or her culture. Barbara Gawin- ski, director of the University of Rochester and Highland Hospi- tal's Medical Family Therapy Internship, identified her plan for immersing doctoral interns in a family medicine residency training program.

When working with students new to a health care setting, I find it essential for them to get a glimpse of how physicians, nurse- practitioners, and others spend their clinical time. The mental health trainee shadows nurse-practitioners and physicians seeing patients. They follow a third-year resident during an inpatient rotation. They also sit in the preceptor's office to hear how faculty and community physicians discuss cases with the nurses and physicians-in-training. The experience helps the mental health professional develop respect for time, pace, and depth in the doctor-patient relationship. One medical family therapy intern reported the experience of watching a resident care for 12 patients in 3 hours. She then understood why it was difficult to obtain all the information she requested of the physician. Sometimes the resident just had little time to get all the questions answered before the next patient was ready.

Gary Bischof, who completed his one-year full-time medical family therapy internship in the University of Rochester's Department of Family Medicine, found immersion to be particularly important.

The part I valued most was the immersion in the day-to-day culture of a family practice, particularly a family medicine residency training setting. I learned through listening to the conversations in the preceptor's office, attending grand rounds, participating in psychosocial and biomedical cores [teaching sessions], and shadowing doctors during hospital rounds. . . . I think I soaked up a lot just about the culture that I wasn't necessarily learning consciously.

Immersion in the culture of medicine and health care is the foundation of any clinical placement. Familiarity with common medical terminology develops with hearing it used regularly (see appendix E). The intern learns the most helpful way to relate to health care professionals by watching their work. Linda Garcia-Shelton, director of Michigan State University's Postdoctoral Fellowship in Primary Care Health Psychology, shares a trainee's story. He immersed himself in the clinical experiences of a physician colleague at the hospital. He shadowed a resident for a week. Finally, he shed his dress shoes and donned sneakers to keep pace with his physician colleague. Recognizing the different meaning that time had for physicians, this fellow then modified the duration of his conversations with his medical colleagues in the office.

In an effort to both improve primary care for their patients and train interdisciplinary teams of providers, the Veterans Administration is providing salary support for more than 1,000 new trainees in areas such as medicine and family medicine, psychology, nursing, social work, pharmacy, and occupational therapy. Last year the PRIME (primary medical education) program funded 37 new psychology internship positions across the country (De Groot, 1994). Douglas Rait, director of the Family Therapy Program at the VA Palo Alto Health Care System, described how this clinic's psychology internship training immerses interns in the clinical setting as well as in academic, didactic experiences. Interns accepted into the primary care/behavioral medicine rotation (half-time, yearlong) are attached to primary care teams, or PACTs (Palo Alto

Care Teams), as members and also carry their own caseload of patients in the behavioral medicine clinic. In addition, their weekly seminars focus on a diverse set of topics presented by interdisciplinary staff: physicians present on different diseases and their medical management; pharmacologists teach about various classes of medication and their side effects; a neuropsychologist trains interns in neuropsychological screening and assessment; a psychologist and nurse from the Family Therapy Program present a series on family-centered primary care and medical family therapy approaches; and the psychologists in the behavioral medicine clinic survey health psychology research and behavioral medicine interventions (e.g., relaxation training, hypnosis, cognitive-behavioral techniques). Rait reports that, having already completed its first year, much energy exists in the Palo Alto program to change the structure and practice of health care delivery for veterans and their families. However, implementing a true interdisciplinary approach will take time.

Modeling

We all feel more confident attempting a new behavior after we have watched it successfully executed by another person. Mental health trainees are no different. During their first few months in training, they learn how to respectfully interact with patients, families, and health care colleagues by watching their trainer's interactions with others in the clinical setting. Modeling encourages trainees to conduct themselves similarly with physicians and health care colleagues. A successful training experience is almost ensured in a setting where trainees witness successful collaboration regularly.

Jeri Hepworth, director of the Master's Practicum Placement at Asylum Hill Family Practice in Hartford, Connecticut, says, "In order for interns to develop their own ability to respect and value the people, they have to feel that from their supervisor too." This generalized support happens only in an environment where the trainer feels supported, respected, and appreciated. Adding a trainee to the environment without this support would be premature.

In describing her role as a supervisor, Hepworth says that modeling was crucial in helping new colleagues understand the role of mental health professionals in a health care setting. "When we are supervising trainees, we are affirming them in their relationships with families. This allows them not only to affirm the family's strengths, but also the relationships that other professionals have with the families."

Besides modeling how to provide mental health care and collaborative care, the trainer must help the trainee to see the important relationship between the health care provider and the patient. "What I think we do not teach people enough," says Hepworth, "is to value the relationship that the physicians already have with patients." The mental health care provider most often becomes a temporary professional added on to a very powerful healing relationship. Neither the physician nor the patient wants to lose the connection. This is a very different role for the traditional mental health professional.

This affirming clinical supervision style moves trainees beyond the therapist-patient/family relationship. It helps them see the therapeutic relationship between the health care provider, the patient, and the family. Finally, therapists include themselves in the existing provider-patient relationship. They need guidance in not assuming too much responsibility for care. Valerie Correa, a master's degree practicum student supervised by Hepworth, says, "Providing mental health care is much less intimidating when I remember what my supervisor told me. I remember that other providers are working with the patient and family too."

Mentoring

We identify four important aspects of mentoring mental health professionals when they are working in health care settings: (1) demystifying the role of the physician, (2) adapting to the emotionally charged nature of the context, (3) addressing the impact of collaboration on the trainee's own health and illness beliefs, and (4) exploring professional development.

Demystifying the Role of the Physician

The first issue is the common belief among new trainees that physicians should be on a pedestal. Some trainees are intimidated by the role alone. Others are anxious relating to health care professionals because of a personal or family illness experience. This reaction makes collaborative practice difficult. The role of the mentor is to demystify the role of the physician. In a friendly environment of collaboration, trainers and trainees develop open conversations with their health care colleagues. Over time the trainees feel more comfortable and confident in their new setting, and their experiences with their health care colleagues become very important and meaningful. They have peak collaborative moments with the patient, the patient's family, and the professionals involved. Through these encounters, the trainees assimilate the power of shared care. Bischof related his experience of mutual respect.

> The doctor referred me a patient, and I started the case in the usual mental health style. I assumed the patient was the consumer or customer for mental health services, but she really was not. She came because her doctor suggested it; she would often cancel. Later my role changed to a consultant to the physician and to the physician-patient relationship. We held joint medical appointments, and I consulted some with the doctor. I shared articles on somatization. After visits, we would talk about feeling overwhelmed and incompetent with this very complex and demanding patient. We talked about ways to use language in the session differently. He had hoped to promote a little bit more positive discussion in the sessions. I really felt helpful in this process, but it was not with the patient directly. This was a major shift for me, because I arrived thinking physicians would be too busy to want to talk with me. I did not realize I had something to offer them too.

The Emotionally Charged Medical Context

The second issue is the emotionally charged nature of the context. Providing care in a medical setting can be scary. Preparing for the death of a family member, witnessing the loss of a pregnancy at full term, managing the adjustment to an HIV-positive diagnosis, and coping with a life of Crohn's disease are among the many serious conditions faced by patients who present for mental health services. Traditional mental health training does not prepare its graduates for this type of clinical and emotional work. Trainees in this context benefit from a mentoring relationship with their supervisor. Trainees agree. Correa related her experience:

> The most helpful part of this experience has been having Jeri [Hepworth] here to guide me through this process. She really directs me and encourages me. She reminds me that you don't have to do this alone. Other players exist and influence this person's life besides you. You are one player of a full team. She knows that coming in is emotionally overwhelming when you have four clients in a row, and having someone who is dying is

scary. Probing their trainees is important for a supervisor. She would discuss how I feel about having a client that has a certain disease or a certain kind of experience. When I listen to them, she would ask what does that bring up for me. I need to have trust with my supervisor.

The total experience of practicing in a health care setting changes therapists' perspective on the mental health care they provide. They realize that patients experience the pain and anguish of their failing bodies. No therapeutic maneuver can change the suffering. The mental health professional works with patients and families to help them live with suffering and pain. This is a kind of work that many trainees never anticipated doing. They address the illness or disease in the collaborative treatment approach, recognizing that the pain may not change. Trainees also may change their own beliefs about health and illness.

Personal Health and Illness Beliefs

This leads to the third issue trainees often explore with a mentor. When mental health professionals enter the health care arena, they begin to attend to their own and their family's issues around personal illness experiences. Long-held beliefs about physicians and health care professionals begin to surface (Rolland, 1994b). A therapist's unresolved or unclarified feelings about death and dying need personal attention before working with patients on those issues. The trainer, having created a safe environment in which to explore these issues, can support the trainee's processing of this realization. At times supervisors may refer their trainees for personal therapy outside the supervision experience.

During a supervision session in the middle of her one-year clinical experience, Speice reflected on her own family.

I come from a family background where business and productivity received the main focus and not emotions. I am beginning to translate my own family experience into different family stories and language. I have not had any acute, tragic medical crisis in my immediate family. We have never talked about what happened before us. This year we have begun to mark the changes in my family. We are beginning to talk. Now we can say that it is just a matter of time before something happens to someone, and we need to be ready to think differently.

Personal Development

The fourth area of mentoring is professional development. Attention to this area includes socializing trainees to a new professional focus while also helping them stay connected to their discipline of origin so as not to feel marginalized. Garcia-Shelton encourages her trainees to complete their postdoctoral training not only by improving their generic clinical skills across the life span but by increasing their ability to work with physicians and other health care professionals and acquiring teaching tools for their next professional position. She encourages her trainees to move in the direction of integrating themselves into other academic medical settings. They begin to research and publish in health care journals as well as traditional mental health journals. This process during training assists the trainee in developing a network of peers in his or her new professional area.

On-site Supervision

The integration of the new mental health trainee into a medical practice takes time, even if the site has accepted trainees for years. For that reason, having a supervisor with experience working in the setting is essential. An on-site supervisor serves three functions: facilitating the other key training elements (modeling, immersion, and mentoring); helping the trainee recognize that patient care also includes navigating a whole new culture; and reducing some of the trainee's anxieties about new clinical experiences.

An on-site supervisor decreases the trainee's sense of isolation in the new culture. In addition, students often need to have access to immediate supervision on cases that may be acutely problematic or emotionally charged for them. Most trainers practice on-site with their trainees for at least part of the time. They provide intensive individual and group supervision at a ratio of one supervision hour for five clinical cases.

The clinical experience in a health care setting differs from other mental health clinical settings in various ways. First, the clinical caseload includes medically related problems that need specialized supervision. Second, the mechanics of referring for mental health counseling and engaging in collaboration will be specific to each context. Some programs have a formalized referral process with written documentation. Other programs orchestrate referral through live case consultation during a medical interview. Still other programs conduct therapy only in joint sessions with the medical provider. Finally, the administrative nuances of the practice are often difficult to navigate during the orientation months. Usually, the intern shares office space, videotaping equipment, and clerical support with the faculty and other trainees. The intern needs guidance in negotiating these issues. Chart documentation is always unique to the context. The on-site supervisor offers assistance to the trainee in translating traditional therapy notes into useful medical chart notes without losing the impact of the session. One final example is the billing system. Methods of documenting that the encounter occurred, may be billed for, and is appropriately supervised vary from setting to setting.

Hepworth recognized the importance of being available to her trainees throughout the day. Because of other professional commitments, sometimes she cannot be available. Consequently, she supplements her supervision by enlisting the support of her on-site physician faculty. Each day the mental health trainee reviews cases with the physician faculty preceptor. Together they discuss the session, current diagnosis, medication, and treatment plan. This true integrated health and mental health supervision demonstrates how to use the strengths of each supervisor on the case.

Students have been training at the University of Connecticut's family medicine residency training site for 12 years. The physician faculty and residents eagerly anticipate the arrival of new mental health trainees each year. This modeling of collaboration in a training setting encourages both the mental health students and the residents to search for or re-create this type of collaborative relationship when they leave the academic setting.

Other sites have multiple supervisors to address medical family therapy, health psychology, and behavioral medicine. At Michigan State University, two family medicine behavioral faculty share supervision of the fellows. Together they offer a wide breadth of on-site supervision in psychology, family therapy, and collaborative health care. An additional faculty supervisor from the local university's psychology department offers traditional supervision. These additional supervision hours are helpful in traditional clinical work. However, the collaboration process, which is specific to the context, is neglected with an off-site supervisor. On-site supervision works best.

Cohort Effect

Being new to the culture of medicine can be a lonely experience. Having the opportunity to discuss the experience with someone at a similar developmental level provides grounding (Shapiro & Schiermer, 1993). Some programs train two or more trainees simultaneously. Michigan State's Garcia-Shelton followed the guidelines of the American Psychological Association when she developed her fellowship program, which requires a minimum of three trainees at any one time. When she was enrolled in the University of Connecticut's family practice residency, Valerie Correa shared one practicum day with her trainee colleague. They also enrolled in common classes in the master's degree program at the university. She said, "I enjoyed having someone from my master's program at Asylum Hill Family Practice. We could bounce things off each other. I found that very helpful."

Other programs use the medical residents to serve as a cohort group, since the level of training is similar. Bischof, who trained in Rochester as a solo medical family therapy intern, joined the residents' professional development group to process his experience with them. Although their practices were different, they addressed similar areas: managing personal and professional boundaries, termination, and emotional responses to the difficulties the patients were enduring. Because he felt closer to the residents socially, he approached them more easily on clinical material. By understanding the differences in their training, he began to recognize the special skills he had to offer them and their patients.

In the first year of the Palo Alto Care Team (PACT), Doug Rait focused on a plan for training psychology interns. "Of the 22 full-time interdisciplinary trainees, psychology received 4 slots. Those 4 interns work with 18 other health care professionals for one year of their training. The other disciplines include internal medicine, psychiatry, nurse-practitioners, physical therapy, occupational therapy, optometry, pharmacy, social work, and speech pathology." The psychology interns work with multiple health care providers on clinical cases, act as consultants to them, and receive consultation from their health care colleagues as well.

In summary, clinical placement offers trainees a year or two of on-site clinical supervision with full immersion into the medical setting. Through modeling and mentoring, the trainer guides the trainee. Some sites offer the experience to more than one trainee, providing the benefits of the cohort effect. Trainees accomplish their clinical tasks and come to a much richer understanding of their work with health care providers. They develop the skills necessary for building a relationship, learn effective ways to communicate, recognize the importance of a common purpose, and develop a paradigm more compatible with that of health care professionals.

Integrated Training Programs

In this section, we focus on training opportunities that blend didactic course work, clinical placement, and, in some instances, cotraining of mental health and health care professionals. These programs may be degree-granting or postdegree in nature. They strive to combine all of the important elements of training for collaboration.

Nova Southeastern University

An example of one school committed to providing mental health training in collaborative health care is Nova Southeastern University's School of Social and Systemic Studies. Sherri Muchnick developed the program by combining organized course work with clinical experience in medical settings. The students earn a clinical specialist degree in the Family Systems Health Care Program. Margo Weiss now directs the new Medical Family Therapy Program. Students can obtain a clinical specialization certificate, a master's degree, or a Ph.D. in marriage and family therapy with a specialization in medical family therapy. The clinical specialization students take six courses. Those students enrolled in a graduate degree program in the general family therapy program select additional courses to prepare them for the clinical placements in medical specialists' offices (Muchnick et al., 1993).

Three classroom courses specifically focused on medical and family therapy collaboration cover the biopsychosocial model, family systems medicine, and medical concepts for nonphysicians. Weiss coordinates a discussion group entitled "Medical Grand Rounds" to which community health professionals are invited to speak. This discussion group has two goals: to have health professionals teach mental health students about health-related topics, and to enable physicians and other health professionals to experience this mental health training setting.

A research course introduces students to qualitative research methods. To demonstrate the use of qualitative and quantitative research methodology, Weiss is developing an interdepartmental research project with the Cleveland Clinic's Department of Gastroenterology. The students also design and conduct their research project on a related health topic. Students present their findings in class and complete a research paper.

The students participate in a two-stage practical clinical experience. Their first year of clinical experience is in a live supervision model on campus. Their second year is in various health care settings. They participate as active members of a health care team in both hospitals and noncontiguous ambulatory care offices. Specialists' offices, such as cardiology, immunology, oncology, and psychiatry, provide clinical training sites. Students are also placed at a chemical dependency inpatient unit, in hospice programs, and at Planned Parenthood. On-site clinicians provide supervision.

Nova faculty conduct weekly group case review meetings at which clinical supervisors encourage trainees to share novel experiences and discuss strategies for overcoming obstacles to collaboration. "Interns supported each other's efforts and added humor and perspective to even the most challenging situations" (Muchnick et al., 1993, p. 277). The advantages of an academic program are (1) structured course work, (2) peer group support, (3) multiple on-site and off-site supervisors, and (4) an ongoing mentoring relationship with the faculty. The next level of training moves to integrate the training in collaboration for both mental health care providers and physicians and other health care providers.

University of San Diego

The University of San Diego Marriage and Family Therapy Training Program, under the direction of Jo Ellen Patterson and Joseph Scherger, a Sharp HealthCare Family Medicine Residency Program faculty member, are working together to create collaborative models of training, provide clinical services, and develop research initiatives (Patterson, Bischoff, Scherger, & Grauf-Grounds, 1996). The marriage and family therapy faculty provide training services at the Sharp residency programs, and the Sharp faculty teach in the marriage and family therapy program. This cross-discipline training facilitates an integration of the theory and practice of collaboration for both faculty and learners.

Nearly all of San Diego's population receive their health care through managed-care systems. Almost all private health insurance in the area is capitated. Once Medicaid becomes capitated, the county will have completed the evolution to managed care it began in the 1980s. Sharp HealthCare, one of the four delivery systems in San Diego County, provides care for 25% of the population (Patterson et al., in press). The Marriage and Family Therapy Training Program became associated with the Sharp residency program to prepare its graduates more effectively for careers in managed care. Three courses have been added to the curriculum to reflect changes in how health and mental health services are delivered under managed care. Joseph Scherger, a family physician, teaches the first course, entitled "Family and Health Issues." This course uses the biopsychosocial model to discuss issues of health and wellness. A child psychiatrist teaches the second course, entitled "Pharmacology for Family Therapists," which covers the central nervous system, common pharmacological treatments, and a collaborative approach to family therapy and medication (Patterson & Magulac, 1994). A third course, offered by a health psychologist and entitled "Practice Management Issues for Therapists," highlights issues common to managed-care settings, professional issues for the future of family therapists, and basic business skills. Leaders in the field of managed care present various topics throughout the series.

In 1992 Sharp HealthCare started a family medicine residency program to train family physicians who would remain in the region. They selected three sites across San Diego County. A concern for the family medicine residents in these practice sites was the provision of mental health services. Sharp has a carve-out mental health care plan. For the residents, this meant they would need to refer their patients off-site for mental health services or provide primary care counseling themselves. The residency faculty worked with the marriage and family therapy faculty to develop mental health services within the residency program to provide a more acceptable training and care plan.

At each of the three residency sites, marriage and family therapy faculty offer different services. Based on the program's needs and the skill of the faculty member, they assume one or all of the following roles: traditional behavioral science teacher, psychotherapist, supervisor of a psychotherapist, facilitator of a resident support group, educator, or trainer of residents. They also collaborate with the psychiatrists, who assume responsibility for training the residents during inpatient mental health training. One final connection between these two disciplines is the special arrangement made with community mental health outpatient centers. The family medicine residents rotate through these clinics during their psychiatry rotation. The marriage and family therapy students conduct their practical experiences at the centers as well. The therapy students expect the residents to teach the therapy trainees about medical aspects of their patients. They also expect the residents to present a case for psychosocial consultation with the therapist.

The University of Rochester

The University of Rochester School of Medicine and Dentistry proudly recognizes George Engel as an influential leader. As an internist, he has been a faculty member in psychiatry for a half century. His biopsychosocial model is pervasive in the medical school and across many departments. His work has influenced the Departments of Psychiatry and Family Medicine in particular. Both departments share faculty for training, teaching, and provision of clinical services. Physicians and mental health care providers share appointments in both departments.

In 1969 the Department of Family Medicine of Highland Hospital and the University of Rochester started the Family Medicine Residency Program. Under the visionary leadership of Gene Farley, the program established a fundamental commitment to psychosocial education. In 1972 Lyman Wynne, chair of the Department of Psychiatry, developed the Division of Family Programs. In 1983 M. Duncan Stanton and Judith Landau-Stanton founded the Family Therapy Training Program. The program's diversified faculty provide postgraduate training in family therapy. Under the leadership of Judith Landau-Stanton, Susan McDaniel, and Thomas Campbell, the two departments began to integrate training.

The Family Medicine Residency Program offers a three-year psychosocial curriculum with a focus on interviewing skills, family systems, and collaborative care. Residents have a four-month psychiatry rotation with faculty from both the Department of Family Medicine and the Department of Psychiatry. The rotation teaches psychiatric and psychotherapy skills that are applicable to primary care medicine. Part of this rotation includes advanced family systems theory and family consultation, as well as psychotherapy with primary care mental health patients and families. Family therapists who are approved supervisors in the American Association for Marriage and Family Therapy provide supervision. During their third year, residents often elect to enroll in courses offered in the Family Therapy Training Program (Department of Psychiatry).

The Postgraduate Family Therapy Training Program, directed by David B. Seaburn, is an accredited program leading to a certificate in family therapy. One-quarter to one-half of all trainees in the program are physicians or nursing professionals. They work in live supervision teams with mental health professionals seeing a wide range of families, including those dealing with illness. These live supervision groups encourage collaborative clinical care and socialize health care professionals and mental health professionals to each other's worlds. The Family Therapy Training Program also offers courses in family systems medicine and medical family therapy. Both mental health and health care professionals enroll in these courses.

Just as health care professionals can receive training in the family and marriage clinic, family therapy trainees from a wide range of mental health disciplines can elect to do part of their clinical practicum in the Family Medicine Residency Program's clinic. They are supervised on-site by family therapists who help them learn collaborative skills.

The Department of Family Medicine also offers a full-time clinical internship in medical family therapy under the direction of Barbara Gawinski. Trainees in this program work parallel to physicians-in-training. This cotraining environment facilitates the development of relationships across disciplines while sharing patient care. Often this experience sets the stage for the way physicians select or design their future practice. Mental health care providers graduate from the program and search for collaborative relationships with physicians and other health care professionals. Many physician graduates report sharing an office setting with mental health colleagues.

University of Virginia

David Waters is a faculty member in the Department of Family Medicine, University of Virginia Medical School, who teaches residents family counseling skills. In the late 1970s, he developed a 6- to 8-week intensive live supervision model for 15 hours each week. For the first week, the second-year resident physicians observed therapy conducted by experienced mental health care providers on faculty. Then they began to practice their own skills under live supervision. The faculty used a phone to call in suggestions.

When the local psychology departments learned of Waters's live supervision model, they contacted him to train doctoral students, thus creating a cotraining model. Now psychology graduate students and family medicine residents share observations of clinic cases behind a one-way mirror. They watch each other's work and provide support and recommendations from their own areas of expertise. The residents emerge from the experience with the ability to initiate a process of family investigation and to make the appropriate referral. They also develop an appreciation for the work of their mental health colleagues. The psychologists emerge from the one-year internship with an appreciation and respect for what their medical colleagues do when they initiate a referral for counseling, thus preparing them to collaborate differently on such referrals. They learn the fundamentals of medical cases and recognize that their input is valuable to the doctor-patient relationship. According to Waters, the relationship that develops between the physicians and psychologists is a "mutual admiration society" at first. Over the 6- to 8-week period, the psychologists and physicians develop friendships and a support group. The immersion of 15 hours each week in the cotraining model sets the foundation for collaborations after the residents' rotations are ended.

As with any new program, flexibility is the key. These programs constantly update their training programs to meet the needs of the trainees, patients, and families. As health care delivery continues to change across the country, the collaborative models of cotraining at San Diego and Rochester also adjust their curricula to meet the changes of the larger health care system. We believe these innovative collaborative models of teaching, training, and research will provide a guide for others in the future. The ideal model is the combination of cotraining and advanced course work for health and mental health care providers, directly focusing on collaboration between them. The opportunity to successfully work in an interdisciplinary context produces graduates who are confident enough to develop new collaborative relationships in their next location.

KEY COMPONENTS OF COLLABORATIVE TRAINING

In this section, we suggest ways for trainees and trainers to select and set up training programs. These suggestions are not exhaustive but address some of the most commonly cited issues.

Suggestions for Mental Health Professionals Seeking Training

1: *Review the literature on collaboration* (see References). In particular, become familiar with the biopsychosocial model and how it has been integrated into systems thinking.

2: *Enroll in courses at graduate institutions* (see appendix D). Various programs across the country offer courses or graduate degrees to prepare the mental health professional for collaborative practice. Some programs orchestrate on-site collaboration at various health care settings.

3: *Attend conferences on collaboration* (see appendix C). Some conferences encourage a variety of professionals to attend, such as physicians and other health professionals, mental health professionals, administrators, and insurance company representatives.

4: *Consult with continuing medical education offices and join already established local chapters of the Collaborative Family Health Care Coalition* (see chapter 7 and appendix A). Medical education meetings provide the environment for developing some familiarity with health-related issues and relationships with the physicians and other health care providers who attend. The local CFHCC chapters provide professional support for developing collaborative relationships. Case consultations provide the forum for expanding the knowledge base of the group.

5: *Immerse yourself in the culture of health care.* Participant observation is the best way to learn the language (see appendix E) and culture of medicine and health care. Seek on-site placements in medical or health care settings. Learn a system of documentation appropriate to the medical setting (see appendix F). Health care providers use brief notes to convey a great deal of information. Become familiar with medical shorthand and record maintenance systems. Develop a format to communicate with health care providers.

Suggestions for Developing Successful Clinical Training Sites

We believe trainers should invite trainees to their setting only after successfully establishing the organizational framework for a collaborative environment. This often takes time. Successful programs evolve *after* including all important players (faculty, administrators, business managers, support staff) in developing a collaborative training model and carefully selecting a trainee. The trainer should prepare the site by doing the following:

1: *Be sure those at the top of the organizational hierarchy are supportive of collaborative training.* Typically, the body will follow the head. In the absence of initial collaboration with administrators and physicians at the top of the organization, many stumbling blocks will be encountered.

2: *Work with one or more physicians who support the idea of collaboration.* Physician faculty members can support the mental health trainee when the trainer needs to be off-site. The physician can also offer guidance in the medical system when the trainer encounters a new area (administrative, medical, or financial).

3: *Demonstrate to residency educators, physicians, nurses, and administrators several cases where collaborative work decreased physicians' workload and increased patient satisfaction.* When adding a new component to any residency training program, the staff who will be affected by the change need to know how it will help them in their work. Stressing the positive impact of collaboration increases the likelihood that it wil be warmly received.

4: *Organize clerical and receptionist support.* The details can often overwhelm a system. It is essential to coordinate in advance who will type mental health notes, which differ in style from health care providers' notes. Prepare the secretarial staff for the additional phone calls that will come in for the mental health care providers, and train them in managing those calls. Physicians often accept interruptions when a call comes in; mental health care providers usually do not. Will the mental health care provider pick up calls throughout the day? Will the mental health provider schedule his or her own patients or will the secretaries do so? Work out these details in advance.

5: *Secure financial arrangements.* Students arrive at a practice by way of a variety of cost-saving routes. Master's degree students are often free; the supervision they need is offset by the income collected from the clinical care they provide. Doctoral students receive a stipend and hours of supervision. They see more patients and cover their expenses, including stipend, benefits, and some continuing medical education funds. Fellows hold advanced degrees and offer more to the program by generating income in a variety of ways, such as psychological testing, resident teaching, and clinical care.

6: *Design a plan to refer patients for mental health services.* We recommend developing an educational program to teach residents, other health professionals, and faculty the process for referring for in-house mental health services. A short form can be generated to ease the process for the busy health care professional. Health care clinicians appreciate some quick feedback to learn how long the patient will have to wait before being seen.

7: *Develop a method to record mental health encounters in the medical record.* We recommend documenting each encounter in a standard form. We also find it useful to compile a longer summary after the first few visits. This format provides the health care provider with the mental health professional's summary of the history of the problem, assessment, and treatment plan (see appendix F for details).

8: *Coordinate group supervision for cohort support during training.* All trainees enjoy the opportunity to share their experiences with others at the same level of training. The trainees may or may not be of the same discipline. The most useful aspect of this supervision model is being with others who are also struggling with personal and professional issues.

9: *Screen trainees for personal maturity, interest in collaboration, comfort in new environments, enjoyment of challenges, degree of autonomy, and awareness of personal issues.* The success of any program depends on the trainees. The longer a program operates, the more successful the trainers become at screening applicants to fit the context.

CONCLUSION

The time has come for institutions that prepare mental health professionals, physicians, and nurses to integrate a collaborative approach to patient and family care into their core curricula. For mental health professionals in particular, curricula must include education in health care issues and systems, as well as training in engaging and working with health care professionals. In addition, accrediting bodies must recognize and mandate collaborative skills as fundamental to training our next generation of helping professionals.

There are promising trends in collaborative training curricula at every level. At the local level, Dashiff and colleagues (1990) highlight a training model for physicians and nurses collaborating with an indigent population. This parallel training offers a new perspective for both disciplines. At the state level, Bhatara, Fuller, and Unruh (1994) describe a managed cooperation program to educate health and mental health practitioners to collaborate and share care more effectively. At the national level, the Collaborative Family Health Care Coalition offers an annual conference for training health and mental health care providers. Participants attend workshops on designing collaborative care and teaching about collaboration in their own disciplines or in cross-training efforts. On an international level, Martinez (1990) reports that the Nicaraguan Cooperative has advanced training in mental health in its medical school curriculum. Medical students participate in a work-study program that connects theory and practice by focusing on a number of critical issues: the doctor-patient relationship; the mental and physical health of the child; contagious illnesses as related to the individual, family, and society; chronic disease and its relation to employment; and finally, the psychological aspects of mother-child relationships. As Nicaraguan physicians in this program learn to think systemically, programs in the United States could follow its lead by developing a new level of cooperative education for health and mental health care providers.

As medical education makes changes to increase the number of primary health care providers graduating from medical schools, their curricula need to reflect the important psychosocial issues in health care and the value of collaboration across disciplines. Some medical schools have already made curricular changes to model respectful teaching relationships between mental health faculty and medical faculty. At the University of Rochester School of Medicine and Dentistry, first- and second-year medical students experience a two-year curriculum introducing the biopsychosocial model. Lecturing faculty come from various disciplines and specialties. Skills development groups use a coteaching team of a primary care physician and a mental health care provider (Epstein & Guttmacher, 1995). Modeling this collaboration at such an early phase in their education may encourage these physicians-in-training to work with mental health professionals in their future practices. In Ohio, Talen, Graham, and Walbroehl (1994) designed a new curriculum for a multiprofessional group. This training program is a community-based primary and preventive health care service. Schools of medicine, nursing, professional psychology, and allied health are offering courses and designing clinical experiences to foster collaborative attitudes between professionals.

James Griffith of George Washington University's Department of Psychiatry reports that in addition to traditional psychiatry training, GW's program specifically focuses on the skills needed to collaborate effectively with primary care clinicians. This program, which recognizes the future trends for psychiatrists in managed care, also prepares its graduates to be effective group and organizational leaders. At GW they predict that psychiatrists will be working more often on multidisciplinary treatment teams led by primary care clinicians. In this role, the psychiatrist must be able to facilitate each team member's unique contribution to the treatment plan.

To underscore the importance of collaboration and interdisciplinary training for the next generation of mental health and health care professionals, accrediting bodies must recognize the impact that health care changes are having on the needs of professionals-in-training. Some family therapy training settings recognize the importance of preparing family therapists to work in managed care (Patterson & Scherger, 1995). Lareau and Nelson (1994) cite the potential advantages of the mental health and physician team. They encourage all health and mental health professionals, organizations, and licensing boards to join with health insurance companies to prepare for the future. Professional accrediting bodies should adopt this mandate and prepare health and mental health professionals for the changing health care scene. The Commission on Accreditation for Marriage and Family Therapy Education (COAMFTE), for example, is considering requiring specific course work in this area for all accredited degree-granting and postgraduate family therapy training programs.

Without changes in how they are trained, mental health professionals, physicians, and nurses will not be prepared for the demands of new health care systems. Patients and families will receive collaborative care of their multifaceted problems only if the professionals caring for them are trained to provide it.

CHAPTER 15

Predictions for the Future of Collaboration

WE ARE ON THE BRINK of a new age in health care. In the middle of this century, we witnessed unprecedented expansion and privatization of health care expenditures ("the first revolution"). Since then the cost of health care has climbed beyond what people are willing or able to pay. We are now in the midst of a multitude of efforts at cost containment ("the second revolution"). Managed care has "managed" better than other plans to provide affordable care and has successfully invaded the private health insurance system. Now many federal, state, and local governments are turning over much of their responsibility for administering health care to managed-care programs.

This era of cost containment has not been without its casualties. In presumably well-intentioned attempts to provide affordable care, some tough decisions have been made. Some important benefits, like mental health care, have been eliminated or sharply reduced. Some people, including newborn infants, have been sent home from the hospital earlier than is really safe. In the forthcoming age (what Relman [1988] describes as the "third revolution"), we will more carefully assess the needs of patients and the effectiveness of our methods of care in the context of the cost of care. Health care of the future must respect financial imperatives but also transcend a purely bottom-line orientation. The focus will be on value—providing affordable *and* quality care.

This chapter is organized around four interrelated themes. These themes are well established, widely recognized, and built on one another. The first theme is the movement from inpatient to outpatient provision of health care services. This trend has implications for the future training of all varieties of health care practitioners, including mental health professionals. The second theme is the movement from specialty to primary care; we project a transformation to collaborative primary care teams. The third theme is the expansion from individual-based care to population-based care. This shift, a pleasant and surprising result of capitated strategies, is consistent with the community-oriented primary care model and begets an ecosystemic view of health care. The fourth theme, and to our minds the most important, is the elevation of patients and families as partners in care. We broadly define this trend as consumerism.

Each of the four sections on these themes ends with our perspective on how these changes will influence the collaborative mental health professional of the future.

THE MOVEMENT FROM INPATIENT TO OUTPATIENT SERVICES

> Right now, despite our preeminence in the HMO market in our area, we are losing money every day . . . because we cannot close hospitals fast enough.
>
> High-ranking administrator of a large health maintenance organization (personal communication, July 30, 1995).

Let us set the stage for our predictions about the future by briefly describing the recent past leading up to our current state of affairs. The major financial trends in health care over the past 15 years continue to exert considerable pressure today. These pressures are forcing health care to develop in certain directions. It is useful to start with a summary of a few statistics generated by the National Center for Health Statistics (1995).

1. The United States spends a greater proportion of its gross domestic product (GDP) on health care than any other developed nation, and this gap is widening.
2. Between 1980 and 1993, the average annual rate of growth in

health expenditures as a percentage of GDP was 3.2% in the United States, while it averaged 1.2% for the 24 developed countries that are members of the Organization for Economic Cooperation and Development.

3. In 1980 health care accounted for 9.3% of GDP. It was 13.9% in 1993.
4. Forty-four percent of health care is paid for by the government: 32% by the federal government, and 12% by state and local governments.
5. Health care expenditures make up an increasingly large proportion of the federal budget. In 1965 health care amounted to 4% of the total federal budget; in 1980, 12%; and in 1993, 13.5%.

Hospital care, which is largely financed by government (56%) and to a lesser extent by private insurance (36%), accounts for the greatest share of national health expenditures. In spite of the increase in health care expenditures, especially for hospitalization, hospital admissions and lengths of stay have decreased. Since the implementation in 1983–84 of the prospective payment system for Medicare inpatients (diagnosis-related groups [DRGs]), significant changes in hospital utilization have occurred. Between 1983 and 1988, inpatient admissions declined 13%, to 33 million. Between 1988 and 1992, inpatient admissions remained stable; however, average length of stay has shown a steady decline from 1980 to 1993. For example, for inpatients over 75 years of age, the average length of stay was 11.4 days in 1980. This figure progressively declined to 8.2 days in 1993 (American Hospital Association, 1993–94). *Reducing and shortening hospitalization has been a major focus of cost reduction by both government and private insurance* (see chapter 13).

While government has increased its role in funding health care, some dramatic changes have taken place in the composition of the private insurance industry. As a result of their ability to provide less expensive plans to business, health maintenance organizations have grown tremendously and now dominate many markets. Between 1980 and 1995, enrollment in HMOs more than quadrupled, from 9 million to 51 million. In 1995 more than 20% of the U.S. population was enrolled in an HMO (Bernstein et al., 1994), and this figure is expected to grow. There are now a multitude of efforts at all levels of government across the country to transfer patients from government-funded plans to managed-care plans (see chapter 13).

We anticipate that these efforts will continue and be successful. It seems likely that most people will soon be covered by either private or public managed care. One of the most important keys to the success of managed care has been its ability to influence utilization of hospitalization. Managed-care programs have accomplished this by a variety of methods, including preauthorization for admission, utilization review, and capitation. Government and business at all levels have admired managed care's ability to decrease hospital utilization. As a result, more people receive treatment today on an outpatient basis for the illnesses they would have been hospitalized for in the past.

To summarize, this country has spent and continues to spend an enormous amount of money on health care. Much of this money goes toward hospitalization. HMOs have been successful in large part because of their ability to affect utilization of hospitalization. HMOs will increasingly play a role in both government programs and the private insurance sector. The movement is toward more delivery of care on an outpatient basis, to patients who are more severely ill. What are the implications for the collaborative mental health professional with the new emphasis on outpatient care?

Most mental health professionals work primarily in the outpatient setting. Already 86% of psychologists and 78% of social workers work in an outpatient setting—most of them outpatient mental health settings (Thomas, Pot, & Bennett, 1994). With the increasing emphasis on outpatient medical care, mental health professionals' expertise in outpatient care will be invaluable. The ability to tolerate ambiguity and the ability to mobilize families and community resources are essential skills in outpatient management. More severely ill patients have greater psychosocial needs. An increasing psychosocial stress on the family members responsible for their care will follow. Mental health professionals will be more involved with these medically and psychosocially complex patients and will serve as consultants to the family members taking care of them. Talking in a mental health setting about one's physical health or about caring for an ill family member will no longer be considered an avoidance of talking about the "real issues." Illness-related stresses and concerns will be the real issues.

The trend toward increasing outpatient medical services has implications for training both health care practitioners and mental health professionals. More and more, health and mental health care providers will be trained in collaborative outpatient medical settings. Much of this training will be done in the public sector rather than in academic settings. In fact, many HMOs are already establishing their own training programs so that they can better prepare health and mental health professionals to work together in the changing climate of health care. In a sense, mental health and health care professionals will "grow up" together, learning approaches to clinical practice that are mutually inclusive rather than protective of professional differences. This will be a key to collaborative practice in the future.

The collaborative mental health professional of the future will:

- work increasingly in outpatient medical settings;
- play a greater role in providing care alongside primary care providers for people who are severely ill;
- play a greater role in coproviding care for the family members caring for the severely ill; and
- play a greater role in teaching health care practitioners about caring for people with increased psychosocial needs.

FROM SPECIALTY CARE TO PRIMARY CARE TO PRIMARY CARE COLLABORATIVE TEAMS

A major element in the success of managed care has been the use of the primary care practitioner as a gatekeeper. That is, the primary care practitioners (family practitioners, general practitioners, pediatricians, general internists, and the nurse-practitioners and physician's assistants who work with these physicians) regulate access to the health care services provided by all others. These practitioners provide care for up to 90% of all health care needs. Greater than 80% of office-based health care visits in the United States are to primary care providers (Schappert, 1992).

What is primary care? The Institute of Medicine report on the future of primary care (in Donaldson, Yordy, & Vanselow, 1994) defines primary care as "the provision of integrated, accessible health care services by clinicians who are accountable for addressing a large majority of personal health care needs, developing a sustained partnership with patients, and practicing in the context of family and community" (p. 16). Primary care clinicians are more likely to provide preventive and administrative services (Schappert, 1992). The Center for Mental Health Services (1994) states that primary care clinicians are uniquely suited to initiate and coordinate mental health services for persons with mental disorders because of their longitudinal relationships with patients and families, their knowledge of the patient's situational factors and social support, their management and awareness of other relevant medical conditions, and their position as contact and referral point for the health care system. (p. 149)

These definitions could also apply to many who work in the mental health field.

As gatekeepers, primary care practitioners are essential to the provision of mental health services. Primary care practitioners are often the only source of mental health care for many persons with mental disorders (Manderscheid, Rae, Narrow, Locke, & Regier, 1993). An estimated 20–30% of patients presenting in primary care settings have diagnosable mental disorders (Costello, Edelbrock, Costello, Dulcan, Burns, & Brent, 1988; Kessler, Cleary, & Burke, 1985). Most of these problems are anxiety disorders, depression, somatoform conditions, and substance abuse.

In addition to diagnosable disorders, a number of other primary care patients present with psychological distress insufficient to meet *DSM III-R* criteria for a mental disorder (Williams, Tarnopolsky, Hand, & Shepherd, 1978; Zung, Broadhead, & Roth, 1993). These patients may or may not have a co-occurring general medical condition that further complicates diagnosis and management. Some authors believe these "subthreshold" states are even more common than mental disorders in primary care. Garralda and Bailey (1986, 1987) estimated that *approximately 45% of all primary care visits have a significant psychological component.*

What does the future hold? The Center for Mental Health Services (1994) predicts:

The role of primary care services for persons with mental disorders is likely to expand rapidly in the next decade as a growing percentage of the population are enrolled in managed care health plans (Lehman, 1989; Physician Payment Review Commission, 1992). The primary care clinician will have a larger role as increasing incentives are applied to take care of patients in the primary care setting and avoid referral to more expensive specialists. Even more importantly, almost all of these plans will implement some form of primary care "gate keeping" in which the primary care clinician will be required to authorize the use of all specialty services (Physician Payment Review Commission, 1992; Konrad and DeFriese, 1990). In such a system, the primary care clinician's knowledge, attitudes and beliefs about mental health care along with the financial and administrative barriers imposed by the managed care plan are likely to have important effects on a patient's access to specialty mental health care. (pp. 150–151)

Who will provide all this primary care and gatekeeping service? There is a shortage of primary care physicians. Between 1980 and 1993, while the number of active generalist physicians per 100,000 population increased by only 20%, specialist physicians increased by 29%. In 1993, of the 591,000 active physicians, one-third practiced as generalists and two-thirds as specialists. Many organizations, including the Council on Graduate Medical Education and the Physician Payment Review Commission, have recommended the ideal balance to be at least 50–50 (Rivo & Satcher, 1993; Schwartz, Ginsburg, & LeRoy, 1993). To help meet the demand for primary care, the number of primary care providers who are not physicians has increased. There are now 43,000 nurse-practitioners and 6,400 active nurse-midwives. In addition, of the 23,000 active physician's assistants practicing in 1993, almost one-half (46%) were practicing as generalists.

Given the preponderance of mental health problems, the need for addressing psychosocial issues in primary care, the increasing emphasis on primary care for all health services, and the relative shortage of primary care providers, mental health professionals are an obvious choice to compensate for this imbalance in our health care system. The responsibility to provide quality primary care on all fronts—from performing the gatekeeping function to providing mental health services as well as general medical care—is more than our current supply of primary care practitioners can handle. The responsibility needs to be shared with someone, and the mental health professional is the most logical choice.

Like many other places, the Twin Cities in Minnesota provide direct access to mental health services in a managed-care system. In Minnesota and elsewhere, the mental health professional can function as a primary care access point and gatekeeper. These "health psychologists" provide a large percentage of mental health care needs and refer on to mental health specialists when needed. They provide "primary mental health care." This two-pronged approach to primary care and gatekeeping is increasing in popularity among large health maintenance organizations. This is an exciting new direction in linking mental and physical health care services.

Case management has always been limited by financial and operational designs based on the mind/body split. Triage personnel who allocate benefits have been restricted to working within either the biomedical realm or the mental health realm. Case managers of the future will function as members of teams that will be able to authorize benefits covering the entirety of a person's health care.

In this sense, case management involves the use of interdisciplinary collaborative teams to address the multifaceted issues of complex patients. Dietitians, social workers, and physical therapists will work together with primary care providers and specialists on these teams to provide coordinated care. While the team will be responsible for the care of the patient and family, one person from one of the disciplines listed above will ensure that the team impressions translate into a workable health care plan. As such, the primary care team will select a representative with the relationship and health care expertise most useful to the particular patient. The case manager will be able to authorize benefits not normally included in a plan. For example, one common strategy is to "flex" benefits by turning inpatient benefits into outpatient benefits. Case managers would have the power and authority to ensure flexibility in insurance coverage for unique and complicated patients.

Fallon Healthcare System (Blase & Kaufman, 1994) in Massachusetts proposed a useful definition for case management:

> Case Management is a multidisciplinary approach to organize and coordinate care, focusing on selected complex medical and psychosocial needs of patients and families in an effort to access appropriate resources and services, which by their presence, accompanied by ongoing assessment and adjustment, will create improvements in the quality/cost-effectiveness of medical care and the quality of life. (p. 111)

The goals of case management are:

1. Reduce the number of hospital admissions and readmissions.
2. Reduce the number of ambulatory visits required by high utilizers.
3. Educate primary care physicians and their staff with regard to the complex array of services available to manage their panel of patients.
4. Provide a mechanism for the translation of health care needs from one delivery site to another, as defined by the needs of the patient.

5. Establish a measurement of outcomes for those patients requiring health care service management.
6. Ensure that follow-up care is provided in the most appropriate setting.
7. Encourage and support the highest level of patient independence possible. (Blase & Kaufman, 1994, p. 112)

At this time the Fallon Community Health Plan has 160,000 members and three and a half FTE nurses who work as case managers. They have found that "relationship-building with all the members of the health care continuum became a prime focus in the development of case management services. To enhance relationship building among the members of the health care team the primary care physician became the focal point of team building" (Blase & Kaufman, 1994, p. 113).

This primary care case management team is similar to the "collaborative networking" band on the spectrum of collaboration (see chapter 8). The networking team assesses all the resources in the system and connects the patient and family with those resources that best address their needs. With this approach, the old military metaphor of medicine "combating" disease no longer makes sense. The newer market metaphors of providing care at the lowest cost also have their shortcomings. Annas (1995) proposes a shift to ecosystemic metaphors to more aptly capture the spirit of teams working together within a system of limited resources: "Ecologists use words such as integrity, balance, natural, limited (resources), quality (of life), diversity, renewable, sustainable, responsibility (for future generations), community and conservation. The ecological metaphor also naturally leads us to considerations of population health" (p. 747).

The collaborative mental health professional of the future will:

- work closely with primary health care practitioners;
- see patients for shorter visits over a longer period of time (more like primary care practitioners);
- provide "primary mental health care" and refer as needed to specialty mental health care; and
- be an integral part of a case management team.

POPULATION-BASED CARE

The goal of population-based care is to promote health and provide health care services to a population within a framework of limited resources. It contrasts with individual-based care, in which the needs of any one individual are championed against those of all others. Advocating for individuals promotes competition between individuals, often resulting in the expansion of costs beyond the limits of the system. In population-based care, a population is considered a closed system in which every action affects all other parts of the system. The needs of any one individual are balanced against the needs of the community. To reduce competition for limited resources, providers must emphasize the early identification of needs to facilitate proper allocation of resources. Mental health professionals trained in systems theory will be a tremendous asset in the application of population-based care.

Insurance companies are now more attuned to the health of whole communities. HMOs are interested in community benefits such as playgrounds, health clubs, and water quality. To promote health and decrease the need for services, they emphasize education and prevention by increasing access to primary care and providing earlier care to prevent hospitalization. In most HMOs, money is provided up-front so that the system can be proactive about providing health care services and allocating resources. Unprecedented for private health insurance, these practices are reminiscent of the midcentury Peckham Project in England and community-oriented primary care (COPC) in South Africa.

Indeed, the term "population-based care" may be new, but it is conceptually rooted in the notion of community-oriented primary care. COPC began in the 1940s in rural South Africa, where a single comprehensive health clinic was established and then expanded into a network of health centers. The concept grew and flourished in this country with the advent of the community health centers of the 1960s. Now the two concepts have virtually merged and can be used interchangeably. COPC shares three major principles with population-based care: (1) a defined population for which the service is responsible, and defined programs to address community health problems; (2) complementary use of epidemiologic and clinical skills; and (3) a multidisciplinary team (Tollman, 1991).

Patrick O'Connor notes how COPC will work in managed-care settings:

> The community will be defined as all members of a managed care organization. Many of the health problems to be addressed will be precisely identified on the basis of public health statistics, member surveys, marketing data, and accurate internal data on demographics, diagnoses, utilization, lab results, and prescription drug use. Some of the goals will be locally chosen, while others will be adaptations of the Healthy People 2000 goals, with a little local flavor. Examples would be: Raise the pediatric immunization rate from 75% to 95%. Diagnose 95% of all breast cancers at Stage 1 or 2. Find innovative ways to avoid institutionalization of frail members. Identify and develop strategies to combat domestic violence. Reduce teenage pregnancies. The programs needed to achieve these goals will change medical practice but will also go far beyond the medical model to involve restaurant menus, grocery stores, work-site exercise programs, churches, community events, and community organizations. Evaluation will be done together by managers, physicians, and members. (O'Connor, 1995, p. 6)

Certain high-risk groups within a population (e.g., pregnant teens, victims of sexual or physical abuse) may be targeted for more intensive services. Wright (1993) goes on to note that, "as a cybernetic planning process, COPC maximizes such accountability by establishing linkages between needs assessment, resource allocation, and health outcomes" (p. 2547).

Ironically, it is capitation, originally designed primarily as a cost-cutting tool, that will force providers to think about the needs of a defined population instead of just the needs of individuals. Capitated providers receive a flat rate per member per month to care for a panel of patients. The financial incentives under capitation are completely reversed from fee-for-service. Under fee-for-service, the more services one provides, the more one is reimbursed. In capitated designs, the incentive is to provide preventive care early to avoid costly treatment later. Many of the logistical difficulties of reimbursement for collaborative care may actually be eased by a capitated design. No longer is the concern about how to bill for the brief hallway consultation or phone call. Capitation promotes these brief high-care low-service events. As Patterson and Scherger (1995) note, "New models of integrating mental health providers with primary care physicians will be able to flourish under managed care since capitation liberates the providers from having to worry about coding, charges, and reimbursement from a common office" (p. 134).

The collaborative mental health professional of the future will:

- provide expertise in systemic approaches to implementing population-based care;
- work under a capitated system with increased incentives for collaborative care; and
- identify and collaboratively treat certain high-risk groups.

CONSUMERISM AND COLLABORATION WITH PATIENTS AND FAMILIES

A focus on satisfying the consumer is another business principle brought to the health care dialogue by managed care. A successful marketing strategy for HMOs has been to assess and confirm what patients want or need—"consumerism." This approach increases patient satisfaction. Although the motivation has been to solicit commitments to an insurance plan, the result has been that patients feel better about having a voice in how they get health care. One HMO, Ethix, calls all new enrollees, welcomes them to the plan, and uses an eight-question screening instrument to assess potential needs early on.

This attention to customer satisfaction is also consistent with the notion of collaboration with patients and their families. Collaboration with patients and their families has long been part of providing mental health care. Now an increasingly larger part of providing good medical care, collaboration facilitates an accurate assessment of a patient's needs and promotes a clearer sense of who is responsible for what actions. Collaboration promotes success since treatment is codesigned. Collaboration also encourages patients to take responsibility for their own care. Collaboration with families may increase provider satisfaction by redistributing the responsibility of care among providers, patient, and family members.

If quality steadily increases with the cost of health care, value is the point at which high quality is still affordable. Patients, as payers for health care, want the biggest "bang for their buck." Rather than "care at any cost," or even any outcome, the focus has turned to providing truly beneficial care. Much more attention is paid to outcome research so that quality care may be provided. For example, the Jackson Hole Group convened representatives from private and government organizations to eventually form the Foundation for Accountability (FAcct). This group is "united in a demand for greater attention to health care quality and an objective, uniform system for measuring and reporting medical outcomes" (Keister, 1995). It notes that, "in the long term, reform must be based on more than cost. It must be based on value," and that "the consumer must be in the driver's seat" (p. 20). This group, which has developed close ties with the Health Care Financing Organization, will first address performance measures for six conditions: asthma, breast cancer, coronary artery disease, depression, diabetes, and lower back pain. Several other groups are dedicated to like-minded causes: the American Managed Behavioral Healthcare Association, the Health Outcomes Institute, the Institute for Health Services Research, the National Committee for Quality Assurance, and the Regenstreif Institute. Even *Consumer Reports* (1995) evaluated the value of mental health care from the perspective of the consumer.

Consequently, consumer advocacy groups have grown tremendously. "Infracommunity collaboration" groups have been enormously helpful to countless patients by providing support networks and serving as informational clearinghouses for patients and their families. These very large groups have tremendous power. Many patients and families find that collaboration with other patients and families who have "been there" is particularly helpful. Sometimes it is easier to take advice from someone in the same boat than from an "authority." Some of these groups are professionally facilitated, but many are not. One typical example is the National Family Caregivers Association (NFCA, 9621 E. Bexhill Dr., Kensington, MD 20895). NFCA provides a newsletter, a resource guide, a caregiver profile, a toll-free hotline, educational materials for both caregivers and health professionals, a speaker's bureau, respite assistance, and a person-to-person linked network. Collaboration in these circles has come to be synonymous with good health care.

The collaborative mental health professional of the future will:

- help patients and families form and join peer groups;
- play both participatory and advisory roles to consumer advocacy groups;
- identify strengths, competencies, and resources of consumers;
- lend expertise to the process of collaboration between patients and families and insurance carriers (private or government); and
- facilitate patients and families helping (or collaborating with) other patients and families to address health and mental health concerns.

CONCLUSION

Health care in this country is changing and will continue to change. Following a tremendous expansion of services and costs, we are now emerging from an era of cost containment into a new age of value. Managed care has led the way with its emphasis on outpatient care, primary care, population-based care, and collaboration with its insured. Value in health and mental health care will emerge from the capacity of health and mental health practitioners and patients and families to collaborate. Systems designed to support such collaboration will see the merging of cost and quality. For the mental health professional, this will be a whole new world. It may frighten some who are reluctant to change traditional habits of thought and practice. But for those who are bold enough to venture into this new territory, there will be plenty of opportunity to apply their skills and knowledge to promote the overall health of patients and their families.

Collaborative Family Health Care Coalition Chapters

UNITED STATES

Alaska
Nome
Michael Terry
(901) 443–3284

Arizona
Phoenix/Scottsdale
Michael Belus
(602) 481–9042

California
Los Angeles
Johanna Schor
(213) 658–6120

Sacramento
Marlene Fitzwater
(916) 974–8686

San Diego
Claudia Grauf-Grounds
(619) 685–7397

San Francisco
Doug Rait
(415) 493–5000, x4967

Colorado
Denver
Tina Pittman Wagers
(303) 467–5721

Connecticut
Hartford
Stephen Bittner
(203) 838–1810

District of Columbia
Karen Weihs
(202) 994–2408

Florida
Fort Lauderdale/Miami
Margo Weiss
(305) 424–5700

Georgia
Atlanta
Leigh Ann Townes
(706) 542–4486

Illinois
Chicago
John Rolland
(312) 321–6040

Iowa
Ames/Des Moines
Jennifer Harkness
(512) 292–1915

Maine
Portland
Julie Schirmer
(207) 874–2471

Massachusetts
Amherst/Springfield
Alexander Blount
(413) 447–2157

Boston
Barry Dym
(617) 354–7565

Minnesota
Minneapolis/St. Paul
William Doherty
(612) 625–4752

Missouri
St. Louis
Yvonne Fallert
(314) 362–7883

New Hampshire/Vermont
Lebanon/White River Valley
Janet Cramer
(802) 295–8363

New Jersey
Newark
Kathleen Shiota
(201) 871–4996

New York
Buffalo
Frederick Cooley
(716) 691–2800

Long Island
George Meyer
(718) 864–2225

New York
Donald A. Bloch
(212) 675–2477

Rochester
David Seaburn
(716) 442–7470, x224

North Carolina
Chapel Hill/Durham/Raleigh
Bill Gunn
(919) 684–3620, x329

Ohio
Cleveland
Kathy Cole-Kelly
(216) 459–5737

Oregon
Portland
Shannon Fishman
(503) 244–4454

Pennsylvania
Philadelphia
Margaret Cotroneo
(610) 626–4672

Pittsburgh
David Raney
(412) 624–0459

Tennessee
Knoxville
William Conklin
(615) 586–5031

Texas
Houston
James Bray
(713) 798–7751

San Antonio
Mary Wrzesinski Conran
(210) 829–7985

Washington
Seattle
Larry Mauksch
(205) 548–6577

Spokane
Carl Greenberg
(509) 624–2313, x24

Wisconsin
Milwaukee
Eric Weiner
(414) 291–1608

EUROPE

England
London
Robert Bor
44–171–477–8523

Finland
Oalu
Erkki Vaisanen
358–81–3157–7370

Germany
Freiburg
Michael Wirsching
49–61–270–6805/6

Israel
Petach Tikva
Cynthia Carel
972–3–939–3616

Spain
Badajoz
Francisco Vaz
34–24–289–456

APPENDIX B

Eliciting the Patient's and Family's Story

These questions may be asked of the patient individually or of the patient and family together.

HISTORY OF THE ILLNESS/PROBLEM

- How long have you had this problem?
- How did you first notice it?
- How did family and friends react to changes you were going through?
- Who first suggested that you seek medical help?
- How many physicians and other health care providers have been involved in your care? How have they been helpful? Not helpful?
- What tests or procedures were needed to diagnose this problem? Have you been hospitalized? What medications are you taking?
- What is your understanding of the current status of your health?

IMPACT OF THE ILLNESS ON THE INDIVIDUAL

- How has your daily functioning changed?
- What do you miss most from before you were ill?
- What have you learned from this illness that has been useful to you?
- What do you think will happen with the illness in the future?

- How has your view of the future changed? What do you hope for?

IMPACT OF THE ILLNESS ON THE FAMILY

- What changes have occurred in the family since the illness began?
- How are family members coping with this difficulty?
- Do you talk about the illness as a family?
- Who has been most affected? Least affected?
- Who has the greatest responsibility for caring for the ill family member? How does the primary caregiver get support?
- In general, how do you support one another? How do you express emotions?
- Does this experience remind you or your family of other difficulties the family has faced?
- How well do you feel the family is coping? Is there anything the family wishes they could do differently?

MEANING OF THE ILLNESS AND FAMILY RESOURCES

- Why do you think this illness has occurred?
- How long do you think it will last?
- Are there times when the illness seems stronger than you or the family? Are there times when you or the family seem stronger than the illness?
- Do you or your family have religious or spiritual beliefs about this illness? If so, what are they?
- What are the strengths of your family? What keeps you going?

Note. See also *Medical Family Therapy: A Biopsychosocial Approach to Families with Health Problems* (p. 73) by S. H. McDaniel, J. Hepworth, and W. J. Doherty, 1992, New York: Basic Books.

APPENDIX C

Conferences

American Association for Marriage and Family Therapy
113 15th Street, NW, Suite 300
Washington, DC 20005
(202) 452–0109
Fax: (202) 223–2329

American Psychological Association
750 First Street, NE
Washington, DC 20002
Health Psychology Division, Dr. Edward Sarafino: (609) 771–2485
Family Practice, Division 43, Dr. James Bray: (602) 912–5300

Collaborative Family Health Care Coalition
40 West 12th Street
New York, NY 10011–8604
(212) 675–2477
Fax: (212) 727–1126
E-mail: cfhcc@sprynet.com

Medical Family Therapy Institute
University of Rochester—Family Therapy Training Program
300 Crittenden Boulevard
Rochester, NY 14642
(716) 275–2532

Society of Teachers of Family Medicine (Family in Family Medicine Conference)
8880 Ward Parkway
PO Box 8729
Kansas City, KS 64114
(800) 274–2237

Training Program Directory (degree required to participate)

Linda Garcia-Shelton, Ph.D.
Mark Vogel, Ph.D. (postdoctoral fellowship)
Primary Care Health Psychology Postdoctoral Fellowship
Genesys—Michigan State University
Family Practice Residency
302 Kensington Avenue
Flint, MI 48502
(810) 762–8484
Fax: (810) 762–8837
E-mail: 22568mv@msu.edu

Barbara A. Gawinski, Ph.D., Director (predoctoral
    internship/postdoctoral fellowship)
Medical Family Therapy Internship
University of Rochester Medical School
Department of Family Medicine
885 South Avenue
Rochester, NY 14620
(716) 442–7074, x265
Fax: (716) 442–1901
E-mail: BGSK@DB1.CC.Rochester.EDU

Jeri Hepworth, Ph.D. (master's student placement)
University of Connecticut
Department of Family Medicine

99 Woodland Street
Hartford, CT 06105
(203) 548–6526
Fax: (203) 548–5883
E-mail: BITNET HEPWORTH@UCONNVM

JoEllen Patterson, Ph.D. (master's degree program)
University of San Diego, MFCC Division
Counselor Division
5998 Alcala Park
San Diego, CA 92110
(619) 260–4538
Fax: (619) 260–6835

Douglas S. Rait, Ph.D., Director (predoctoral internship)
Palo Alto VA Medical Center (116–B3)
Department of Psychiatry and Behavioral Sciences
Family Therapy Program
3801 Miranda Avenue
Palo Alto, CA 94304
(415) 493–5000, x4697
Fax: (415) 852–3445
E-mail: DRAIT@FORSYTHE.STANFORD.EDU

John Rolland, M.D. (postgraduate training program)
Chicago Center for Family Health
445 East Illinois Street, Suite 651
Chicago, IL 60611
(312) 321–6040

David Seaburn, M.S., Director (postgraduate training program)
University of Rochester School of Medicine
Department of Psychiatry
Family Therapy Training Program
300 Crittenden Boulevard
Rochester, NY 14642–8409
(716) 275–2532
Fax: (716) 271–7706
E-mail: DBSN@DB1.CC.Rochester.EDU

David Waters, Ph.D. (predoctoral internship)
University of Virginia Medical School

Department of Family Medicine
Box 404
Charlottesville, VA 22908
(804) 924–5348
Fax: (804) 982–4306

Margo Weiss, Ph.D., Director (master's, Ph.D., and specialization
   programs)
Nova Southeastern University
School of Social and Systemic Studies
Medical Family Therapy Program
3301 College Avenue
Fort Lauderdale, FL 33314
(954) 424–5700/(800) 262–7978
Fax: (954) 424–5711
E-mail: Margo@ssss.nova.edu

Medical Terminology

ADD—attention deficit disorder
ADHD—attention deficit disorder with hyperactivity
ASA—aspirin
bf—boyfriend
CABG—coronary artery bypass grafting
CF—cystic fibrosis
c/o—complains of
CP—cerebral palsy
CPE—complete physical exam
CPS—Child Protective Services
CVA—cerebral vascular accident (stroke)
d/c—discontinue
DM—diabetes mellitus
DSS—Department of Social Services/Department of Social
    Security
d/t—due to
ED—emergency department
EtOH—alcohol
FDIU—fetal death in utero (dead fetus)
FOB—father of baby
GERD—gastroesophageal reflux disease
GOMER—get out of my emergency room
HA—headache
h/o—history of
HTN—hypertension (high blood pressure)
HX—history
IM—intramuscular
MGF—maternal grandfather
MGM—maternal grandmother

MI—myocardial infarction (heart attack)
MS—multiple sclerosis
PC—phone call
PGF—paternal grandfather
PGM—paternal grandmother
re—regarding
RX—therapy/prescription
SSI—social security income
SX—symptoms
SZ—seizure
U/A—urinalysis

Mental Health Record-Keeping for Medical Settings

REFERENCES

American Academy of Family Physicians, Commission on Health Care Services. (1994). *White paper on the provision of mental health services by family physicians.* AAFP Order #714. Kansas City, MO: Author.

American Academy of Family Practice. (1995). *Facts about family practice.* Leawood, KS: Nielson Printing.

American Hospital Association. (1993–94). *Hospital statistics.* Chicago: Author.

Anderson, H., & Goolishian, H. A. (1988). Human systems as linguistic systems: Preliminary and evolving ideas about the implications for clinical theory. *Family Process, 27,* 371–393.

Annas, G. J. (1995). Reframing the debate on health care reform by replacing our metaphors. *New England Journal of Medicine, 332*(11), 744–747.

Auerswald, E. (1968). Interdisciplinary versus ecological approach. *Family Process, 7,* 202–215.

Axinn, J., & Levin, H. (1975). *Social welfare: A history of the American response to need.* New York: Dodd, Mead and Co.

Baggs, J. G. (1994). Collaboration between nurses and physicians: What is it? Does it exist? In J. C. McCloskey & H. K. Grace (Eds.), *Current issues in nursing* (pp. 580–585). St. Louis: Mosby.

Baggs, J. G., & Schmitt, M. H. (1988). Collaboration between nurses and physicians. *Image, 20,* 145–149.

Bakan, D. (1966). *The duality of human existence: Isolation and communion in Western man.* Boston: Beacon Press.

Baldwin, D. C. (1994). *The role of interdisciplinary education and teamwork in primary care and health care reform.* Department of Health and Human Services, Public Health Service, Health Resources and Services Administration, Bureau of Health Profession, Office of Research and Planning, 5600 Fishers Lane, Room 8–47, Rockville, MD 20857, Order #92–1009(P).

Baldwin, D. C., & Baldwin, M. A. (1979). Interdisciplinary education and health team training: A model for learning and service. In A. D. Hunt &

L. E. Weeks (Eds.), *Medical education since 1960: Marching to a different drummer* (pp. 190–221). East Lansing: Michigan State Foundation.

Beck, A. T. (1976). *Cognitive therapy and emotional disorders.* New York: International University Press.

Beckman, H., Markakis, K., Suchman, A., & Frankel, R. (1994). The doctor-patient relationship and malpractice: Lessons from plaintiff depositions. *Archives of Internal Medicine, 154,* 1365–1370.

Beeson, P. (1990). Mental health services in rural America. *State Health Reports, 58,* 4–14.

Belar, C. D. (1995). Collaboration in capitated care: Challenges for psychology. *Professional Psychology: Research and Practice, 26,* 139–146.

Bennett, M. J. (1983). Focal psychotherapy—terminable and interminable. *American Journal of Psychotherapy, 37,* 365–375.

Bennett, M. J. (1993). View from the bridge: Reflections of a recovering staff model HMO psychiatrist. *Psychiatric Quarterly, 64,* 45–75.

Bennett, M. J. (1994). Are competing psychotherapists manageable? *Managed Care Quarterly, 2,* 36–42.

Berger, P. L., & Luckmann, T. (1966). *The social construction of reality.* New York: Doubleday.

Berkman, B., Bedell, D., Parker, E., McCarthy, L., & Rosebaum, C. (1988). Preadmission screening: An efficacy study. *Social Work in Health Care, 13,* 35–51.

Bernstein, A., Bergsten, C., Whitmore, H., Dial, T., & Gabel, J. (1994). *1994 HMO performance report.* Washington, DC: Group Health Association of America.

Bhatara, V. S., Fuller, W. C., & Unruh, E. R. (1994). The case for managed cooperation (not competition): South Dakota mental health linkage project. *South Dakota Journal of Medicine, 47,* 307–311.

Blase, N. J., & Kaufman, J. M. (1994). Case management in a vertically integrated health care system. *HMO Practice, 8,* 110–114.

Bleich, M. (1995, July 22). *Collaboration in hospitals and special settings.* Plenary address at the Collaborative Family Health Care Coalition Conference, Washington, DC.

Bloch, D. A. (1988). The partnership of Dr. Biomedicine and Dr. Psychosocial. *Family Systems Medicine, 6,* 2–4.

Bloch, D. A. (1993a). The generic health care team. *Family Systems Medicine, 11,* 119–120.

Bloch, D. A. (1993b). Editorial: Family and psychosocial medicine. *Family Systems Medicine, 11,* 231–234.

Blount, A., & Bayona, J. (1994). Toward a system of integrated primary care. *Family Systems Medicine, 12,* 171–182.

Bly, R. (1990). *Iron John.* Reading, MA: Addison-Wesley.

Board of Trustees, American Medical Association (1932a). The Committee on the Cost of Medical Care. *Journal of the American Medical Association, 99,* 1950–1952.

Board of Trustees, American Medical Association (1932b). The Committee on the Cost of Medical Care. *Journal of the American Medical Association, 99*, 2034–2035.

Bogdewic, S. P., Garr, D., Miller, M. C., & Myers, P. (1994). Characteristics and job satisfaction of nonphysician full-time family medicine faculty members. *Family Medicine, 26*, 79–84.

Boszormenyi-Nagy, I., & Spark, G. M. (1973). Invisible loyalties: Reciprocity in intergenerational family therapy. New York: Harper & Row.

Botelho, R., & Harp, J. (in preparation). *Reflective practitioners in health care: Learning from challenging experiences.* Unpublished manuscript.

Bowen, M. (1978). *Family therapy in clinical practice.* New York: Jason Aronson.

Boyd-Franklin, N. (1982). Afro-American families and the victim system. In M. McGoldrick, J. K. Pearce, & J. Giordano (Eds.), *Ethnicity and family therapy* (pp. 78–80). New York: Guilford Press.

Boyd-Franklin, N. (1989). *Black families in therapy: A multisystems approach.* New York: Guilford Press.

Bray, J. H., & Rogers, J. C. (1995). Linking psychologists and family physicians for collaborative practice. *Professional Psychology: Research and Practice, 26*, 132–138.

Brickman, P. (1982). Models of helping and coping. *American Psychologist, 37*, 368–384.

Bridges, K., & Goldberg, K. (1985). Somatic presentation of *DSM-III* psychiatric disorders in primary care. *Journal of Psychosomatic Research, 29*, 563–569.

Brown, T. (1989). Cartesian dualism and psychosomatics. *Psychosomatics, 30*, 322–331.

Brownell, K., Hecherman, C., Westlake, R., Hayes, S., & Monti, P. (1978). The effects of couples training and partner cooperativeness in the behavioral treatment of obesity. *Behavioral Research and Therapy, 16*, 323–333.

Budd, M. A., & Gruman, J. C. (1995). Behavioral medicine: Taking its place in the mainstream of primary care. *HMO Practice, 9*, 51–52.

Burlingame, G. M., Lambert, M. J., Reisinger, C. W., Neff, W. M., & Mosier, J. (1995). Pragmatics of tracking mental health outcomes in a managed care setting. *Journal of Mental Health Administration, 22*, 226–236.

Burns, B., Goldberg, I., Hankin, J., Hoeper, E., Jacobson, A., & Regier, D. (1982). Uses of ambulatory health/mental health utilization data in organized health care settings. *Health Policy Quarterly, 2*(3), 169–179.

Campbell, T. L., & Patterson, J. (1995). The effectiveness of family interventions in the treatment of physical illness. *Journal of Marital and Family Therapy, 21*, 545–582.

Caplan, G., & Caplan, R. B. (1993). *Mental health consultation and collaboration.* San Francisco: Jossey-Bass.

Cassata, D., & Kirkman-Liff, B. (1981). Mental health activities of family physicians. *Journal of Family Practice, 12*, 683–692.

Cave, D. G. (1995). Vertical integration models to prepare health systems for capitation. *Health Care Management Review, 20,* 26–39.

Cecchin, G. (1987). Hypothesizing, circularity, and neutrality revisited: An invitation to curiosity. *Family Process, 26,* 405–413.

Center for Mental Health Services. (1994). *Mental health, United States, 1994.* R. W. Manderscheid & M. A. Sonnenschein (Eds.), DHHS Pub. No. (SMA) 94–3000. Washington, DC: Government Printing Office.

Christie-Seely, J. (Ed.). (1984). *Working with the family in primary care: A systems approach to health and illness.* New York: Praeger.

Cleary, P. (1991). Patients evaluate their hospital care: A national survey. *Health Affairs, 10,* 254–267.

Cohen, S., & Syme, S. (Eds.). (1985). *Social support and health.* Orlando, FL: Academic Press.

Cole-Kelly, K., & Hepworth, J. (1991). Training sketch: Performance pressures: Saner responses for consultant family therapists. *Family Systems Medicine, 9,* 159–164.

Coleman, J., Patrick, D., Eagle, J., & Hermalin, J. (1979). Collaboration, consultation, and referral in an integrated health-mental health program of an HMO. *Social Work in Health Care, 5,* 83–96.

Combrinck-Graham, L. (1990). *Giant steps: Therapeutic innovations in child mental health.* New York: Basic Books.

Congressional Committee on Managed Care. (1975). Health maintenance organizations: Text of HMO Act of 1973—Proposed and Adopted Regulations. *Medicare and Medicaid, 146,* 57–61.

Consumer Reports. (1995, November). Mental health: Does therapy help? Pp. 734–739.

Costello, E. J., Edelbrock, C., Costello, A. J., Dulcan, M. K., Burns, B. J., & Brent, D. (1988). Psychopathology in pediatric primary care: The new hidden morbidity. *Pediatrics, 82,* 415–424.

Crouch, M., & Roberts, L. (Eds.). (1987). *The family in medical practice.* New York: Springer-Verlag.

Dashiff, C., Greiner, D., & Cannon, N. (1990). Physicians and nurse collaboration in a medical clinic for indigent patients. *Family Systems Medicine, 8,* 57–70.

DeGroot, G. (1994). VA encourages psychologists to be part of medical team. *American Psychological Association Monitor, 25*(7), 59.

DeGruy, F. (1995, Fall). Overview of collaborative research. *Working Together* [newsletter of the Collaborative Family Health Care Coalition, New York, NY], 3–4.

Democritus. (1922). Fragment B3. In H. Diels (Ed.), *Die Fragmente der Vorsokratiker* (4th ed.). Berlin: Weidmann.

DeShazer, S. (1982). *Patterns of brief family therapy: An ecosystemic approach.* New York: Guilford Press.

Devers, K. J., Shortell, S. M., Gillies, R. R., Anderson, D. A., Mitchell, J. B., & Erickson, M. L. K. (1994). Implementing organized delivery systems:

An integration scorecard. *Health Care Management Review, 19,* 7–20.

Devine, E., & Cook, T. (1986). Clinical and cost-saving effects of psycho-educational interventions with surgical patients: A meta-analysis. *Research in Nursing and Health, 9,* 89–105.

Doherty, W. J. (1986). A missionary at work: A family therapist in a family medicine department. *Family Therapy Networker, 10,* 65–68.

Doherty, W. J. (1995). The whys and the levels of collaboration. *Family Systems Medicine, 13,* 275–281.

Doherty, W. J., & Baird, M. A. (1983). *Family therapy and family medicine.* New York: Guilford Press.

Doherty, W. J., & Baird, M. A. (1986). Developmental levels in family-centered medical care. *Family Medicine, 18,* 153–156.

Doherty, W., & Baird, M. (Eds.). (1987). *Family-centered medical care: A clinical casebook.* New York: Guilford Press.

Doherty, W. J., Baird, M., & Becker, L. (1987). Family medicine and the biopsychosocial model: The road to integration. *Marriage and Family Review, 10,* 51–70.

Doherty, W. J., & Campbell, T. L. (1988). *Families and health.* Newbury Park, CA: Sage.

Donaldson, M., Yordy, K., & Vanselow, N. (Eds.). (1994). *Defining primary care: An interim report.* Committee on the Future of Primary Care, Division of Health Care Services, Institute of Medicine. Washington, DC: National Academy Press.

Duer, S., Schwenk, T. L., & Coyne, J. C. (1988). Medical and psychological correlates of self-reported depressive symptoms in family practice. *Journal of Family Practice, 27,* 609–614.

Dym, B. (1986). Collaborative work: The primary care health team. *Working Together, 1,* 9.

Dym, B. (1987). The cybernetics of physical illness. *Family Process, 26,* 35–48.

Dym, B., & Berman, S. (1986). The primary health care team: Family physician and family therapist in joint practice. *Family Systems Medicine, 4,* 9–21.

Endicott, J., & Spitzer, R. (1978). A diagnostic interview: The schedule for affective disorders and schizophrenia. *Archives of General Psychiatry, 35,* 837–844.

Engel, G. L. (1977). The need for a new medical model: A challenge for biomedicine. *Science, 196,* 129–136.

Engel, G. L. (1980). The clinical application of the biopsychosocial model. *American Journal of Psychiatry, 137,* 535–544.

Epstein, R., & Guttmacher, L. (1995). *Biopsychosocial Medicine I: Part 1. Introduction to the patient-physician relationship.* Unpublished faculty manual for the University of Rochester School of Medicine, Rochester, NY.

Fawzy, F., Cousins, N., & Fawzy, N. (1990). A structured psychiatric intervention for cancer patients: Changes over time in methods of coping and affective disturbance. *Archives of General Psychiatry, 47,* 720–725.

Fink, A., Siu, A., Brook, R., Park, R., & Soloman, D. (1987). Assuring the quality of health care for older persons: An expert panel's priorities. *Journal of the American Medical Association, 258,* 1905–1908.

Finney, J., Riley, A., & Cataldo, N. (1991). Psychology in primary health care: Effects of brief targeted therapy on children's medical care utilization. *Journal of Pediatric Psychology, 16,* 447–461.

Follette, W., & Cummings, N. (1967). Psychiatric services and medical utilization in a prepaid health plan setting. *Medical Care, 5,* 25–36.

Freud, S. (1965). *The Interpretation of Dreams* (A. A. Brill, Trans.). New York: Modern Library. (Original work published 1900)

Freud, S. (1990). *The Standard Edition* (J. Strachey, Ed. and Trans.). New York: Norton. (Original work published 1887–1938)

Garralda, M. E., & Bailey, D. (1986). Psychological deviance in children attending general practice. *Psychological Medicine, 16,* 423–429.

Garralda, M. E., & Bailey, D. (1987). Psychosomatic aspects of children's consultations in primary care. *European Archives of Psychiatry and Neurological Sciences, 237,* 319–322.

Geertz, C. (1973). *The interpretation of cultures.* New York: Basic Books.

Gergen, K. (1985). The social constructionist movement in modern psychology. *American Psychologist, 40,* 266–275.

German, M. (1994). Effective case management in managed mental health care: Conditions, methods, and outcomes. *HMO Practice, 8,* 34–40.

Gerteis, M., Edgman-Levitan, S., Daley, J., & Delbanco, T. (Eds.). (1993). *Through the patient's eyes.* San Francisco: Jossey-Bass.

Glenn, M. (1985a). Putting the pieces together: The therapist in medical practice. *Family Therapy Networker, 9*(1), 30, 32–33, 36.

Glenn, M. (1985b). Toward collaborative family-oriented health care. *Family Systems Medicine, 3,* 466–475.

Glenn, M. (1987a). *On diagnosis: A systemic approach.* New York: Brunner/Mazel.

Glenn, M. L. (1987b). *Collaborative health care: A family-oriented model.* New York: Praeger.

Gonzales, J., & Norquist, G. (1994). Mental health consultation-liaison interventions in primary care. In J. Miranda, A. Hohmann, C. Atkinson, & D. Larson (Eds.), *Mental disorders in primary care* (pp. 347–377). San Francisco: Jossey-Bass.

Gonzalez, S., Steinglass, P., & Reiss, D. (1989). Putting the illness in its place: Discussion groups for families with chronic medical illnesses. *Family Process, 28,* 69–87.

Goolishian, H. A., & Anderson, H. (1990). Understanding the therapeutic process: From individuals and families to systems in language. In F. Kaslow (Ed.), *Voices in family psychology* (pp. 91–113). Newbury Park, CA: Sage.

Graham, H., Senior, R., Dukes, S., Lazarus, M., & Mayer, R. (1993). The introduction of family therapy to British general practice. *Family Systems Medicine, 11,* 363–373.

Grieco, A., Garnett, S., Glassman, K., Valoon, P., & McClure, M. (1990). New York University Medical Center's Cooperative Care Unit: Patient education and family participation during hospitalization—The first ten years. *Patient Education and Counseling, 15,* 3–15.

Griffith, J. L., & Griffith, M. E. (1994). *The body speaks: Therapeutic dialogues for mind-body problems.* New York: Basic Books.

Grimaldi, P. (1995). Risk sharing to avert decapitation. *Nursing Management, 26,* 12–16.

Guttmacher, L. B. (1988). *Concise guide to somatic therapies in psychiatry.* Washington, DC.: American Psychiatric Press.

Haley, J. (1973). *Uncommon therapy.* New York: Norton.

Haley, J. (1976). *Problem-solving therapy.* San Francisco: Jossey-Bass.

Hays, R. D., Wells, K. B., Sherbourne, C. D., Rogers, W., & Spritzer, K. (1995). Functioning and well-being outcomes of patients with depression compared with chronic general medical illness. *Archives of General Psychiatry, 52,* 11–19.

Hepworth, J., Gavazzi, S. M., Adlin, M. S., & Miller, W. L. (1988). Training for collaboration: Internships for family-therapy students in a medical setting. *Family Systems Medicine, 6,* 69–79.

Hepworth, J., & Jackson, M. (1985). Health care for families: Models of collaboration between family therapists and family physicians. *Family Relations, 34,* 123–127.

Hewson, M. G. (1992). Clinical teaching in the ambulatory setting. *Journal of General Internal Medicine, 7,* 76–82.

Hippocrates. (1988). *Epidemics I.* In P. Potter (Ed.), *Hippocratic medicine* (p. 43). Quebec: Les Éditions du Sphinx.

Hooley, J. M., Orley, J., & Teasdale, J. D. (1986). Levels of expressed emotion and relapse in depressed patients. *British Journal of Psychiatry, 148,* 642–647.

House, J., Landis, K., & Umberson, D. (1988). Social relationships and health. *Science, 241,* 540–545.

Howard, G. (1991). Culture tales: A narrative approach to thinking, cross-cultural psychology, and psychotherapy. *American Psychologist, 46,* 187–191.

Hoyt, M. F. (1994). Promoting HMO values and the culture of quality: "Doing the right thing" in an HMO mental health department. *HMO Practice, 8,* 122–126.

Huebel, E. (1993, March). *One-stop shopping.* Unpublished report to the Department of Public Health in Madison, Wisconsin.

Hunter, R. M. (1991). *Doctors' stories: The narrative structure of medical knowledge.* Princeton, NJ: Princeton University Press.

Huygen, F. J. A. (1978). *Family medicine: The medical life history of families.* New York: Brunner-Mazel.

Imber-Black, E. (1988). *Families and larger systems.* New York: Guilford Press.

Jacobsen, A., Regier, D., & Burns, B. (1978). Factors relating to the use of mental health services in a neighborhood health center. *Public Health Reports, 93,* 232–239.

Jaffe, D. T. (1986). The inner strains of healing work: Therapy and self-renewal for health professionals. In C. Scott and J. Hawk (Eds.), *Heal thyself: The health of health care professionals* (pp. 122–135). New York: Brunner/Mazel.

James, W. (1890). *Principles of psychology.* New York: Dover.

James, W. (1961). *The varieties of religious experience: A study in human nature.* New York: Collier. (Original work published 1902)

James, W. (1970). *The Meaning of Truth.* Ann Arbor, MI: Ann Arbor Press. (Original work published 1909)

James, W. (1971). *Essays in radical empiricism* and *A pluralistic universe.* New York: Dutton. (Original work published 1905–7)

James, W. (1974). *Pragmatism* and *Four essays from The meaning of truth.* New York: New American Library. (Original works published 1907 and 1909)

Jansen, M. (1986). Emotional disorders and the labor force. *International Labor Review, 125,* 605–615.

Johnson, B., Jeppson, E., & Redburn, L. (1992). *Caring for children and families: Guidelines for hospitals.* Bethesda, MD: Association for the Care of Children's Health.

Jones, K., & Vischi, T. (1979). Impact of alcohol, drug abuse, and mental health treatment on medical care utilization. *Medical Care, 17,* 1–82.

Karpel, M. (1986). *Family resources: The hidden partner in family therapy.* New York: Guilford Press.

Kathol, R., Harsch, H., Hall, R., Shakespeare, A., & Cowart, F. (1992). Categorization of types of medical/psychiatry units based on level of acuity. *Psychosomatics, 33,* 376–386.

Katon, W., & Gonzales, J. (1994). A review of randomized trials of psychiatric consultation-liaison studies in primary care. *Psychosomatics, 35,* 268–278.

Katon, W., Kleinman, A., & Rosen, G. (1982). Depression and somatization: A review. *American Journal of Internal Medicine, 72,* 127–135.

Katon, W., Von Korff, M., Lin, E., Bush, E., Russo, J., Lipscomb, P., & Wagner, E. (1992). A randomized trial of psychiatric consultation with distressed high utilizers. *General Hospital Psychiatry, 14,* 86–98.

Katon, W., Von Korff, M., Lin, E., Lipscomb, P., Wagner, E., & Polik, E. (1990). Distressed high utilizers of medical care: DSM-IIIR diagnosis and treatment needs. *General Hospital Psychiatry, 12,* 355–362.

Katon, W., Von Korff, M., Lin, E., Walker, E., Simon, G. E., Bush, T., Robinson, P., & Russo, J. (1995). Collaborative management to achieve treatment guidelines: Impact on depression in primary care. *Journal of the American Medical Association, 273,* 1026–1031.

Keister, L. W. (1995, October). With health costs finally moderating, employers' focus turns to quality. *Managed Care,* 20–24.

ler, L., Cleary, P., & Burke, J. (1985). Psychiatric disorders in primary are. *Archives of General Psychiatry, 42,* 583–587.

einman, A. (1988). *The illness narratives: Suffering, healing, and the human condition.* New York: Basic Books.

Kleinman, A., Eisenberg, L., & Good, B. (1978). Culture, illness, and care: Clinical lessons from the anthropologies and cross-cultural research. *Annals of Internal Medicine, 88,* 251–258.

Klerman, G. L., Weissman, M. M., Rounsaville, B. J., & Chevron, E. (1984). *Interpersonal psychotherapy of depression.* New York: Basic Books.

Konrad, T. R., & DeFriese, G. H. (1990). Impact of financial and organizational changes on primary care. In J. Mayfield & M. L. Grady (Eds.), *Primary care research: An agenda for the 90's* (pp. 97–106). Rockville, MD: U.S. Department of Health and Human Services.

Kuhn, T. (1970). *The structure of scientific revolutions.* Chicago: University of Chicago Press.

Landau-Stanton, J., & Clements, C. (1993). *AIDS, health, and mental health: A primary sourcebook.* New York: Brunner/Mazel.

Lareau, M., & Nelson, E. (1994). The physician and licensed mental health professional team: Prevalence and feasibility. *Family Systems Medicine, 12,* 37–45.

Lehman, A. F. (1989). Capitation payment and mental health care: A review of the opportunities and risks. *Journal of Child Psychiatry, 30,* 449–458.

Lehrer, P., Sargunaraj, D., & Hochron, S. (1992). Psychological approaches to the treatment of asthma. *Journal of Consulting and Clinical Psychology, 60,* 639–643.

Levenson, D. (1984). *Montefiore: The hospital as a social instrument.* New York: Farrar, Straus.

Like, R., Breckenridge, M., Swee, D., & Lieberman III, J. (1993). Family health science and the new generalist practitioner. *Family Systems Medicine, 11,* 149–161.

Longlett, S., & Kruse, J. (1992). Behavioral science education in family medicine: A survey of behavioral science educators and family physicians. *Family Medicine, 24,* 28–35.

Madanes, C. (1981). *Strategic family therapy.* San Francisco: Jossey-Bass.

Magner, L. (1992). *History of medicine.* New York: Marcel Dekker.

Manderscheid, R. W., Rae, D. S., Narrow, W. E., Locke, B. Z., & Regier, D. A. (1993). Congruence of service utilization estimates from the epidemiologic catchment area project and other sources. *Archives of General Psychiatry, 50,* 108–114.

Martinez, I. M. (1990). Mental health: The history of an internationalist cooperation with Nicaragua. *Family Systems Medicine, 8,* 327–337.

Maturana, H. R., & Varella, F. S. (1988). *The tree of knowledge: The biological roots of human understanding.* Boston: Shambhala Press.

Mauksch, L. B., & Heldring, M. (1995). Behavioral scientists' views on work environment, roles, and teaching. *Family Medicine, 27,* 103–108.

Mauksch, L., & Leahy, D. (1993). Collaboration between primary care medicine and mental health in an HMO. *Family Systems Medicine, 11,* 121–135.

McDaniel, S. (1992). Implementing the biopsychosocial model: The future for psychosocial specialists. *Family Systems Medicine, 10,* 277–281.

McDaniel, S., & Campbell, T. (1986). Physicians and family therapists: The risks of collaboration. *Family Systems Medicine, 4,* 4–8.

McDaniel, S. H., Campbell, T. L., & Seaburn, D. B. (1990). *Family-oriented primary care: A manual for medical providers.* New York: Springer-Verlag.

McDaniel, S. H., Hepworth, J., & Doherty, W. J. (1992). *Medical family therapy: A biopsychosocial approach to families with health problems.* New York: Basic Books.

McGoldrick, M., & Gerson, R. (1985). *Genograms in family assessment.* New York: Norton.

McGuire, T. G. (1994). Predicting the cost of mental health benefits. *Milbank Quarterly, 72,* 3–23.

Mechanic, D. (1994). Establishing mental health priorities. *Milbank Quarterly, 72,* 501–515.

Mechanic, D., Schlesinger, M., & McAlpine, D. D. (1995). Management of mental health and substance abuse services: State of the art and early results. *Milbank Quarterly, 73,* 19–55.

Medalie, J. H. (Ed.). (1978). *Family medicine: Principles and applications.* Baltimore: Williams & Wilkins.

Medalie, J., & Cole-Kelly, K. (1993). Behavioral science and family medicine collaboration: A developmental paradigm. *Family Systems Medicine, 11,* 15–64.

Melosh, B. (1982). *"The physician's hand": Work, culture, and conflict in American nursing.* Philadelphia: Temple University Press.

Mengel, M. (1987). Physician ineffectiveness due to family-of-origin issues. *Family Systems Medicine, 5,* 176–190.

Miller, R. H., & Luft, H. S. (1994a). Managed care plans: Characteristics, growth, and premium performance. *Annual Review of Public Health, 15,* 437–459.

Miller, R. H., & Luft, H. S. (1994b). Managed care plan performance since 1980: A literature analysis. *Journal of the American Medical Association, 271,* 1512–1519.

Minuchin, S. (1974). *Families and family therapy.* Cambridge, MA: Harvard University Press.

Minuchin, S., & Fishman, C. (1981). *Family therapy techniques.* Cambridge, MA: Harvard University Press.

Molinari, E., Taverna, A., Gasca, G., & Constantino, A. L. (1994). Collaborative team approach to asthma: A clinical study. *Family Systems Medicine, 12,* 47–59.

Morisky, D., Levine, D., Green, L., Shapiro, S., Russell, R., & Smith, C.

(1983). Five-year blood pressure control and mortality following health education for hypertensive patients. *American Journal of Public Health, 73,* 153–162.

Muchnick, S., Davis, B., Getzinger, A., Rosenberg, A., & Weiss, M. (1993). Collaboration between family therapy and health care: An internship experience. *Family Systems Medicine, 11,* 271–279.

Mumford, E., Schlesinger, H., & Glass, G. (1982). The effects of psychological intervention on recovery from surgery and heart attacks: An analysis of the literature. *American Journal of Public Health, 72,* 141–151.

Mumford, E., Schlesinger, H., Glass, G., Patrick, C., & Cuerdon, T. (1984). A new look at evidence about reduced cost of medical utilization following mental health treatment. *American Journal of Psychiatry, 141,* 1145–1158.

National Center for Health Statistics. (1995). *Health, United States, 1994.* Hyattsville, MD: Public Health Service.

Navarro, V. (1976). *Medicine under capitalism.* New York: Prodist.

Naylor, M. (1990). Comprehensive discharge planning for hospitalized elderly: A pilot study. *Nursing Research, 39,* 156–161.

Neher, J. O., Gordon, K. C., Meyer, B., & Stevens, N. (1992). A five-step "microskills" model of clinical teaching. *Journal of the American Board of Family Practice, 5,* 419–424.

Nelson, S. Z., Mensing, C., Baines, B., & Smith, J. (1995). An integrated continuum of care. *HMO Practice, 9,* 40–43.

Nightingale, F. (1860). *Notes on nursing: What it is, and what it is not.* New York: Appleton.

O'Connor, P. (1995). Community-oriented primary care in managed care organizations. *Copacetic, 2*(2), 2–6.

Olfson, M., & Pincus, H. A. (1994). Outpatient psychotherapy in the United States: Part 1. Volume, costs, and user characteristics. *American Journal of Psychiatry, 151,* 1281–1288.

Ormel, J., Von Korff, M., Ustan, B., Pini, S., Korten, A., & Oldehinkel, T. (1994). Common mental disorders and disability across cultures: Results of the WHO collaborative study on psychological problems in general health care. *Journal of the American Medical Association, 272,* 1741–1748.

Pallak, M. S., Cummings, N. A., Dorken, H., & Henke, C. J. (1994). Medical costs, Medicaid, and managed mental health treatment: The Hawaii study. *Managed Care Quarterly, 2,* 64–70.

Patterson, J., Bischoff, R., Scherger, J. E., & Grauf-Grounds, C. (1996). University family therapy training and a family medicine residency in a managed-care setting. *Family, Systems, and Health, 14,* 5–16.

Patterson, J., & Magulac, M. (1994). The family therapist's guide to psychopharmacology: A graduate-level course. *Journal of Marital and Family Therapy, 20,* 151–174.

Patterson, J., & Scherger, J. E. (1995). A critique of health care reform in the

United States: Implications for the training and practice of marriage and family therapy. *Journal of Marital and Family Therapy, 21,* 127–135.

Patterson, J. M., McCubbin, H. I., & Warwick, W. J. (1990). The impact of family functioning on health changes in children with cystic fibrosis. *Social Science Medicine, 31,* 159–164.

Pearce, J., Lebow, M., & Orchard, J. (1981). Role of spouse involvement in the behavioral treatment of overweight women. *Journal of Consulting and Clinical Psychology, 49,* 236–244.

Pearse, I. H., & Crocker, L. H. (1943). *The Peckham experiment.* London: Allen & Unwin.

Peek, C. J., & Heinrich, R. L. (1995). Building a collaborative healthcare organization: From idea to invention to innovation. *Family Systems Medicine, 13,* 327–342.

Physician Payment Review Commission. (1992). Managing care: Beyond the rhetoric. In *Physician Payment Review Commission annual report* (pp. 313–342). Washington, DC: Author.

Preston, J., O'Neal, J. H., & Talaga, M. C. (1994). Handbook of clinical psychopharmacology for therapists. Oakland, CA: New Harbinger.

Price, J. (1894). Obstetrical asepsis. *Boston Medical and Surgical Journal, 131,* 40–42.

Pyle, T. O., & Brunk, G. (1995, January). The reformation of the health care system. *The Internist,* 13–16.

Quirk, M. P., Rubenstein, S., Strosahl, K., & Todd, J. (1993). Quality and customers: A planning approach to the future of mental health services in a health maintenance organization. *Journal of Health Care Administration, 20,* 1–7.

Quirk, M. P., Strosahl, K., Todd, J. L., Fitzpatrick, W., Casey, M. T., Hennessy, S., & Simon, G. (in press). Quality and customers: Type 2 change in mental health delivery within health care reform. *Journal of Mental Health Administration.*

Ransom, D. C. (1993). The family in family medicine: Reflections on the first 25 years. *Family Systems Medicine, 11,* 25–29.

Regier, D., Goldberg, I., & Taube, C. (1978). The defacto U.S. mental health services system: A public health perspective. *Archives of General Psychiatry, 35,* 685–693.

Regier, D. A., Narrow, W. E., Rae, D. S., Manderscheid, R. W., Locke, B. Z., & Goodwin, F. K. (1993). The de facto U.S. mental and addictive disorders service system. *Archives of General Psychiatry, 50,* 85–94.

Relman, A. (1988). Assessment and accountability: The third revolution in medical care. *New England Journal of Medicine, 319,* 1220–1222.

Reverby, S., & Rosner, D. (Eds.). (1979). *Health care in America: Essays in social history.* Baltimore: Temple University Press.

Rinaldi, R. (1985). Positive effects of psychosocial interventions on total health care: A review of the literature. *Family Systems Medicine, 3,* 417–426.

Rivo, M., & Satcher, D. (1993). Improving access to health care through physician work force reform: Directions for the 21st century. *Journal of the American Medical Association, 270,* 1074–1078.

Robins, L., Helzer, J., Croughan, R., & Ratcliffe, K. (1981). National Institute of Mental Health Diagnostic Interview Schedule: Its history, characteristics, and validity. *Archives of General Psychiatry, 38,* 381–389.

Rogers, J. C., & Holloway, R. L. (1993). Professional intimacy: Somewhere between collegiality and personal intimacy? *Family Systems Medicine, 11,* 263–271.

Rogers, W. H., Wells, K. B., Meredith, L. S., Sturm, R., & Burnam, A. (1993). Outcomes for adult outpatients with depression under prepaid or fee-for-service financing. *Archives of General Psychiatry, 50,* 517–525.

Rolland, J. S. (1994a). *Families, illness, and disability: An integrative treatment model.* New York: Basic Books.

Rolland, J. S. (1994b). Working with illness: Clinicians' personal and interface issues. *Family Systems Medicine, 12,* 149–169.

Rorty, R. (1979). *Philosophy and the mirror of nature.* Princeton, NJ: Princeton University Press.

Ross, J., & Doherty, W. J. (1988). Systems analysis and guidelines for behavioral scientists in family medicine. *Family Medicine, 20,* 46–50.

Ross, M., & Scott, M. (1985). An evaluation of the effectiveness of individual and group cognitive therapy in the treatment of depressed patients. *Journal of Royal College of General Practitioners, 35,* 239–242.

Rubenstein, L. (1984). Effectiveness of a geriatric evaluation unit: A randomized clinical trial. *New England Journal of Medicine, 311,* 1664–1670.

Saccone, A., & Israel, A. (1978). Effects of experimental versus significant other controlled reinforcement and choice of target behavior on weight loss. *Behavior Therapy, 9,* 271–278.

Safran, C., & Phillips, R. (1989). Interventions to prevent readmission: The constrains of cost and efficacy. *Medical Care, 2,* 204–211.

Schappert, S. M. (1992). National ambulatory medical care survey: 1989 summary. National Center for Health Statistics. *Vital Health Statistics, 13*(110).

Schlesinger, J., Mumford, E., Glass, G., Patrick, C., & Sharfstein, S. (1983). Mental health treatment and medical care utilization in a fee-for-service system: Outpatient mental health treatment following the onset of a chronic disease. *American Journal of Public Health, 73,* 422–429.

Schrage, M. (1990). *Shared minds: The new technologies of collaboration.* New York: Random House.

Schurman, M., Kramer, P., & Mitchell, J. (1985). The hidden mental health network: Treatment of mental illness by nonpsychiatrist physicians. *Archives of General Psychiatry, 42,* 84–94.

Schwartz, A., Ginsburg, P., & LeRoy, L. (1993). Reforming graduate medical education: Summary report of the Physician Payment Review Commission. *Journal of the American Medical Association, 270,* 1079–1082.

Seaburn, D. B. (1988). *Medical stuff.* Rochester, NY: University of Rochester Media Center.

Seaburn, D. B. (1994). Consulting to a health care system in transition: The case of hemophilia. *Family Systems Medicine, 12,* 183–196.

Seaburn, D. B. (1995). Language, silence, and somatic fixation. In S. H. McDaniel (Ed.), *Counseling families with chronic illness* (pp. 49–66). Alexandria, VA: American Counseling Association.

Seaburn, D. B., Gawinski, B. A., Harp, J., McDaniel, S. H., Waxman, D., & Shields, C. (1993). Family systems therapy in a primary care medical setting: The Rochester experience. *Journal of Marital and Family Therapy, 19,* 177–190.

Seaburn, D. B., Landau-Stanton, J., & Horwitz, S. (1995). Core techniques in family therapy. In R. Mikesell, D-D. Lusterman, & S. McDaniel (Eds.), *Integrating family therapy: Handbook of family psychology and systems theory* (pp. 5–26). Washington, DC: American Psychological Association Press.

Seaburn, D. B., Lorenz, A., & Kaplan, D. (1992). The transgenerational development of chronic illness meanings. *Family Systems Medicine, 10,* 385–394.

Senge, P. (1990). *The fifth discipline: The art and practice of the learning organization.* New York: Doubleday/Currency.

Shapiro, J. (1980). A revisionist theory for the integration of behavioral science into family medicine departments. *Journal of Family Practice, 10,* 275–282.

Shapiro, J. (1990). Parallel process in the family medicine system: Issues and challenges for resident training. *Family Medicine, 22,* 312–319.

Shapiro, J., & Schiermer, D. C. (1993). Clinical training of psychologists in family practice settings: An examination of special issues. *Family Medicine, 25,* 443–446.

Shemo, J. (1985). Cost-effectiveness of providing mental health services: The offset effect. *International Journal of Psychiatry in Medicine, 15,* 19–30.

Shepherd, M., Cooper, B., Brown, A., & Kalton, G. (1966). *Psychiatric illness in general practice.* London: Oxford University Press.

Shields, C. G., Wynne, L. C., McDaniel, S. H., & Gawinski, B. A. (1994). The marginalization of family therapy: A historical and continuing problem. *Journal of Marital and Family Therapy, 20,* 117–138.

Shortell, S., Gillies, R., & Devers, K. (1995). Reinventing the American hospital. *Milbank Quarterly, 73,* 131–159.

Shryrock, R. (1959). *The history of nursing: An interpretation of the social and medical factors involved.* London: Saunders.

Shusterman, A. J. (1995). Why HMOs need specialized partners for behavior health care. *HMO Magazine, 36,* 51–52.

Sjodin, I. (1983). Psychotherapy in peptic ulcer disease: A controlled outcome study. *Acta Psychiatrica Scandinavica, 6,* 307.

Sloan, D., & Chamel, M. (1991). *The quality revolution and health care: A primer for purchasers and providers.* New York: American Society for Quality Control.

Smilkstein, G., Kleinman, A., Chrisman, N., Rosen, G., & Katon, W. (1981). The clinical social science conference in biopsychosocial teaching. *Journal of Family Practice, 12,* 347–353.

Smith, C., Monson, R., & Ray, D. (1986). Psychiatric consultation in somatization disorder. *New England Journal of Medicine, 314,* 1407–1413.

Smith, D., & Mahoney, R. (1990). *McDonnell Douglas Corporation employee assistance program financial offset study: 1985–1989.* Westport, CT: Alexander and Alexander Consulting Group.

Smith, R., Rost, K., & Kashner, M. (1995). A trial of the effect of a standardized psychiatric consultation on health outcomes and costs in somatizing patients. *Archives of General Psychiatry, 52,* 238–243.

Society of Teachers of Family Medicine Behavioral Science Task Force. (1985). Behavioral science in family medicine residencies: Part 1. Teachers and curricula. *Family Medicine, 17,* 64–69.

Society of Teachers of Family Medicine Behavioral Science Task Force. (1986). *Core competency objectives in behavioral science education.* Kansas City, MO: Society of Teachers of Family Medicine.

Spiegel, D., Bloom, J., & Kramer, H. (1989). Effects of psychosocial treatment on survival of patients with metastatic breast cancer. *Lancet, 2,* 888–891.

Sprenkle, D. H., & Bischof, G. P. (1994). Contemporary family therapy in the United States. *Journal of Family Therapy, 16,* 5–23.

Starr, B., & Findlay, S. (1994, November). Mental health: Solving the quality problem. *Business and Health,* 23–28.

Stein, H. F., & Apprey, M. (1990). *Clinical stories and their translation.* Charlottesville: University Press of Virginia.

Stephens, G. (1982). *The intellectual basis of family practice.* Kansas City, MO: Society of Teachers of Family Medicine/Winter Publishing.

Strathdee, G. (1987). Primary care–psychiatry interaction: A British perspective. *General Hospital Psychiatry, 9,* 102–110.

Strosahl, K. (1994). New dimensions in behavioral health–primary care integration. *HMO Practice, 8,* 176–179.

Svedlund, J. (1983). Psychotherapy in irritable bowel syndrome: A controlled outcome study. *Acta Psychiatrica Scandinavica, 67,* 306.

Talen, M. R., Graham, M. C., & Walbroehl, G. (1994). Introducing multiprofessional team practice and community-based health care services into the curriculum: A challenge for health care educators. *Family Systems Medicine, 12,* 353–360.

Temkin, O. (1991). *Hippocrates in a world of pagans and Christians.* Baltimore: Johns Hopkins University Press.

Thomas, R., Pot, L., & Bennett, W. (1994). *Health care book lists, 1993.* Winter Park, FL: PMD Publishers Group.

Thompson, T., Stoudmire, A., & Mitchell, W. (1982). Effects of a psychiatric liaison program on internists' ability to assess psychosocial problems. *International Journal of Psychiatry in Medicine, 12,* 153–160.

Tillich, P. (1948). *The shaking of the foundations.* New York: Scribner's.

Tollman, S. (1991) Community-oriented primary care: Origins, evolution, application. *Society and Scientific Medicine, 32,* 633–642.

U.S. Department of Commerce (1980). *Statistical abstracts of the United States.* 101s.d. 1S.P.–25, N.802,888. Washington, DC: Government Printing Office.

Vaughn, C. E., & Leff, J. B. (1976). The influence of family and social factors on the course of psychiatric illness: A comparison of schizophrenic and depressed youth. *British Journal of Psychiatry, 129,* 125–137.

Venters, M. (1981). Familial coping with chronic and severe childhood illness: The case of cystic fibrosis. *Social Science Medicine, 15A,* 289–297.

Von Korff, M. (1990). *GHC Center for Health Studies: August 1990 data* (informed estimate based on a range of studies).

Von Korff, M., Katon, W., Lin, E., & Wagner, E. (1987). Evaluation of psychiatric consultation-liaison in primary care settings. *General Hospital Psychiatry, 9,* 118–125.

Wagner, E. R. (1993). Types of managed care organizations. In P. R. Kongstvedt (Ed.), *The Managed Health Care Handbook* (2nd ed., pp. 12–21). Gaithersburg, MD: Aspen Publications.

Waitzkin, H. (1985). Information giving in medical care. *Journal of Health and Social Behavior, 26,* 81–101.

Walsh, F. (Ed.). (1993). *Normal family processes* (2nd ed.). New York: Guilford Press.

Wamboldt, M. (1994). Current status of child and adolescent medical-psychiatric units. *Psychosomatics, 35,* 434–444.

Wells, K. B., Hays, R. D., Burnam, A. M., Rogers, W., Greenfield, S. G., & Ware, J. E. (1989). Detection of depressive disorder for patients receiving prepaid or fee-for-service care. *Journal of the American Medical Association, 262,* 3298–3302.

Wells, K. B., Manning, Jr., W. G., Duan, N., Newhouse, J. P., & Ware, J. (1987). Cost-sharing and the use of general medical physicians for outpatient mental health care. *Health Services Research, 22,* 1–17.

Wells, K. B., Stewart, A., Hays, R. D., Burnam, A. M., Rogers, W., Daniels, M., Berry, S., Greenfield, S., & Ware, J. (1989). The functioning and well-being of depressed patients. *Journal of the American Medical Association, 262,* 914–919.

Westberg, J., & Jason, H. (1993). *Collaborative clinical education: The foundation of effective health care.* New York: Springer.

White, M., & Epston, D. (1990). *Narrative means to therapeutic ends.* New York: Norton.

Williams, P., Tarnopolsky, A., Hand, D., & Shepherd, M. (1978). *Psychological medicine. Minor psychiatric morbidity and general practice consultation: The West London study.* London: Cambridge University Press.

Wilson, G., & Brownell, K. (1978). Behavior therapy for obesity: Including family members in the treatment process. *Behavior Therapy, 9,* 943–945.

Winslow, R. (1989, December 13). Spending to cut mental health costs. *Wall Street Journal,* 8–9.

Wittgenstein, L. (1953). *Philosophical investigations.* New York: Oxford University Press.

Wright, L. H., & Leahey, H. (1994). *Nurses and families: A guide to family assessment and intervention* (2nd ed.). Philadelphia: F. A. Davis.

Wright, L. M., & Leahey, M. (1987a). *Families and chronic illness.* Springhouse, PA: Springhouse Corp.

Wright, L. M., & Leahey, M. (1987b). *Families and life-threatening illness.* Springhouse, PA: Springhouse Corp.

Wright, L. M., & Leahey, M. (1987c). *Families and psychosocial problems.* Springhouse, PA: Springhouse Corp.

Wright, R. A. (1993). Community-oriented primary care: The cornerstone of health care reform. *Journal of the American Medical Association, 269,* 2544–2547.

Wynne, L. C., McDaniel, S. H., & Weber, T. T. (Eds.). (1986). *Systems consultation: A new perspective for family therapy.* New York: Guilford Press.

Wynne, L. C., Shields, C. G., & Sirkin, M. I. (1992). Illness, family theory, and family therapy: Part 1. Conceptual issues. *Family Process, 31,* 3–18.

Zung, W. W. K., Broadhead, W. E., & Roth, M. E. (1993). Prevalence of depressive symptoms in primary care. *Journal of Family Practice, 37,* 337–344.

INDEX